IADVL

User's Manual of
Systemic and
Topical Steroids

IADVL
1973
INDIAN ASSOCIATION OF DERMATOLOGISTS, VENEREOLOGISTS & LEPROLOGISTS

IADVL
User's Manual of
Systemic and
Topical Steroids

Chief Editor
Neena Khanna MD
Professor
Department of Dermatology and Venereology
All India Institute of Medical Sciences
New Delhi

Associate Editors

Abhishek De MD FAGE
Associate Professor
Department of Dermatology
Calcutta National Medical College
Kolkata

Neetu Bhari MD DNB MNAMS
Assistant Professor
Department of Dermatology and Venereology
All India Institute of Medical Sciences
New Delhi

Assistant Editors

Eswari L MD DVL
FRGUHS (Dermatosurgery)
FAADV (Dermatopathology)
Associate Professor
Department of Dermatology
Bangalore Medical College and
Research Institute
Currently Joint Secretary
Bangalore Dermatology Society
Bengaluru

Meghana Phiske MD DNB DVD DDV
Associate Professor
Department of Dermatology
TNMC and BYL Ch. Nair Hospital
Mumbai

Vishal Gupta MBBS MD
Assistant Professor
Department of Dermatology
and Venereology
All India Institute of Medical
Sciences
New Delhi

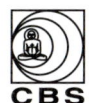

CBS

CBS Publishers & Distributors Pvt Ltd

New Delhi • Bengaluru • Chennai • Kochi • Kolkata • Mumbai

Bhopal • Bhubaneswar • Hyderabad • Jharkhand • Nagpur • Patna • Pune • Uttarakhand • Dhaka (Bangladesh) • Kathmandu (Nepal)

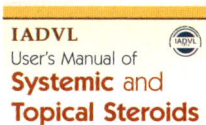

ISBN: 978-93-88725-63-7

Copyright © IADVL
IADVL does not endorse any of the product/s appearing in this publication.

First Edition: 2020

Published by Satish Kumar Jain and produced by Varun Jain for

CBS Publishers & Distributors Pvt Ltd
4819/XI Prahlad Street, 24 Ansari Road, Daryaganj, New Delhi 110 002, India.
Ph: 011-23289259, 23266861, 23266867   Fax: 011-23243014   Website: www.cbspd.com
e-mail: delhi@cbspd.com; cbspubs@airtelmail.in
Corporate Office: 204 FIE, Industrial Area, Patparganj, Delhi 110 092
Ph: 011-49344934   Fax: 011-49344935   e-mail: publishing@cbspd.com; publicity@cbspd.com

Branches

- **Bengaluru:** Seema House 2975, 17th Cross, K.R. Road,
  Banasankari 2nd Stage, Bengaluru 560 070, Karnataka
  Ph: +91-80-26771678/79   Fax: +91-80-26771680   e-mail: bangalore@cbspd.com
- **Chennai:** 7, Subbaraya Street, Shenoy Nagar, Chennai 600 030, Tamil Nadu
  Ph: +91-44-26680620, 26681266   Fax: +91-44-42032115   e-mail: chennai@cbspd.com
- **Kochi:** 68/1534, 35, 36 Power House Road, Opp. KSEB, Kochi 682018, Kerala
  Ph: +91-484-4059061-65   Fax: +91-484-4059065   e-mail: kochi@cbspd.com
- **Kolkata:** 6/B, Ground Floor, Rameswar Shaw Road, Kolkata 700 014, West Bengal
  Ph: +91-33-22891126, 22891127, 22891128   e-mail: kolkata@cbspd.com
- **Mumbai:** 83-C, Dr E Moses Road, Worli, Mumbai 400018, Maharashtra
  Ph: +91-22-24902340/41   Fax: +91-22-24902342   e-mail: mumbai@cbspd.com

Representatives

• **Bhopal**	0-8319310552	• **Bhubaneswar**	0-9911037372	• **Hyderabad**	0-9885175004	• **Jharkhand**	0-9811541605
• **Nagpur**	0-9421945513	• **Patna**	0-9334159340	• **Pune**	0-9623451994	• **Uttarakhand**	0-9716462459
• **Dhaka (Bangladesh)**	01912-003485	• **Kathmandu (Nepal)**	977-9818742655				

Printed at: Nutech Print Services, Faridabad, India

Foreword

It was fashionable to quote that "steroid thy home is dermatology" at the time when very few medications were available for dermatotherapy. Now, dermatologists have a variety of therapeutic options in their armamentarium, but steroid still enjoys key position in dermatotherapeutics.

Because of its anti-inflammatory, immunosuppressive, anti-allergic and vasoconstrictive effects, topical and systemic steroids are widely prescribed as a palliative treatment in management of dermatoses of diverse origin. It is crucial that every steroid prescriber must know its pharmacologic nuances and nitty-gritty.

My proposal as a National President, 2017 to come out with *"IADVL User's Manual of Systemic and Topical Steroids"* was readily accepted. I felt very comfortable when Dr Neena Khanna consented to assume responsibility as a Chief Editor. Her team was very strong, having Dr Neetu Bhari and Dr Abhishek De as associate editors. My heartfelt appreciation to one and all involved in this project.

The manual contains a wide range of topics related to topical, intralesional, systemic and pulse steroid therapy. Complications, special precautions, role of steroids in dermatologic emergencies and steroid abuse are aptly discussed. Inclusion of a chapter on "evidence-based use of steroids" adds a lot of value to the manual.

User's manual on steroids was a felt need and this manual will definitely fill the void.

Yours in scientific and academic pursuit.

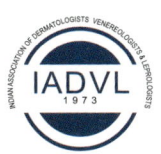

Yogesh S Marfatia
Immediate Past National President, IADVL

Foreword

IADVL proudly presents this manual which in detail explains use and misuse of both topical and systemic steroids. All the topics are discussed in detail which will help our dermatologists in practice.

On behalf of IADVL, I congratulate the team headed by Prof Neena Khanna. We hope that this book will enrich our knowledge about steroids.

Thanks and regards!

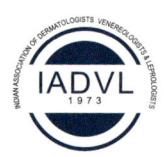

Ramesh Bhat M
President, IADVL (National), 2018

Foreword

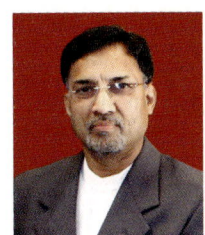

The advent of corticosteroids is such a significant and seminal event in the management of skin disorders that the history of dermatology can be divided into "pre- and post-corticosteroid" era. Such being the importance of these wonderful molecules in the dermatological therapeutic armamentarium, there is a need have a ready reference book on the use of systemic and topical corticosteroids in dermatology for all concerned. And this *"IADVL User's Manual of Systemic and Topical Steroids"* is a commendable effort to fulfill that need. The chapters included in this manual outline their use in most situations in dermatological practice, both systemic as well as topical preparations. It is noteworthy that there are chapters on "complications of systemic corticosteroids" apart from chapters on "topical corticosteroids abuse" and "steroid misuse" in this user manual. The inclusion of a chapter on "evidence-based use of steroids" makes the information comprehensive.

The editorial team headed by Dr Neena Khanna did a wonderful job in planning and compiling these chapters and the content. I am sure, it will a ready-reckoner for all practitioners and would find a place on their desktop.

P Narasimha Rao MD PhD
President, IADVL, 2019

Foreword

Corticosteroids, both topical and systemic are the standard of care treatment for many dermatological dermatoses. Despite being in use in their treatment for more than 65 years, the indications and modalities of treatment continue to be modified. The current focus is on responsible prescription of both topical and systemic steroids and mechanisms to minimize the well known toxicities. This is especially relevant in therapy of many inflammatory and autoimmune diseases, that require long-term treatment with corticosteroids. The misuse of these drugs by many is also creating scenarios of modified infectious and inflammatory dermatoses leading to many cutaneous adverse reactions and delay in diagnosis or inappropriate therapy. The need for an updated detailed text on this topic is therefore obvious. The IADVL, therefore, is happy to present a synopsis in the form of this *"IADVL User's Manual of Systemic and Topical Steroids"* that can serve as a ready-reckoner for the practical aspects of usage of topical and systemic corticosteroids including the indications, methods of prescriptions, withdrawal, monitoring and modalities of dealing with adverse effects. We are confident that the book will serve the needs of all students, physicians or researchers who would like to keep updated about the current knowledge status of the role of corticosteroids in dermatology.

We on behalf of the IADVL academy, commend the editorial team with Prof Neena Khanna as Chief Editor, for this superlative effort.

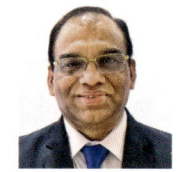

KA Seetharam
IADVL Academy

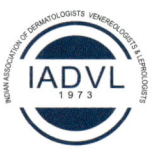

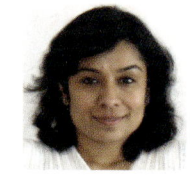

Deepika Pandhi
IADVL Academy

Preface

The *IADVL User's Manual of Systemic and Topical Steroids* covers various aspects of steroid use in dermatology practice. Since systemic and topical steroids are frequently used for a myriad of skin diseases, we hope this book will serve as a ready reference as it includes details of indications of steroids, different formulations, appropriate dosing and guidelines for proper monitoring and expected adverse effects.

The IADVL Academy Chairperson, Dr KA Seetharam and Convener, Dr Deepika Pandhi came up with the idea of this book. We feel honoured to have been assigned this task. The contents were approved by the IADVL Academy and Dr Yogesh Marfatia.

The manual begins with chapters on topical and intralesional steroids describing their structure, classification, mechanism of action and appropriate indications. The potential adverse effects of these formulations are discussed in detail in a separate chapter on "complications of topical steroids". In subsequent chapters, we have discussed systemic and pulsed steroids, their indications and basic principles of treatment. Complications of systemic steroids and how to manage them are discussed in a separate chapter. Topical steroid abuse has become rampant in India, and an entire chapter has been dedicated to this public health issue. Use of systemic steroids in emergency dermatoses and evidence-based use of steroids in steroid responsive dermatoses are also discussed in separate chapters. We have attempted to cover broadly all aspects of steroid usage in dermatology, including practical tips on how to use steroids safely and effectively. Correct use of topical and intralesional steroids has been illustrated by schematic diagrams. We thank our authors for their wonderful contributions.

Our special thanks to Mr SK Jain CMD, CBS Publishers & Distributors Pvt. Ltd., and Mr YN Arjuna, Senior Vice-President—Publishing, Editorial and Publicity, Mrs Ritu Chawla General Manager—Production and their team for their support throughout the entire process.

We hope the readers will find this manual an asset in their daily dermatology practice.

The Editorial Team

Contributors

Aarti Sarda MD
Consultant Dermatologist
Wizderm Skin and Hair Clinic
Kolkata

Abhishek De MD
Associate Professor
Department of Dermatology
Calcutta National Medical College
Kolkata

Deepika Yadav MD
Senior Resident
Department of Dermatology
All India Institute of Medical Sciences
New Delhi

Eswari L MD
Assistant Professor
Department of Dermatology
Bangalore Medical College and Research Institute
Bengaluru

Kerkar Sulaksha Surya MD
Junior Resident
Bangalore Medical College and Research Institute
Bengaluru

Manik Aggarwal MBBS
Junior Resident
Department of Dermatology
All India Institute of Medical Sciences
New Delhi

Monika Khemka MBBS
Junior Resident
Department of Dermatology
Calcutta National Medical College
Kolkata

Neena Khanna MD
Professor
Department of Dermatology
All India Institute of Medical Sciences
New Delhi

Neetu Bhari MD
Assistant Professor
Department of Dermatology
All India Institute of Medical Sciences
New Delhi

Neha Taneja MD
Senior Resident
Department of Dermatology
All India Institute of Medical Sciences
New Delhi

Nikhil Mehta MBBS
Junior Resident
Department of Dermatology
All India Institute of Medical Sciences
New Delhi

Savera Gupta MD
Senior Resident
Department of Dermatology
All India Institute of Medical Sciences
New Delhi

Sonal Singh MBBS
Junior Resident
Department of Dermatology
Calcutta National Medical College
Kolkata

Sujata Sinha MBBS
Junior Resident
Department of Dermatology
Calcutta National Medical College
Kolkata

Vishal Gupta MD
Assistant Professor
Department of Dermatology
All India Institute of Medical Sciences
New Delhi

Contents

Topical Corticosteroids

Abhishek De, Sonal Singh, Aarti Sarda, Savera Gupta, Neena Khanna

SUMMARY

- All steroids have a basic 4-ring structure with 3 hexane rings (designated A to C) and one pentane ring (designated D) with hydroxyl (OH) group at C11, a double bond at C4–5 and ketone moiety on C3. However, parts of the ring and side chains can be modified to increase penetration, potency and specificity of action and reduce side effects.
- Therapeutic effects (anti-inflammatory, antiproliferative and atrophogenic effects) of topical corticosteroids (TCS) are mediated by classical genomic and non-genomic pathways.
- Two important systems of classification of TCS on the basis of potency are British system (classes I to IV) and American system (classes I to VII), with class I being the most potent. However, apart from the structure of the steroid, clinical potency (hence efficacy and side effect profile) of TCS depends on other factors including concentration, formulation, method of application (with occlusion/hydration), site of use and background condition of skin.
- Dermatological conditions can be divided on the basis of their response to steroids into highly responsive, moderately responsive and least responsive.
- TCS are the first-line treatment for dermatitis including atopic dermatitis (AD) which is a highly steroid-responsive dermatoses. Once control of AD is achieved with a daily regimen of TCS, long-term remissions can be sustained in a subset of patients with twice weekly applications of potent TCS in order to reduce TCS-induced adverse effects. In children with extensive disease, diluted TCS under wet wrap dressings may be used to avoid systemic administration of steroids.
- TCS are of established value in psoriasis. Potent and very potent TCS are the most commonly used topical therapy for localized disease. In widespread disease, mild or moderate potency TCS are used as an adjunct to systemic therapy. Mild-to-moderate potency TCS are also first line of therapy in flexures. If lesions are thick, then TCS are often combined with salicylic acid in ointment base. Soaking of the affected part prior to TCS application is of particular value in palmoplantar psoriasis.

- Vitiligo is moderately steroid-responsive dermatoses and TCS are the first-line therapy for localized disease. Compared with PUVA, which promotes a predominantly perifollicular pattern of repigmentation, TCS result in more diffuse repigmentation, which occurs more quickly but is less stable.
- TCS and topical antifungals, either alone or in combination, are the mainstay of therapy in seborrheic dermatitis. In very hyperkeratotic lesions over scalp, TCS in lotion formulation are used and the scalp can be occluded with a shower cap overnight.
- Potent and very potent TCS are the first-line therapy in pompholyx.
- Potent and very potent TCS, when used under supervision and for finite duration, are the first line of treatment for lichen sclerosus in adults as well as in children in both sexes.
- Treatment of lichen simplex chronicus is aimed at interrupting the itch-scratch-itch cycle and the first-line measures to control itch include use of potent or very potent TCS and antihistamines. Petrolatum can be applied to the surrounding skin to avoid perilesional hypopigmentation and atrophy.
- TCS may be used in aphthous stomatitis to hasten healing and reduce the associated pain.
- TCS, particularly the potent ones when used for at least 3 months, have shown efficacy in some studies of localized alopecia areata, although the results are variable and they do not appear to be effective in alopecia totalis/universalis.
- Potent and very potent TCS have emerged as first-line therapy for limited bullous pemphigoid. In extensive disease, TCS are invariably used as an adjunct to systemic therapy but may be used even as a standalone therapy of very potent TCS as whole body twice a day application in patients who cannot use systemic steroids. Such use is, however, limited by practical factors (time needed, compliance and cost).
- TCS are required in most patients of allergic contact dermatitis for rapid alleviation of symptoms, along with other measures including use of emollients and antihistamines.
- TCS are the cornerstone of initial therapy for patients with limited discoid lupus erythematosus and is one of the few conditions warranting use of potent steroids on the face.
- Although TCS are widely accepted and are practically almost always used as first-line treatment in lichen planus (LP), there is paucity of scientific evidence supporting this conventional therapeutic modality. A potent TCS once daily application is used until remission in cutaneous LP. For oral LP, potent TCS may be applied three times daily with a gloved finger in symptomatic patients.
- Optimal use of TCS includes choosing the right potency formulated in appropriate vehicle, used inappropriate concentration and amount for an adequate duration.

- The choice of potency of TCS used depends on the dermatoses to be treated, type of lesion, site of lesion and the body surface area involved. It is recommended that therapy should be initiated with lowest potency of TCS to sufficiently control the disease and once partial disease control is achieved, a lower potency TCS is introduced.
- Once daily application is as efficacious as more frequent applications of very potent steroid and sudden discontinuation should be avoided after prolonged use to prevent rebound phenomenon.
- Simple practical guides to the quantity of a topical medication to apply are provided by the fingertip unit (FTU). As a thumb rule no more than 50 g/week of potent and 100 g/week of mild or moderate potent TCS should be used in an adult.
- Prior hydration of the skin helps in optimising results with TCS and they may be used under occlusion (by bandage, gloves and socks, cling film) for thick or lichenified lesions.

INTRODUCTION

- Even after 65 years of their initial discovery, steroids remain the most commonly prescribed anti-inflammatory agents in dermatology and are used in a large number of dermatological conditions.
- Safe and effective use of topical corticosteroids (TCS) requires knowledge of the various molecules formulations and potencies.
- TCS have a long list of potential side effects and newer molecules are being introduced, to improve efficacy and circumvent the adverse effects.

HISTORY AND EVOLUTION OF TCS

- Kendall and his team in 1948 isolated the extract of bovine adrenal glands and marked the compounds from A to F. Of these six compounds, E (cortisone) and F (hydrocortisone) were found to be medically effective. The team received the Nobel prize in 1950 for the discovery and elucidating the structure and biological effects of glucocorticoids.
- Sulzberger and associates first time reported the use of steroids in dermatology. However, it was a challenge to use corticosteroids topically, as corticosteroids with—O group at the C11 position (e.g. cortisone) had to be reduced to 11-hydroxyl analogs (e.g. hydrocortisone) to be effective, and this change does not happen in skin. This group created history in 1952 by successfully treating eczematous eruptions with topical hydrocortisone. Decades of research and widespread use led to the development of a variety of TCS preparations and formulations.

STRUCTURE[1]

- All steroids have a basic 4-ring structure with 3 hexane rings (designated A to C) and one pentane ring (designated D; Fig. 1.1a) with hydroxyl (OH) group at C11, a double bond at C4–5 and ketone moiety on C3. However, parts of the ring and side chains can be modified to:
  - Increase penetration
  - Increase potency
  - Increase specificity of action
  - Reduce side effects.
- Hydrocortisone is the prototype TCS molecule (Fig. 1.1b) and modifications done to the basic molecule include:
  - *Esterification*: Esterification at 16-, 17-, 21-positions result in:
    - Improved penetration: As it increases lipid solubility.
    - Decreased systemic side effects: Because of increased de-esterification resulting in formation of inactive metabolites.
    - Increased potency of molecule, e.g. esterification at 17-position of betamethasone (Fig. 1.1c) results in formation of betamethasone-17-valerate (Fig. 1.1d), which is 125 times more potent than betamethasone because of greater binding to glucocorticoid receptor (GCR). In contrast esterification at 21-position results in formation of betamethasone-21-valerate, which binds less tightly to GCR, but is more lipophilic, so has better percutaneous absorption.
  - *Halogenation*: Halogenation at 6-, 9- or 21-position increases potency especially antiproliferative effect which can be utilised as targeted therapy in psoriasis and chronic lichenified eczema:
    - Chlorination at 21-position produces clobetasol propionate (Fig. 1.1e) which has increased binding to GCR and this chlorination also inhibits de-esterification at 17-position resulting in significantly increased potency.
    - Fluorination at 6- and/or 9-position increases potency (e.g. difluorosone diacetate) by inhibiting de-esterification.
  - *Hydroxylation*: Addition of hydroxyl group at 16-position reduces mineralocorticoid activity, e.g. triamcinolone acetonide.
  - *Others*:
    - Addition of methyl group at 16-position reduces mineralocorticoid activity.
    - A double-bond in 1–2 position increases glucocorticoid activity.
    - Some topical steroid molecules have OH groups at 11-, 17- and 21-positions or ketone groups at 3- and 20-positions or a double-bond at 4-position of the glucocorticoid nucleus.

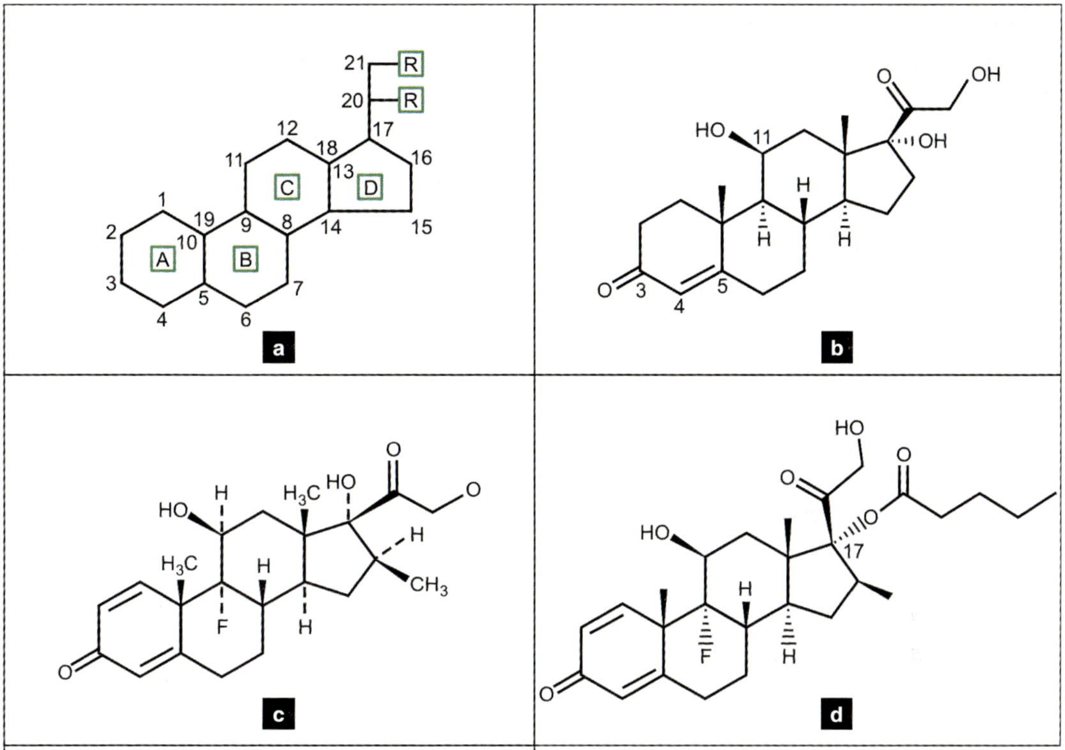

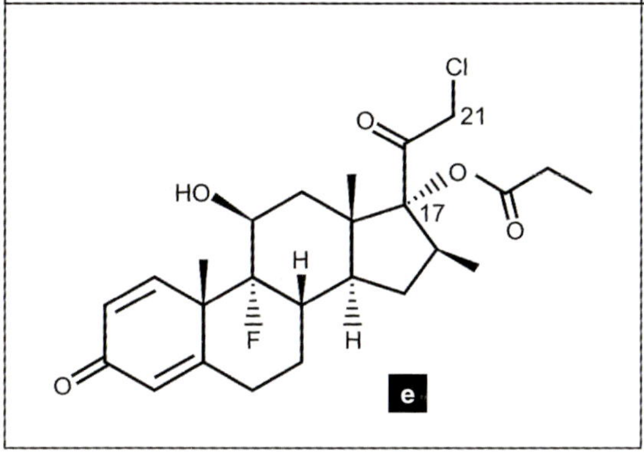

Fig. 1.1: (a) Corticosteroid basic structure: Made of 3 hexane (A–C) and 1 pentane (D) ring; **(b) Hydrocortisone:** Prototype TCS molecule; **(c) Betamethasone; (d) Beta-methasone valerate:** Esterification at 17-position increases binding to GCR; **(e) Clobetasol propionate:** Chlorination at 21-position increases binding to GCR and inhibits de-esterification.

MECHANISM OF ACTION OF TCS[2]

TCS diffuse through the stratum corneum barrier (a rate-limiting step in drug delivery) and through plasma membrane (easily pass due to their lipophilic structure) to reach the cytoplasm of cells in the epidermis and dermis. In the cytoplasm they bind to a specific receptor, the glucocorticoid receptor (GCR) and binding to these receptors (based on their chemical structure) determines potency of corticosteroids.

Therapeutic effects of steroids are mediated by:
- Classical genomic effects.
- Non-genomic effects.

Classical Genomic Mechanism of TCS Action

- *Glucocorticoid receptor GCRα[a]:* It is a protein which belongs to the same receptor superfamily as receptors for other steroids, thyroid hormone, calcitriol, etc. The unligated cytosolic GCR (cGCR) is located in cytoplasm as a multi-protein complex (composed of HSP 70, HSP 90, chaperone immunophilins).
- *Molecular mechanism:* TCS bind to GCR to form GC-GCR complex, with disassociation from HSP 90 (capping protein) from the GCR. Thereafter GC-GCR complex translocates to the nucleus and binds to the GC response elements (GRE) in DNA, causing alteration in transcription and translation of proteins.

Non-genomic Mechanism of TCS Action

Rapid anti-inflammatory and immunosuppressive actions of TCS (actually both of topical and oral steroids) are mediated by three different mechanisms:

- *Non-specific interactions with cellular membranes:* TCS have several effects on plasma and mitochondrial membranes of immune cells.
- *Non-genomic effects mediated by GCR:* When GCR binds to its ligand, it dissociates from the multi-protein complex and many of these molecules are responsible for rapid GC effects. So GCR is not only important as a nuclear regulator of gene transcription, but is also involved in rapid non-genomic GCR-induced effects.
- *Specific interactions with a membrane-bound GCR (mGCR):* Apart from cytoplasm (cGCR), GCRs are also present on cell membrane (mGCR) and several kinases are rapidly inhibited *in vitro* and *in vivo* by treatment with TCS, mediated *via* a mGCR-dependent pathway.

EFFECTS OF TCS[2]

Anti-inflammatory Effects

Direct Effects

TCS have several direct effects which help to reduce inflammation immediately:

- *Stabilization of cell membrane and lysosomal membrane* thereby preventing release of lysosomal contents and phospholipid precursors required for synthesis of prostaglandins and platelet activating factor (PAF) which are mediators of inflammation.
- *Vasoconstriction:* This is mediated by—
  - Potentiating vascular response to catecholamines.
  - Reducing sensitivity of vascular smooth muscle to vasodilators like histamine, bradykinin and nitric oxide (NO).

---

[a]**GCRα:** Consists of 3 different domains with various functions—N terminal domain containing transactivation functions, a DNA binding domain and a ligand binding domain. A GCR β-isoform does not bind to GC, but is believed to regulate transcriptional activity and so is an endogenous inhibitor of GC action and may be an important marker of steroid insensitivity.

- *Effect on mast cells*:
  - Inhibit mast cell sensitization induced by IgE.
  - Inhibit release of mast cell mediators like histamine.

GCR-mediated Effects

TCS induce synthesis of several anti-inflammatory proteins mediated through GCR and these effects are delayed. The proteins include:

- *Lipocortins*:
  - Prevent formation of potent inflammatory mediators (prostaglandins, leukotrienes, 12-HETE, and 15-HETE).
  - Prevent PAF-induced wheal and flare reactions and leukocyte chemotaxis.
  - Decrease vascular permeability.
- *Vasocortin*: Inhibits histamine release from mast cells.
- *Vasoregulin*: Decreases vascular permeability.

Anti-inflammatory Effect on Specific Cells

This action is mediated both directly and through GCR. Cells affected include:

- *Polymorphonuclear leukocytes*:
  - Reduced ability to adhere to vascular endothelium.
  - Reduced migration to sites of inflammation.
  - Reduced number at sites of inflammation.
  - Reduced phagocytosis, bactericidal activity, release of acid hydrolases and pyrogens.
  - Cause abnormal nitroblue tetrazolium test *in vitro*.
- *Monocytes*:
  - Reduced number at sites of inflammation.
  - Reduced fungicidal activity and clearance of opsonized particles.
  - Reduced response to macrophage activating factor and decreased chemotaxis.
  - Reduced response to mixed leukocyte reaction.
- *Lymphocytes*:
  - Reduced response of lymphocytes to concanavalin A-induced T cell blastogenesis, and to tetanus toxoid and streptodornase-streptokinase.
  - Reduced antibody-dependent cell-mediated cytotoxicity.
  - Reduced natural killer cell activity.
- *Langerhans' cells*:
  - Moderate potency TCS decrease expression of Fc receptor, C3b receptor, and HLA DR positivity, with no alteration in CD1a antigen expression.
  - Very potent TCS cause loss of cells expressing Langerhans cell markers.
- *Effects on immune cytokine production*:
  - Reduce production of IL-1, IL-2, interferon-γ, tumor necrosis factor and granulocyte monocyte colony-stimulating factor.

Antiproliferative and Atrophogenic Effects

Epidermis

- *Effects of TCS on epidermis*:
  - Reduced thickness of stratum corneum.
  - Reduced or absent granular layer.
  - Flattened basal layer with reduced mitoses.
  - Suppressed keratinocyte growth factors.
  - Reduced production of melanin by melanocytes.
  - Normal keratinocyte ultrastructure (keratin filaments, keratohyalin granules, membrane-coating granules).
  - Unaffected basement membrane.
- *Mediators*: TCS reduce levels of molecules (opioid peptides, enkephalins), which modulate epidermal differentiation and inflammatory processes.

Dermis

- *Early atrophy*: Changes seen include:
  - Reduction in dermal volume:
    - Reduction of amount of glycosaminoglycans (GAGs).
    - Decreased water content (due to loss of GAGs and TCS-induced vasoconstriction).
  - Hypoactive fibroblasts:
    - Suppression of procollagen transcription.
    - Reduced activity of prolyl 4-hydroxylase and lysyl oxidase.
    - Decreased hyaluronate synthetase activity.
  - Collagen and elastic fibers unchanged.
- *Late atrophy*:
  - Dermal volume reduced.
  - Collagen and elastic fibers diminished (starts within 3 days of administration but manifests late) and abnormally aggregated.
  - Hypoactive fibroblasts.
  - Dermal vessels become fragile, due to loss of fibrous tissue and ground substance support.

Vasoconstriction

TCS cause constriction of superficial dermal capillaries thus reducing erythema but the mechanism of TCS induced vasoconstriction is not yet completely known. It is thought to be related to inhibition of release of natural vasodilators such as histamine, bradykinins and prostaglandins and endothelial NO.

Systemic Effects

Effects following systemic absorption on metabolic and other areas are similar to those seen with systematic corticosteroids.

POTENCY

Factors Determining Potency

Potency of TCS reflects intensity of clinical effects and depends on several factors:

- *Structure of TCS:* TCS molecules have inherent differences in potency based on their structure which determine the following.
  - *Lipophilicity*: Thereby increased percutaneous absorption due to their ability to penetrate the stratum corneum, e.g. esterification at 21-position of betamethasone results in formation of betamethasone-21-valerate which is more lipophilic so has better percutaneous absorption.
  - *Affinity to GCR*:
    - Esterification at 17-position of betamethasone results in formation of betamethasone-17-valerate, which is 125 times more potent than betamethasone because of greater binding to GCR.
    - Chlorination at 21-position produces clobetasol propionate which has increased binding to GCR.
  - *Metabolism in skin*: TCS get metabolized mainly by intraepidermal de-esterification. It may be one of the causes for tachyphylaxis. Reduced de-esterification at 17-position increases potency, e.g. by chlorination at 21-position in clobetasol propionate and by fluorination at 6- and 9-position in difluorosone diacetate.
  - *Specificity for a particular action*: Halogenation at 6-, 9- or 21-position increases potency especially antiproliferative effect which can be utilised as targeted therapy in psoriasis and chronic lichenified eczema, e.g. clobetasol propionate.
- *Concentration of TCS:*
  - This is logical. The target for TCS is the viable epidermis and dermis and clinical response to a formulation is directly proportional to the concentration of TCS achieved at target site. A comparative study of skin concentrations after topical *vs* oral corticosteroid treatment found that most TCS have the potential to achieve greater effective drug levels in the superficial layers of skin than achieved by standard dose of oral prednisolone. Therefore, the apparent greater efficacy of oral corticosteroids may be due in part to poor patient compliance with topical therapy.
  - Stratum corneum also act as a reservoir for TCS which is TCS potency dependant. Experimental studies in rabbit skin have shown a reservoir effect of:
    - 4 days for clobetasol propionate 0.5% and mometasone furoate 0.1%.
    - 2 days for fluticasone propionate 0.005% and betamethasone valerate.
    - 1 day for hydrocortisone butyrate 0.1%.[3]
- *Vehicle and formulations*: Active TCS molecule is dissolved in a vehicle to allow easy dispersion and adequate release of the drug. They alter therapeutic and adverse actions of TCS by modulating their pharmacokinetics.
  - Several formulations of TCS are available including cream, ointment, foam, shampoo, lotion and gel. Oil-in-water preparations such as creams and lotions

are created with emulsifying agents. Emulsifiers help to distribute the drug evenly on the skin surface.

- Occlusive vehicles like ointments enhance a TCS molecule's percutaneous absorption by increasing hydration[b] of stratum corneum. This makes ointment more potent than a cream.
- Humectants are added in oil-in-water preparations to maintain the optimal water content.
- Solvents are used in lotions, solutions, gels, and sprays to decrease viscosity. Solvents such as propylene glycol and ethanol (which have high solubility for TCS molecule) enhance potency by increasing percutaneous absorption.

• *Occlusion:* Penetration of TCS is greatly increased (up to 10 times) by occlusion. Methods of occlusion include bandages, gloves and socks, cling films and wet wraps. Hydrocolloid dressings and paste bandages with TCS incorporated are also available. However, whole body occlusion of TCS has fallen out of favor because of adverse effects.

• *Site of use:* Different sites have different levels of absorption of TCS, correlating inversely with thickness of stratum corneum and directly with vascularity of the area (Table 1.1).

Table 1.1: Site related absorption of TCS	
Site	Relative levels of absorption
Fore arm	1
Palm	0.8
Axilla	3.6
Sole	0.1
Ankle	0.4
Back	1.7
Scalp	3.5
Eyelids	56
Forehead	06
Scrotum	42

• *Condition of skin:*
- Inflamed skin (e.g. eczematous skin) tends to absorb TCS more readily while thick hyperkeratotic lesions absorb TCS less readily (e.g. lichen simplex chronicus).
- Sites which are naturally occluded (axillae, groin) also are more susceptible to developing side effects because of greater percutaneous absorption (due to hydration and occlusion).

Assessing Potency

Though there are several assays available to compare the potency of TCS, the most frequently used is the vasoconstriction assay and usually a second assay (like efficacy in a skin disease, e.g. psoriasis) is used to validate it (Table 1.2).

Classification of Potency TCS[4]

There are two important systems of classification of potency of TCS:

• *British system:* Classifies TCS into 4 classes. According to British National Formulary class I is the most potent and class IV the least potent[c] (Table 1.3).

---

[b]Hydration enhances absorption by four times.
[c]However, in continental Europe, class IV is regarded as the most potent and class I as the least potent.

- *American system*: Classifies TCS into 7 classes with class I being the most potent and class VII being the least potent (Table 1.4).

Table 1.2: Methods of assessing potency of TCS

Using laboratory animals/cell cultures	Using human volunteers

Assays of anti-inflammatory potency
• *Mitotic index suppression*: Hairless mouse
• *Antigranuloma assay*: Rat
• *Croton oil inflammation assay*: Rat
• *6-chloro-2–4-dinitrobenzene inflammation*: Guinea pig
	• *Vasoconstrictor assay*[d]
	• *Artificially induced inflammation*
	  – Tape stripping
	  – Ultraviolet light
	  – Mustard oil
	  – Nitric acid
	  – Tetrahydrofurfuryl alcohol
	  – Nickel-induced positive patch tests
	  – Dimethyl sulfoxide
	  – Sodium hydroxide
	• *Efficacy in skin disease*: Psoriasis

Assays of atrophogenicity • Inhibition of fibroblast growth *in vitro* • Neutral red release assay • Mouse tail epidermis • Transgenic mouse model expressing human elastin promoter/chloramphenicol acetyl transferase • Guinea pig epidermis	• Micrometer calipers • Histopathologic examination of skin biopsies • X-ray radiography • Pulsed ultrasound • Optical coherence tomography

[d]**Vasoconstriction assay:** It is the assay of choice because it correlates well with clinical efficacy and is reproducible by same and other observers in completely different settings, locations, climates, and subjects. *Disadvantages*: It is subjective and only measures one aspect of TCS effects and there is no 'hard copy' for subsequent comparison, analysis, and validation. *Method*: Formulation of test corticosteroid in 95% alcohol is applied to volar surface of a normal volunteer's forearm and test area is covered with an occlusive dressing for 16 hours after alcohol is allowed to evaporate. The tested area is assessed for vasoconstriction 2 hrs later on a blind basis by an experienced investigator using a multiple unit scale (0–3 or 0–4). *Exceptions*: Aclometasone ointment and hydrocortisone valerate cream, both demonstrate greater vasoconstrictive activities than clinical efficacy.

Table 1.3: British national formulary classification of potency of TCS

Class	Potency	Drugs	Conc	Formulation
Class I	Very potent	Clobetasol propionate	0.05%	Cream, ointment, lotion
Class II	Potent	Betamethasone dipropionate	0.05%	Cream, ointment, lotion
		Betamethasone valerate	0.1%	Cream, ointment, lotion
		Beclomethasone dipropionate	0.025%	Cream, ointment, lotion
		Fluocinolone acetonide	0.025%	Cream, ointment, lotion
		Fluticasone propionate	0.05%	Cream
		Fluticasone propionate	0.005%	Ointment
		Mometasone furoate	0.1%	Cream, ointment, lotion
Class III	Moderate	Desonide	0.05%	Cream, lotion
		Clobetasone butyrate	0.05%	Cream
Class IV	Mild	Hydrocortisone acetate	1.0%	Cream
		Hydrocortisone aceponate	0.127%	Cream

Table 1.4: American system of classification of TCS

Steroid	Concentration	Formulations
Class I (Superpotent)		
• Clobetasol propionate	0.05%	All formulations except scalp solution
• Betamethasone dipropionate	0.05%	Ointment, gel
• Halobetasol propionate	0.05%	Cream, ointment
• Diflorasone diacetate	0.05%	Ointment
Class II (Potent)		
• Clobetasol propionate	0.05%	Scalp solution
• Betamethasone dipropionate	0.05%	Cream, ointment
• Desoximetasone	0.25%	Cream
• Mometasone furoate	0.1%	Ointment
• Triamcinoloe acetonide	0.5%	Ointment
• Halcinonide	0.1%	Cream, gel, ointment, solution
• Fluocinonide	0.5%	Gel
Class III (Upper mid potency)		
• Betamethasone dipropionate	0.05%	Cream
• Betamethasone valerate	0.1%	Ointment
• Fluticasone propionate	0.005%	Ointment
• Triamcinolone acetonide	0.1%	Ointment
	0.5%	Cream
Class IV (Mid potency)		
• Betamethasone valerate	0.12%	Foam
• Desoximetasone	0.05%	Cream
• Fluocinolone acetonide	0.025%	Ointment
• Hydrocortisone valerate	0.2%	Ointment
• Mometasone furoate	0.1%	Cream
Class V (Lower mid potency)		
• Betamethasone dipropionate	0.05%	Lotion
• Betamethasone valerate	0.1%	Cream
• Fluticasone propionate	0.05%	Cream, lotion
• Fluocinolone acetonide	0.25%	Cream
• Hydrocortisone butyrate	0.1%	Ointment, cream, lotion
• Hydrocortisone valerate	0.2%	Cream
• Triamcinolone acetonide	0.025%	Ointment
	0.1%	Lotion
Class VI (Mild potency)		
• Desonide	0.05%	Gel, ointment, cream, lotion, foam
• Fluocinolone acetonide	0.01%	Cream, solution
• Betamethasone valerate	0.1%	Lotion
• Triamcinolone acetonide	0.025%	Cream, lotion
Class VII (Least potent)		
• Hydrocortisone acetate	1%	Cream, ointment, foam
• Dexamethasone sodium phosphate	0.1%	Cream
• Methylprednisolone acetate	0.25%	Cream

INDICATIONS

TCS are one of the most commonly used dermatological drugs with good evidence to support their use in several skin disease (Table 1.5).

Atopic Dermatitis (AD)[6]

- Patient education about skin care is the cornerstone of management of AD. TCS are the first line for treating inflammation and pruritus associated with AD that is unresponsive to appropriate skin care and moisturizers. Table 1.6 provides a brief summary of a few recent randomized trials on TCS in dermatitis including AD.
- In practice, there is a huge variation in prescribing habits of TCS (e.g. quantity, frequency and duration of therapy) among dermatologists. The various strategies used include:
  - Using prolonged treatment with mild potency steroid preparations, because AD is a highly steroid responsive dermatoses.
  - Starting treatment with potent TCS in order to induce rapid remission, followed by a relatively quick tapering down of potency, as the dermatitis improves.
  - Using short bursts of potent TCS followed by moisturizers alone until relapse occurs.
  - However, recent studies suggest that once control of AD is achieved with a daily regimen of TCS, long-term remissions can be sustained in a subset of patients with twice weekly applications of potent TCS (fluticasone) to areas that have healed but are prone to developing eczema (Fig. 1.2), with patients/caretakers being instructed to follow instructions carefully to avoid potential side effects.[7]

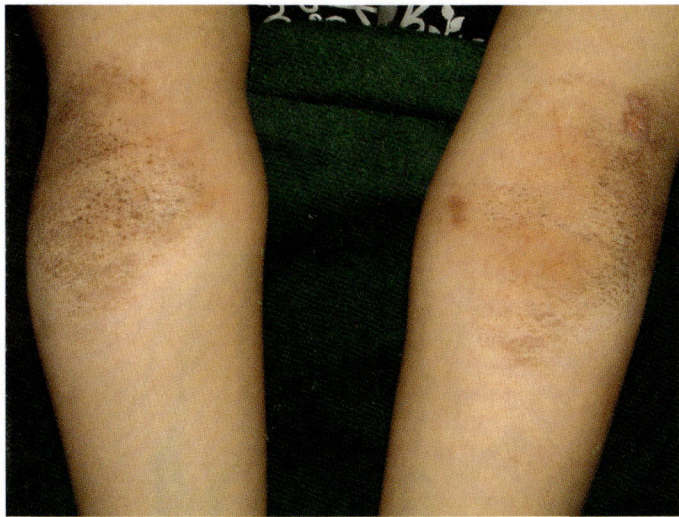

Fig. 1.2: TCS are the first line agents for treating inflammation and pruritus associated with AD that is unresponsive to good skin care and moisturizers. In this patient, the acute flare of AD was controlled with a daily regimen of betamethasone valerate cream and long-term remission was sustained with twice weekly applications of diluted betamethasone (with cold cream 1:1) to areas prone to developing eczema immediately after a bath while the skin was still moist.

Table 1.5: Grade of evidence and potency of TCS used in dermatological diseases[5]

Evidence grade	Indication	Potency of TCS (British)
A: Double blind RCTs	Atopic dermatitis	Mild, moderate, potent
	Psoriasis	Mild, moderate, potent, very potent
	Vitiligo	Potent, very potent
	Seborrheic dermatitis	Mild, moderate
	Pompholyx	Potent, very potent
	Lichen sclerosus	Potent, very potent
	Lichen simplex	Potent, very potent
	Aphthous stomatitis	Potent
B: Clinical trials	Alopecia areata	Potent, very potent
	Bullous pemphigoid	Potent, very potent
	Allergic contact dermatitis	Moderate, potent
	Cutaneous T cell lymphoma	Moderate, potent
	Discoid lupus erythematosus	Potent, very potent
	Polymorphic eruptions of pregnancy	Potent
		Mild, moderate
	Pruritus ani	Moderate, potent
	Pruritus valvae	
C: Small trials or >20 cases	Actinic prurigo	Potent, very potent
	Chronic actinic dermatitis	Moderate, potent
	Chronic irritant dermatitis	Mild, moderate, potent, very potent
	Nummular dermatitis	Potent, very potent
	Geographical tongue	Potent
	Hailey Hailey disease	Mild, moderate, potent
	Juvenile planter dermatosis	Moderate, potent
	Lichen planus	Potent, very potent
	Pemphigus gestationis	Potent, very potent
	Pretibial myxedema	Potent
	Sarcoidosis	Potent
	Sweet's syndrome	Potent
	Urticaria pigmentosa	Potent, very potent
D: At least 5 cases	Grover's disease	Potent
	Lichen planopilaris	Potent, very potent
	Necrobiotic lipoidica	Potent
	Pyoderma gangrenosum	Potent, very potent
	Scleromyxoedema	Potent
	Infantile hemangioma	Very potent
	Subcorneal pustular dermatosis	Moderate, potent
	Prurigo nodularis	Potent, very potent
E: <5 cases reported	Granuloma annulare	Potent, very potent
	Granuloma faciale	Moderate, potent
	Lichen nitidus	Potent
	Lymphocytoma cutis	Potent
	Lymphomatoid papulosis	Potent, very potent
	Morphoea	Potent
	Pityriasis rosea	Moderate, potent
	Subacute cutaneous lupus erythematosus	Moderate, potent

Table 1.6: Summary of a clinical trials on use of TCS in AD

Authors, year of publication	Drugs	Result
Prado de Oliveira et al, 2002	Mometasone furoate 0.1% BD vs Desonide 0.5% OD	Mometasone group showed better response
Hanifin et al, 2002	Intermittent fluticasone propionate or vehicle, OD 4 d/wk × 4 weeks followed by OD 2 d/wk	AD relapse 7.7 times less likely with twice-a-week fluticasone propionate than with emollients alone
Torok et al, 2003	Clocortolone pivalate 0.1% + tacrolimus 0.1% BD vs Clocortolone pivalate 0.1% BD vs Tacrolimus 0.1% BD	Combination therapy was superior to TCS or tacrolimus alone arms
Kirkup et al, 2003	Fluticasone propionate vs Hydrocortisone 1% cream vs Hydrocortisone butyrate 0.1% cream	Fluticasone propionate was more effective than hydrocortisone 1% in both acute and maintenance treatment of AD
Beattie and Lewis-Jones, 2004	Hydrocortisone 1% OD as wet wrap vs Hydrocortisone 1% BD	Twice a day hydrocortisone + emollients not statistically significantly inferior than wet wrap therapy in moderate AD
Hebert et al, 2007	Desonide 0.05% vs Vehicle BD	Desonide 0.05% was statistically significantly better than vehicle
Peserico et al, 2008	Emollient ± methylpredni-solone aceponate 0.1% cream twice weekly	Treatment with methylprednisolone aceponate twice weekly + emollient had a 3.5 fold lower risk of relapse than treatment with emollients alone
Glazenburg et al, 2009	Fluticasone propionate 0.005% ointment BD vs Placebo	87% children had remission in 4 week period; twice weekly fluticasone propionate reduced risk of relapse in moderate-severe AD
Rubio et al, 2013	Fluticasone propionate cream 0.05% BD vs Vehicle cream BD	Fluticasone group had 2.7 times lower risk of relapse than vehicle group

- Another technique of TCS application is wet wrap dressings, used specially in cases with severe extensive disease to avoid systemic administration of steroids. In children with severe refractory AD, 5%, 10%, and 25% dilutions of fluticasone propionate 0.05% cream proved highly efficacious, irrespective of dilution, when applied under wet-wrap dressings. Improvement occurred mainly during the first week, and the only significant adverse effect was folliculitis.[8]
- Regarding frequency of application, a systematic review found no clear differences in outcomes between once-daily and more frequent application of TCS.[9]

- A systemic review on safety of TCS in AD found that although some systemic exposure does occur, clinically significant changes appear to be uncommon, and systemic complications are rare when medications are used properly.[10]

Nummular Dermatitis

- Management of nummular dermatitis (Fig. 1.3) is similar to other dermatitis and TCS along with emollients are the mainstay of treatment.
- Moderate-potency to potent TCS (sometimes along with topical antibiotics) are used at least initially and may be weaned with topical immunomodulators like tacrolimus or pimecrolimus as the patient responds.
- Severely pruritic and chronic lichenified lesions respond better to potent agents, but this seems a safe option as the lesions are limited and rarely affect thin skin sites such as face or flexures.

Psoriasis[6]

TCS are of established value in psoriasis. Potent and very potent TCS are the most effective topical monotherapy for localized disease based on their cost-effectiveness (Table 1.7).

- *Indications:*
  - *Chronic plaque psoriasis*:
    - Localized diseases: As a standalone therapy a potent (or very potent if lesions are thick) TCS is used carefully on the lesions (Fig. 1.4a and b).
    - Widespread disease: Mild or moderate potency TCS is used as an adjunct to systemic therapy.

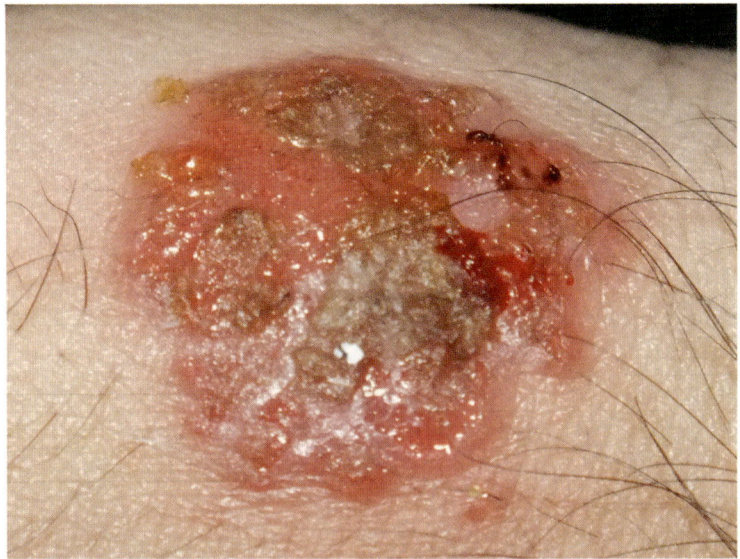

Fig. 1.3: TCS are first line of treatment for nummular dermatitis. In this patient a moderate potency steroid antibiotic combination was used for 3 weeks. Always rule out underlying atopy in these patients.

Table 1.7: Summary of clinical trials on use of TCS in chronic plaque psoriasis

Authors, year of publication	Drugs	Result
Stein et al, 2001	Betamethasone valerate foam vs Placebo BD	Betamethasone valerate foam was superior to placebo
Green & Sadoff, 2001	Tazarotene 0.1% vs Tazarotene + high-potency TCS (fluocinonide 0.05%, mometasone 0.1% or diflorasone 0.05%) vs Tazarotene + mid-high potency TCS (betamethasone 0.05% or fluticasone 0.005%, or diflorasone 0.05%). All applied OD	Betamethasone 0.05% was best performing steroid. Mometasone + tazarotene was best tolerated option
Gottlieb et al, 2003	CP foam 0.05% BD vs Placebo	In CP group, 68% achieved PGA 0/1 vs 21% in placebo group (p <0.001)
Decroix et al, 2004	CP lotion vs Vehicle BD	CP lotion was efficient, safe and well tolerated
Lowe et al, 2005	CP lotion vs CP emollient cream vs Vehicle	CP lotion was comparable to CP emollient cream and significantly more effective than vehicle
Koo et al, 2006	CP foam + calcipotriene ointment vs CP foam vs Calcipotriene ointment	Combination therapy was better than either agent. Weekend maintenance with CP was better than maintenance with placebo
Jarratt et al, 2006	CP spray 0.05% vs Vehicle	CP spray 0.05% was effective and safe
Angelo et al, 2007	Tazarotene 0.1% vs CP 0.05%	At 12 weeks, there was 100% response in CP group vs 88% in tazarotene group.
Mraz et al, 2008	CP 0.05% spray vs CP foam	There was 64% reduction in BSA involvement with CP spray vs 25% with CP foam (p <0.01), indicating spray was better than foam

Note: CP: Clobetasol propionate.

- *Hyperkeratotic and lichenified psoriasis*: Salicylic acid (3–6%) is often added to potent/very potent TCS to treat thick hyperkeratotic (Fig. 1.5) and lichenified psoriasis.
- *Scalp psoriasis:* Potent and very potent TCS are also the most effective therapy for scalp psoriasis[11] (Fig. 1.6a). If lesions are thick, then TCS are often combined with salicylic acid (3–6%) and occlusion improves response.
- *Palmoplantar psoriasis:* Potent and very potent TCS are also the most effective therapy for palmoplantar psoriasis (Fig. 1.6a), but it is necessary to ask the patient to hydrate the skin by soaking the affected part and immediately applying the medication carefully, avoiding inadvertent rubbing of the excess medication on dorsal aspect (Fig. 1.6b), otherwise this overzealous treatment results in hypopigmentation of dorsal aspect of digits (Fig. 1.6c).

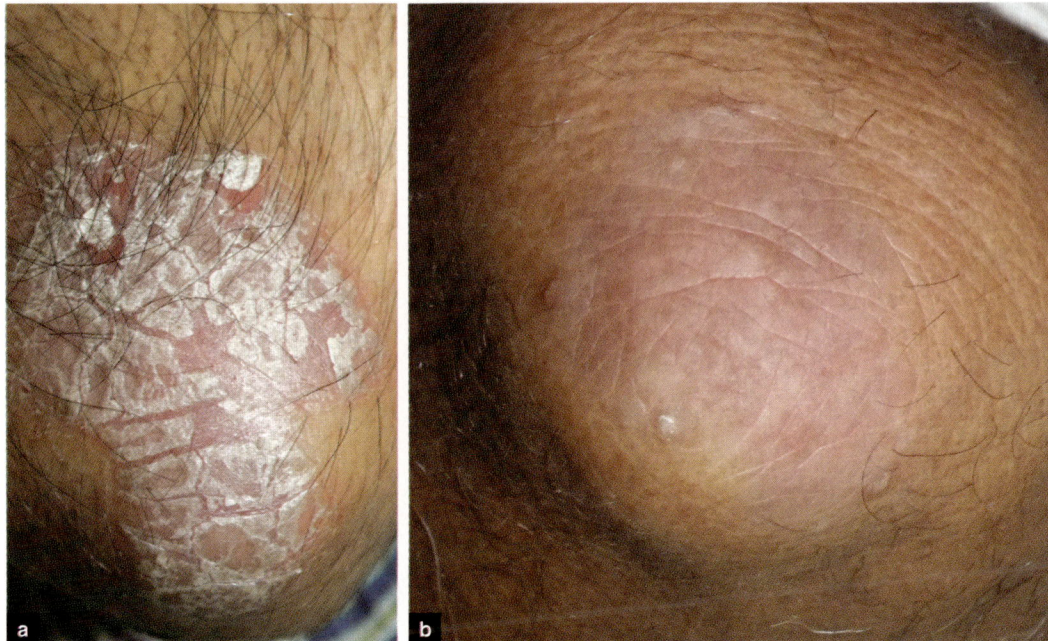

Fig. 1.4: Localized psoriasis: (a) Pre-treatment: In this patient, who had localized but recurrent disease (when ever he stopped therapy) involving only elbows and knees, a very potent steroid (clobetasol propionate 0.05%, in ointment base) was used taking care to avoid application to surrounding skin. **(b) Post-treatment:** Improvement was seen in 4 weeks and patient was maintained on weekend therapy with betamethasone valerate with no relapses. Such a patient can also be treated with a combination of calcipotriol and TCS.

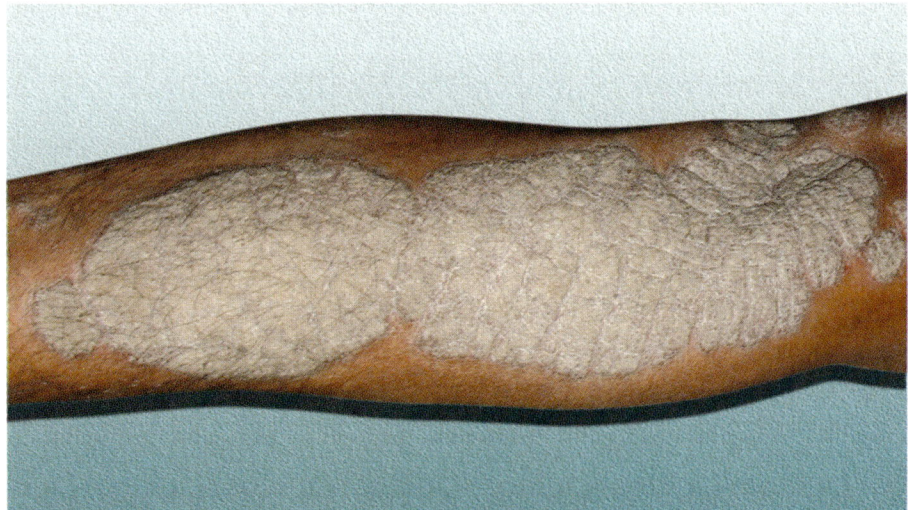

Fig. 1.5: Hyperkeratotic psoriasis: This patient, who had a localized hyperkeratotic lesion was treated with a combination of a very potent TCS (clobetasol propionate 0.05%)—salicylic acid (3%) combination in ointment base used carefully to avoid application to surrounding normal skin after moistening the lesion using a wet towel. Lesion flattened in 4 weeks and potency of steroid was reduced to a moderate potency formulation. Improvement was achieved in 8 weeks and patient was maintained on weekend therapy with betamethasone valerate.

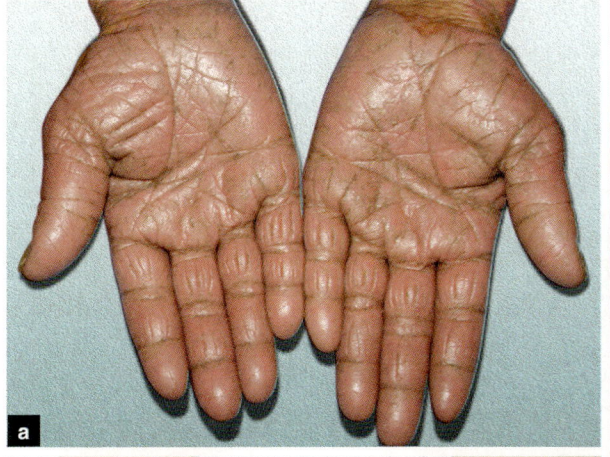
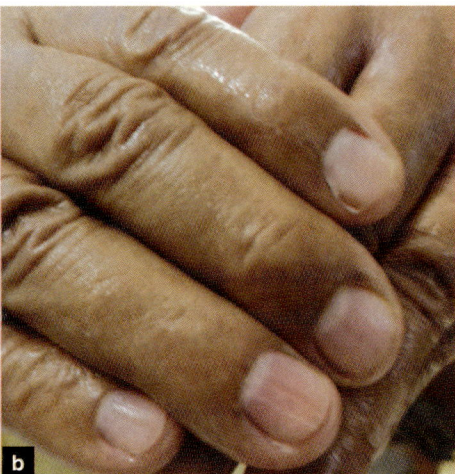
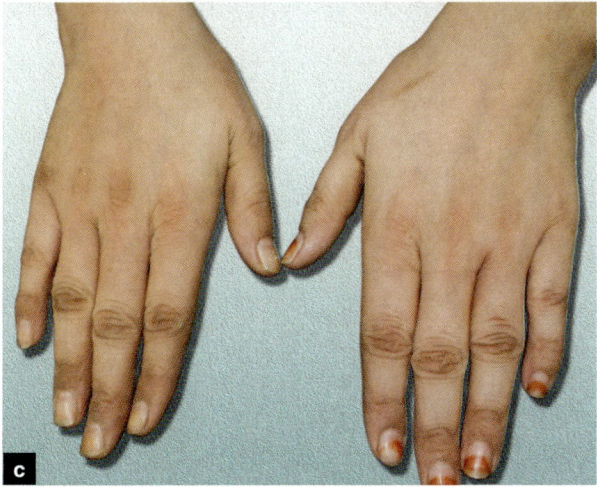

Fig. 1.6: Palmoplantar psoriasis: (a) Potent and very potent TCS in ointment base are the most effective therapy for palmoplantar psoriasis. If lesions are thick, then TCS are often combined with salicylic acid (3–6%). This patient with palmoplantar psoriasis was asked to soak the affected part in saline, and immediately apply a combination of clobetasol propionate + 3% salicylic acid, after patting dry the skin **(b)** Patients are often overzealous with the application of medication, inadvertently rubbing the excess ointment on dorsal aspect of hands. **(c)** This results in hypopigmentation of dorsal aspects of digits.

- *Flexural psoriasis:* Mild-to-moderate potency TCS are also first line of therapy in flexures (Fig. 1.7a) and genitalia where other topical treatments may irritate. Very potent TCS should not be used in flexures as it may lead to side effects like dermatophytic infections and striae (Fig. 1.7b).
- *Unstable, erythrodermic and generalized pustular psoriasis*: Mild TCS or TCS diluted with emollients are often used as adjunct to systemic therapy.
- *Resistant psoriasis*: Intralesional CS can be used in small resistant plaques, for instance on the backs of hands and knuckles and the effect may be long lasting and repetition of the injection unnecessary for several months. In the treatment of psoriasis of the fingernails, the nail fold can be injected, but results are often disappointing and the procedure may be painful.

- *Formulations:*
  - Potent and very potent steroids in cream/ointment formulation (depending on thickness of lesions) are the most effective treatment for localised psoriasis, but may be associated with side effects.

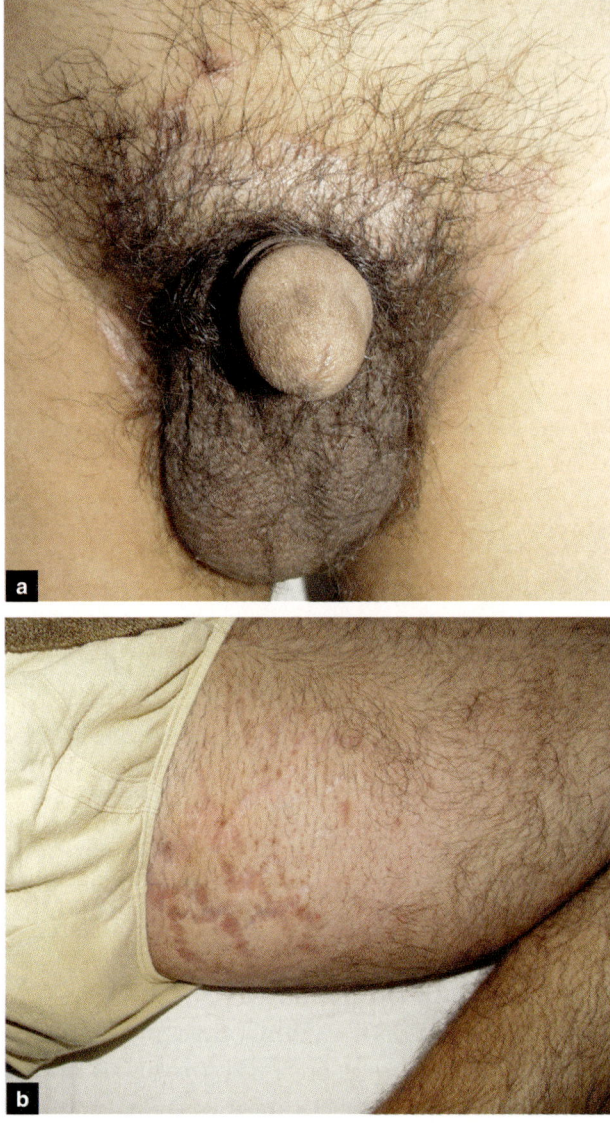

Fig. 1.7: Flexural psoriasis: (a) Mild to moderate potency TCS are first line of therapy at sites such as flexures and genitalia where other topical treatments can induce irritation. **(b)** Very potent TCS should not be used in flexures as it may lead to side effects like striae.

- Mild-to-moderate potency TCS are the treatment of choice for psoriasis on the face and neck.
- Newer formulations of TCS, particularly foams, are easier to apply than traditional creams or ointments and can be used for scalp, truncal or limb psoriasis.
- *Dosing:* It remains unclear whether once or twice daily applications should be recommended. However, it is generally agreed that use of very potent TCS should be limited to 2–4 weeks and less than 50 g/week. Very potent TCS should not be occluded and should not be used on the face or intertriginous sites.

- *Response:* Improvement is usually achieved within 4–6 weeks but patients usually require maintenance treatment consisting of intermittent applications (often restricted to the weekends). But frequency, as well as duration, should be tapered down in maintenance phase because of cutaneous and systemic adverse effects of TCS.
- *Advantages:* TCS generally lack irritancy, do not stain skin or clothing and have the merits of ease of application and are frequently combined with other topical agents to counteract irritancy.
- *Disadvantages:*
  - *Side effects:* Potential side effects of TCS are well known and include cutaneous atrophy (risk less in psoriasis than in AD) and systemic absorption, although there is a lack of data about the magnitude of these risks. However, it is prudent to limit the use of potent TCS to stable plaque psoriasis affecting limited areas.
  - *Psoriasis specific disadvantages:*
    - Tachyphylaxis to treatment with TCS is a suspected, but debatable phenomenon in psoriasis.
    - Potent TCS also do not induce a lasting remission, unlike tar or dithranol.
    - Another concern is that when TCS are discontinued, patients may rebound, sometimes with disease worse than it was prior to treatment (pustular lesions).
- *Combination therapy:*
  - *Salicylic acid*: TCS are often combined with salicylic acid 3–6% in an ointment formulation to treat thick hyperkeratotic and lichenified psoriasis and palmoplantar lesions. Similar combination in a lotion formulation is used to treat scalp psoriasis.
  - *Calcipotriol*: Combination of a potent TCS with calcipotriol provides the most effective strategy for topical treatment of limited plaque psoriasis over a short period of time.

Vitiligo

- *Indications:* TCS are the first-line therapy for localized vitiligo and are highly recommended for small lesions and for use in children (Table 1.8).
- *Dosing:* Vitiligo is a moderately steroid responsive dermatoses and a potent/very potent TCS (e.g. clobetasol propionate ointment, 0.05%) is used once daily for 4 weeks and application gradually tapered to a lower potency TCS (e.g. hydrocortisone butyrate, 0.1% cream).[12]
- *Advantages*: Ease of application, high compliance rate, and low cost are advantages of using TCS. Compared with PUVA, which promotes a predominantly perifollicular pattern of repigmentation, TCS result in more diffuse repigmentation (Fig. 1.8) which occurs more quickly but is less stable.

Table 1.8: Summary of a clinical trials on use of TCS in vitiligo

Authors, year of publication	Drugs	Result
Lim-Ong et al, 2005	CP 0.05% and NB-UVB vs Placebo and NB-UVB	CP + NBUVB induced earlier repigmentation but over all repigmentation comparable in both groups.
Sanclemente et al, 2008	Betamethasone 0.05% vs Topical catalase/dismutase superoxide	Good repigmentation in both groups at 10 months
Sassi et al, 2008	308 nm laser phototherapy twice weekly + hydrocortisone 17-butyrate cream BD vs 308 nm laser phototherapy twice weekly alone	At 12 wks laser phototherapy twice weekly + hydrocortisone 17-butyrate cream BD superior in repigmentation and PGA scores ($p = 0.0087$)
Kose et al, 2010	Mometasone 0.1% vs Pimecrolimus 1%	Mometasone cream effective in vitiligo on any part of body, while pimecrolimus was effective only on face
Akdeniz et al, 2014	Calcipotriol + NB-UVB + betamethasone vs NB-UVB + calcipotriol vs NB-UVB	Combination of topical calcipotriol + NB-UVB + betamethasone showed superior repigmentation (63.3%) vs NB-UVB alone (46.7%)

Note: CP: Clobetasol propionate.

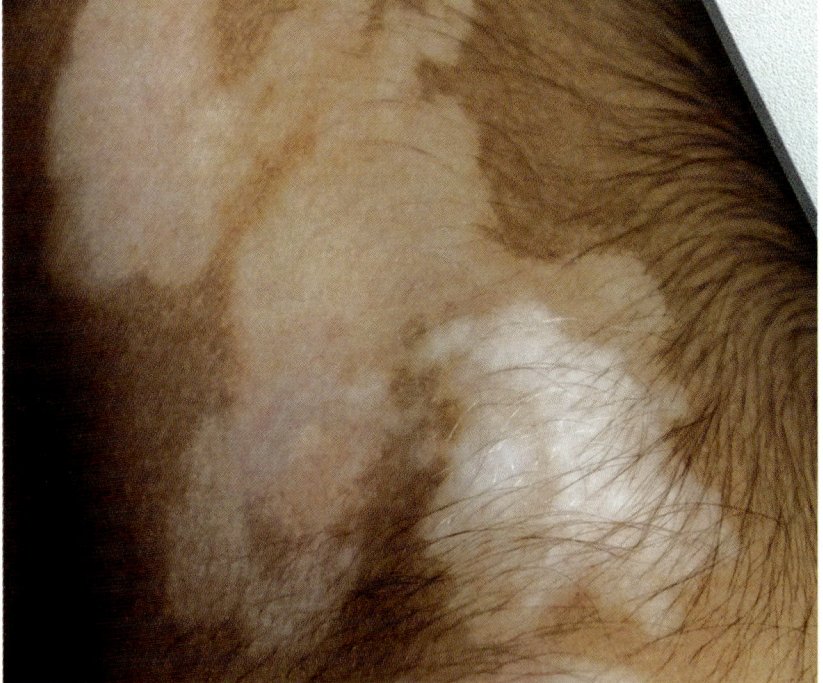

Fig. 1.8: Vitiligo: TCS are the first-line therapy for localized vitiligo and are highly recommended for small lesions and for use in children. TCS result in more diffuse repigmentation, which occurs more quickly but is less stable.

Steroid-treated repigmented vitiligo skin showed marked repopulation by functional melanocytes which appear dendritic and DOPA-positive, and contain many melanosomes of normal size and shape.[13]

- *Disadvantages:*
  - Caution is necessary when using TCS around the eyelids, as they can increase intraocular pressure and exacerbate glaucoma.
  - TCS induced pigmentation is less stable and recurrence after cessation of treatment is not uncommon.
  - TCS induced other side effects.
- *Combination therapy:* TCS + UVB, TCS + calcineurin inhibitors, TCS + vitamin D analogs may be beneficial in some cases, as two agents act synergistically on pigment restoration and on immune suppression, at lower individual doses, thus potentially minimizing side effects.

Seborrheic Dermatitis (SD)

- TCS and topical antifungals, either alone or in combination, are the mainstay of therapy in SD. When topical antifungal monotherapy fails, it is recommended that a short course of mild to moderately potent TCS be added to control acute flares and improve results.
- SD of scalp is frequently treated with combination of TCS (even clobetasol propionate) and salicylic acid in a lotion formulation, applied at night with shampooing the next morning. In very hyperkeratotic lesions (Fig.1.9a), patient is asked to apply TCS in lotion (initially even an ointment, though cumbersome to use) formulation and occlude the scalp with a shower cap overnight (Fig.1.9b).
- The side effects of TCS preclude their long (even short term) use over face especially in thin-skin areas such as eyelids and therefore, topical calcineurin inhibitors (tacrolimus and pimecrolimus) though not yet approved for use in SD are emerging as effective alternatives.[14]

Pompholyx

- Potent and very potent TCS are the first line therapy. They are often more effective if used under occlusion, although this approach may increase the chance of side effects.
- Overzealous or inadvertent application of the TCS on the dorsal aspect of hands often results in hypopigmentation and atrophy of these areas.

Lichen Sclerosus (LS)

- Potent and very potent TCS, when used under supervision and for finite duration, are the first line of treatment for LS in adults as well as in children in both sexes.[15]
- There are no RCTs comparing formulations or frequency of application of TCS in LS, but the general recommendation is to use clobetasol propionate 0.05%

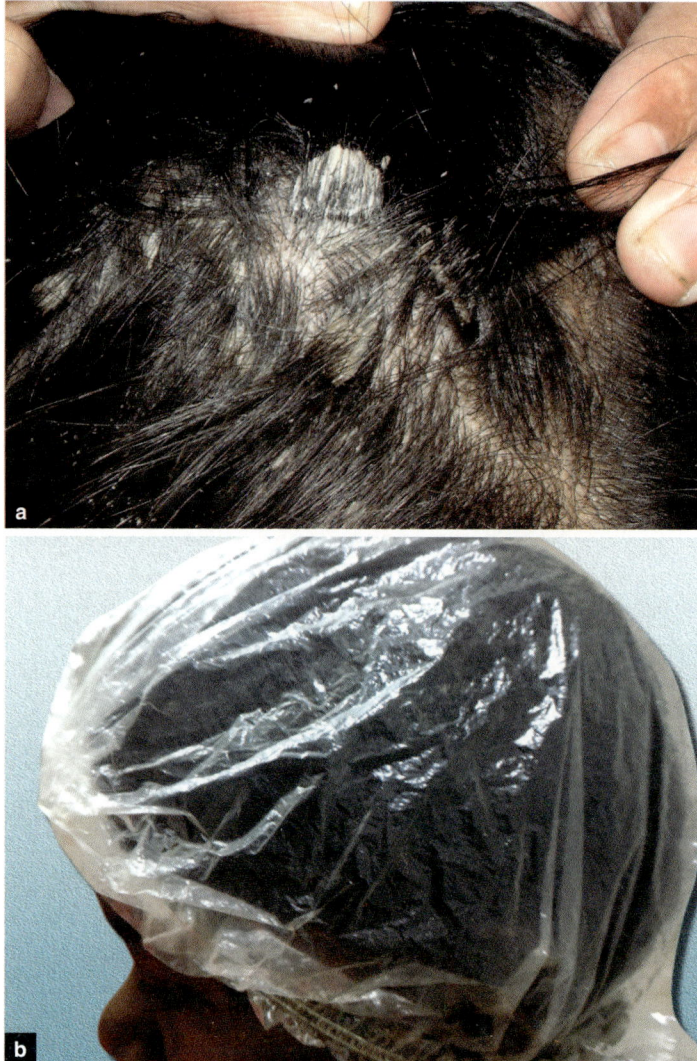

Fig.1.9: Seborrheic dermatitis of scalp. (a) This patient had hyperkeratotic lesions (pityriasis amiantacea) which is frequently treated with combination of clobetasol propionate and salicylic acid in a lotion (initially even ointment) formulation, applied over night with shampooing of scalp next morning. **(b)** To improve the efficacy, TCS can be applied on scalp under occlusion using a shower cap.

ointment once a day for a month, on alternate days for a month, and then twice weekly for a further month, with a 30 gram tube lasting at least 3 months in an adult and 6 months in a child. Patient can thereafter be weaned off to a less potent steroid or topical calcineurin inhibitor.

- Complications of use of TCS in genital LS include development of anogenital warts (Fig.1.10) and reactivation of genital herpes (GH), along with secondary candidal and bacterial infection. It is recommended that those with history of GH should be prescribed prophylactic acyclovir.[16]

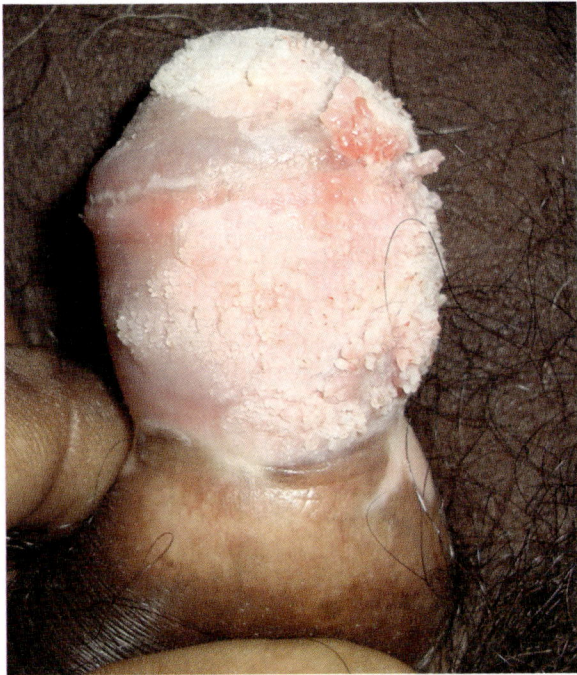

Fig. 1.10: Genital lichen sclerosus: Potent and very potent TCS are the first line of treatment for genital LS but need to be used under supervision and for finite duration. This patient with genital LS had used very potent TCS for several years and developed condyloma acuminatum-like lesions. Other infections which can develop in this scenario include reactivation of GH and secondary candidal and bacterial infection.

Lichen Simplex Chronicus (LSC)

- Treatment of LSC is aimed at interrupting the itch-scratch-itch cycle and the first-line measures to control itch include use of potent or very potent TCS and antihistamines.[17]
- It is important to ask the patient to use the TCS within the margin of the lichenified plaque and protect the surrounding skin with petrolatum to avoid perilesional hypopigmentation and atrophy (Fig. 1.11).

Aphthous Stomatitis[18]

- *Indications:* Though the natural history of aphthous stomatitis is of spontaneous remission, many dermatologists do prescribe TCS to hasten healing and reduce the associated pain, which is often very severe.
- *Use:* Response to TCS in oral mucosa can be enhanced by cotton tip applications for 30 seconds and avoidance of eating or drinking for 30–60 minutes thereafter.
  - For mild disease, TCS such as fluocinonide, hydrocortisone, triamcinolone (as an oral paste) can be used to up to four times daily.
  - For severe aphthosis, potent TCS such as clobetasol (gel formulation) are used twice a day.

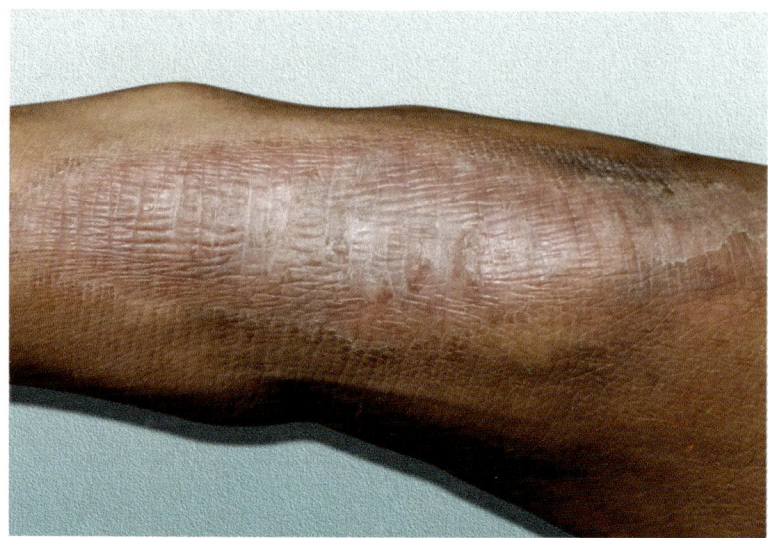

Fig.1.11: Lichen simplex chronicus: The first-line treatment to control itch include use of potent TCS and antihistamines. It is important to ask the patient to use the TCS within the margin of the lichenified plaque and protect the surrounding skin with petrolatum to avoid perilesional hypopigmentation and atrophy as seen in this patient.

- Betamethasone/dexamethasone elixir 0.5 mg/5 ml three times daily can also be used as a swish and spit mouthwash.
- Intralesional triamcinolone in concentration of 3–10 mg/ml repeated over 2–4 weeks intervals are useful in treatment of major aphthae.
- TCS formulated in aerosol sprays can be used to target ulcers on the soft palate or oropharynx.
- *Side effects:* When used for less than 3 weeks, systemic absorption and HPA axis suppression are unlikely.

Alopecia Areata (AA)
- *Indications:* Localized AA.
- *Use:*
  - TCS, particularly the potent ones when used for at least 3 months, have shown efficacy in alopecia areata (few lesions) in some studies, although the results are variable and they do not appear to be effective in alopecia totalis/universalis.[19]
  - Intralesional corticosteroids: May be used in resistant patches.
- *Advantages:* Practical to use in the form of lotion and foam.
- *Side effects:* Transient folliculitis is the main side effect (Fig.1.12).

Bullous Pemphigoid (BP)
- *Indications:*
  - *Localized disease:* Potent and very potent TCS have emerged as first line therapy for limited disease.

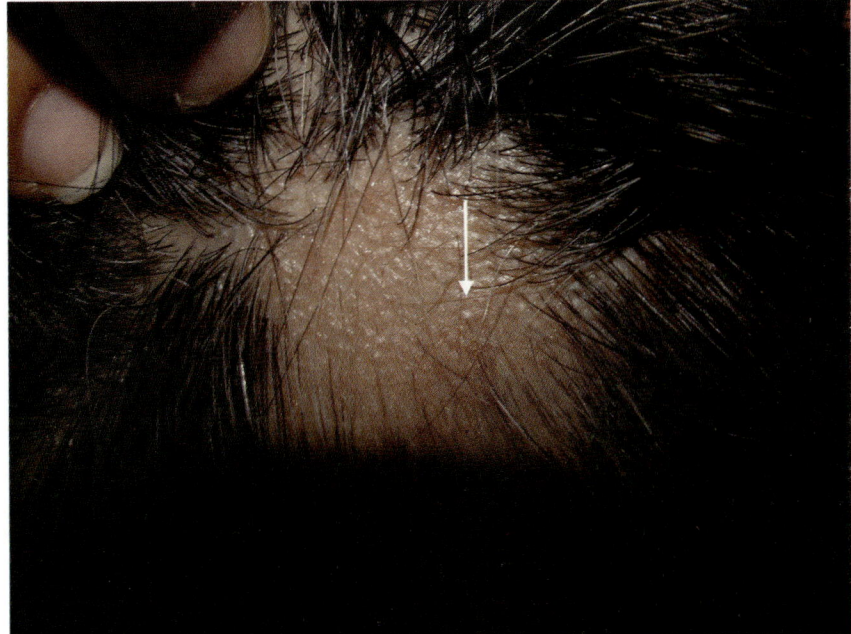

Fig. 1.12: Alopecia areata. Potent TCS as a lotion or foam are routinely used in the treatment of alopecia areata, when few lesions are present. Transient folliculitis (arrow) is the main side effect.

- *Moderate or extensive disease:* TCS are invariably used as an adjunct to systemic therapy in BP (Table 1.9) and may be used as a standalone therapy in patients who cannot use oral steroids and other immunosuppressives.
- *Use:* Very potent TCS (clobetasol propionate cream, 0.05%) applied twice a day (up to 40 g/day) to the whole body in extensive disease and to lesions in limited disease may be used as standalone therapy for 3 weeks. Even lower dose (10–30 g/day) is effective and is associated with fewer side effects.
- *Disadvantages:* However, the use of TCS in extensive disease may be limited by practical factors (time consuming, compliance and cost).

Table 1.9: Summary of a clinical trials on use of TCS in bullous pemphigoid[6]		
Authors, year of publication	*Drugs*	*Result*
Joly *et al*, 2002	CP 0.05% cream BD *vs* Prednisone (0.5 mg/kg for moderate disease and 1 mg/kg for severe disease)	At 3 wks, CP cream was superior to oral prednisone in extensive bullous pemphigoid (*P* = 0.02), while both groups showed 100% disease control in moderate disease.
Joly *et al*, 2009	CP was given depending on disease severity and body weight as mild regimen (10–30 g/day) *vs* Standard regimen (40 g/day)	Though disease control was excellent in both groups, there was 2-fold decrease in risk of death or life-threatening adverse events with mild regimen *vs* Standard regimen (*P* = 0.039).

Allergic Contact Dermatitis (ACD)

- *Indications:* Though avoidance of the allergen is the mainstay of therapy in acute ACD, TCS are required in most patients for rapid alleviation of symptoms, along with other measures (barrier creams, emollients and antihistamines). In extensive chronic ACD (like airborne contact dermatitis), TCS are frequently used as adjunct to systemic therapy.
- *Use:* Potency of TCS used depends on site and morphology of lesions (less potent steroids for face, flexures and more potent steroids for chronic lichenified lesions) and duration of use depends on response (longer for lichenified lesions). For extensive disease (like in airborne contact dermatitis), patient may need a short course of oral steroids and maintenance with oral immunosuppressive agents.

Cutaneous T Cell Lymphoma

TCS have been used in the treatment of mild, patch stage MF with good results, but unfortunately, evidence in favor of using them is lacking. The current evidence-based recommendation is that the moderately potent or potent TCS are effective in temporarily clearing patches and plaques in some patients with early-stage IA/IB MF.[20]

Discoid Lupus Erythematosus

- *Indications*: TCS are the cornerstone of initial therapy for patients with limited involvement and are an important adjunct to systemic therapy in extensive disease.
- *Use:*
  - There is limited data comparing one molecule over another, but in general potent and very potent TCS appear to be more effective and DLE is one of the few conditions warranting use of potent steroids on the face. Occlusion may further help.[21]
  - Intralesional steroids give good response in patients with hypertrophic lesions.
- *Side effects:* Side effect of atrophy is probably not a concern in DLE which is a scarring dermatoses in itself.

Pruritic Urticarial Papules and Plaques of Pregnancy (PUPPP)

- *Indications:* Since the patient is very symptomatic, most patients need to be treated with frequent application of potent TCS like betamethasone/mometasone and emollients, usually with antihistamines.[22]
- *Response:* New lesions usually stop appearing within a few days and subsequently the frequency of applications can be tapered (Fig. 1.13a and b).

Pruritus Ani

- *Indications:* Cleansing and application of TCS are the mainstay therapy for chronic or idiopathic pruritus ani.

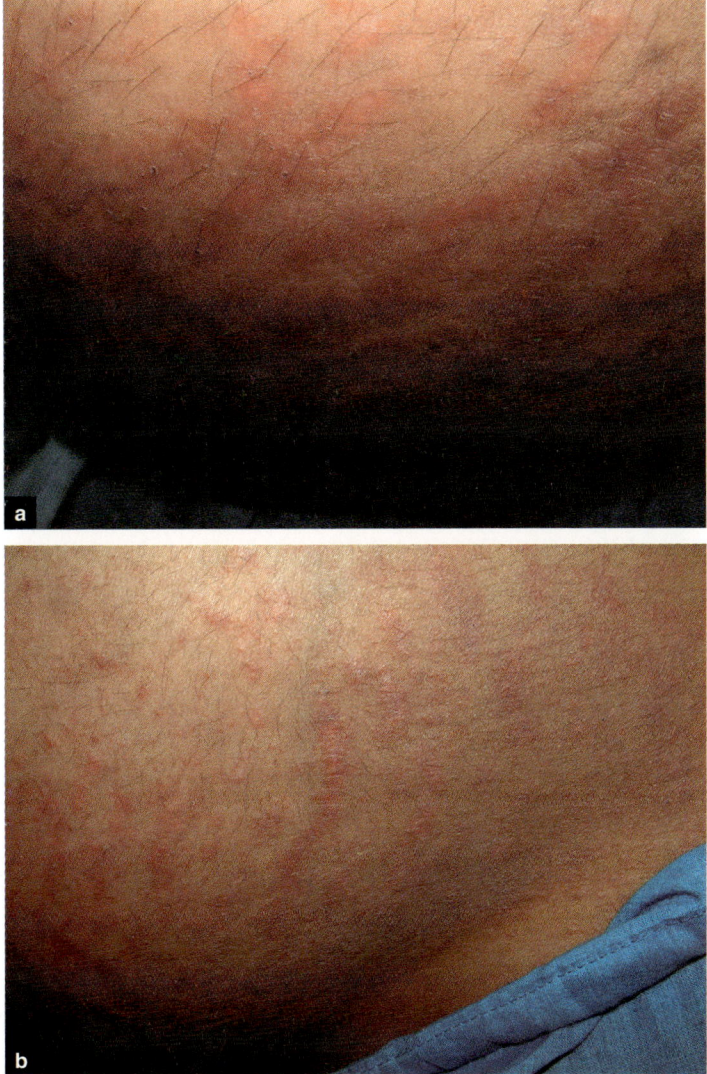

Fig. 1.13: Pruritic urticarial papules and plaques of pregnancy. (a) This extremely symptomatic patient in third trimester of pregnancy was treated with moderate potency TCS in cream base along with antihistamines and emollients. **(b)** Ten days later not only was she symptomatically better but lesions were conspicuously less erythematous and flatter.

- *Use:* A short course of mild to moderately potent TCS is recommended for a few weeks, followed by reduction in potency as symptoms improve.[23]
- *Side effects:* Caution must be taken with prolonged use of potent agents as the area is particularly prone to atrophy.

Pruritus Vulvae

- *Indication an basis of use:* Identification and elimination of the suspected allergens and irritants is important in the treatment for pruritus vulvae. TCS along with emollients are used to control the inflammation to provide symptomatic relief and interrupt the vicious itch-scratch cycle.

- *Use:*
  - Moderately potent TCS ointment is preferred in pruritus vulvae as other formulations may contribute to allergic or irritant contact dermatitis.
  - Small quantity of ointment is used once a day (along with emollients several times a day) under close supervision to limit side effects such as striae, folliculitis, and atrophy.[24]

Actinic Prurigo

- *Indications:* TCS are invariably used as adjunct to photoprotection in actinic prurigo.
- *Use:*
  - *For acute disease*: Potent/very potent TCS along with photoprotection.
  - *Recurrent disease:* Springtime phototherapy is administered, often with application of moderate potency TCS to the affected areas prior to session of phototherapy to reduce the risk of flare.[25]

Chronic Actinic Dermatitis (CAD)

- *Indications:* TCS are invariably used as adjunct to photoprotection in CAD.
- *Use:* Along with photoprotection, the treatment of active disease involves the use of potent TCS. For acute flares which are not sufficiently controlled with TCS, systemic steroids can be administered (tapered over weeks) and with continued use of TCS for maintenance of control often along with other immunosuppressives.[26]

Irritant Chronic Dermatitis (ICD) of Hands

- *Indications:* Though avoidance of irritants, liberal use of moisturisers and appropriate hand care is the primary strategy in management of ICD, TCS are often used to control inflammation and relieve symptoms.
- *Use:* Potency of TCS used in ICD depends on the severity of irritant dermatitis, but usually mild-moderate potency TCS used once or twice a day is usually sufficient.
- *Disadvantages:* TCS induced secondary compromise in barrier function of skin must be considered. Topical calcineurin inhibitors may be used as alternative to low potency TCS in selective patients with mild inflammatory changes who do not experience a burning sensation when the product is applied.[27]

Geographical Tongue

- *Indications:* For patients who continue to remain symptomatic despite consevative measures (gentle brushing and saline rinses, avoidance of hot, spicy food and harsh mouthwashes), TCS may be prescribed.
- *Use:* TCS are to be applied on tongue at bedtime and after meals till patient is symptomatically better.[28]

Hailey-Hailey Disease

- *Indications:* Apart from controlling friction and infection, TCS along with anti-infective agents may be needed.
- *Use:* Combining anti-infective therapy with potent TCS is effective in controlling the disease flare when used promptly.
- *Disadvantages:* However, caution must be exercised as lesions are predominantly seen in flexures (axillae and groin) which are particularly susceptible to side effects of TCS.[29]

Juvenile Plantar Dermatosis

- *Indications:* Changing to non-occlusive, open, leather footwear and cotton socks is the primary treatment strategy. TCS may be beneficial, if there is an inflammatory component.
- *Use:* A moderate or potent TCS applied once a day is usually sufficient, if patient is complying with other measures.[30]

Lichen Planus (LP)

Although TCS are widely accepted and are practically almost always used as first line treatment in LP, there is paucity of scientific evidence supporting this conventional therapeutic modality.

- *Indications:*
  - *Oral LP:* There are several RCTs (Table 1.10) and one Cochrane review[31] indicating the efficacy of TCS in oral LP but they should only be used if the patient is symptomatic.[32]
  - *Cutaneous LP:* There are only few RCTs assessing the usefulness of TCS. However, the majority of these trials are small, have used unvalidated outcome measures with high risk of bias. Unfortunately for genital LP, nail LP, lichen planopilaris and other lichenoid disorders there are no RCTs which have assessed the efficacy of TCS.
- *Use:*
  - *Cutaneous LP*: A potent TCS once daily application is used until remission, while in hypertrophic LP very potent TCS under occlusion is used initially and potency is titrated as patient responds.
  - For oral LP, potent TCS may be applied three times daily with a gloved finger. Efficacy of TCS in oral lesions can be enhanced by using an oral paste (steroids formulated in orabase) or gel formulation, using cotton tip application for 30 seconds and avoiding eating or drinking for 30–60 minutes thereafter. Also, mouthwash swish and rinse can be done with 5 mg prednisolone/2 mg betamethasone dissolved in 15 ml water three times a day. Oral candidiasis is a frequent complication of TCS treatment of oral LP and so these treatments are frequently combined with prophylactic weekly fluconazole, 150 mg.

Table 1.10: Summary of a clinical trials on use of TCS in oral lichen planus[6]		
Authors, year of publication	*Drugs*	*Result*
Campisi *et al*, 2004	CP 0.025% microsphere *vs* CP 0.025% as lipophilic ointment in hydrophilic phase	New drug delivery system increased symptom remission and compliance
Conrotto *et al*, 2006	CP 0.025% BD *vs* Topical ciclosporin 1.5% both in hydroxyethyl cellulose BD	CP more effective in inducing clinical improvement but associated with more side effects
Yoke *et al*, 2006	Triamcinolone acetonide 0.1% in orabase TDS *vs* Topical ciclosporin 0.1% solution TDS	Triamcinolone group showed better clinical response and symptom relief than ciclosporin at week 4.
Laeijen decker *et al*, 2006	Triamcinolone acetonide 0.1% in hydroxyethyl cellulose *vs* Tacrolimus 0.1% ointment both applied 4 times daily	Topical tacrolimus 0.1% ointment induced a better initial therapeutic response at 6 weeks, but was associated with frequent relapses at 3–9 weeks
Gorouhi *et al*, 2007	Triamcinolone acetonide 0.1% paste QID *vs* Pimecrolimus 1% QID	Both groups showed significant clinical response at 4 months (P-0.86), with no prominent adverse effects
Carbone *et al*, 2009	Topical clobetasol 0.025% *vs* Topical clobetasol 0.05% both in hydroxyethyl cellulose BD	Both showed significant clinical improvement (87% and 73%, with clobetasol 0.025% and clobetasol 0.05%, respectively), without any statistically significant difference after 2 months of treatment
Ghabanchi *et al*, 2009	Triamcinolone acetonide 0.1% paste TID *vs* Mucoadhesive prednisolone tablet (5 mg) BD	A fair to good response was seen in both groups at 2 weeks

Pemphigoid Gestationis

- *Indications:* Management depends on the severity of disease with the goal of treatment being to suppress blister formation and to relieve intense pruritus.
  - *Mild cases*: Potent TCS along with systemic antihistamines.
  - *Severe cases:* Systemic steroids along with TCS and systemic antihistamines.

Pretibial Myxedema

- *Indications:* TCS are indicated in patients with significant dermopathy.
- *Use:* Potent TCS with or without occlusion are used for at least 2 months. Using compression bandage may offer additional benefit in resistant cases. If symptoms persist, intralesional steroids may be tried. Systemic steroids have been shown to improve lesions in several patients, but their use is limited by systemic side effects.

Sarcoidosis

- *Indications:* Localized disease, usually in single/few plaques.
- *Use:* Although high level scientific evidence is lacking, very potent TCS have been used successfully in localized cutaneous disease.

Sweet's Syndrome

- *Indications:* Addressing underlying associated condition (malignancy, inflammatory bowel disease, infection, medication, radiation and pregnancy) may lead to resolution of skin lesions. Standard treatment of idiopathic Sweet's syndrome is systemic steroids but for localized disease, potent TCS may be tried.
- *Use:*
  - *Limited/mild disease:* Very potent TCS and intralesional corticosteroids may be useful as monotherapy.
  - *Extensive disease:* As adjuvant treatment.

Mastocytosis

Indications: Although the resolution of mastocytomas may occur with or without treatment, resolution is faster with TCS.

CHOOSING APPROPRIATE TCS

Potency of TCS

The choice of potency of TCS used depends on several factors but it is recommended that therapy should be initiated with lowest potency of TCS to sufficiently control the disease and once partial disease control is achieved, a lower potency TCS is introduced. The factors which determine the potency of steroid to be chosen depends on:

- *Dermatoses to be treated:* Dermatological conditions can be divided on the basis of their response to steroids (Table 1.11) into:
  - *Highly responsive,* which respond to mild to moderately potent steroids.
  - *Moderately responsive,* which respond to moderately potent to potent steroids.
  - *Least responsive,* which would need treatment with potent to very potent steroids.
- *Type of lesions:* Potency of TCS chosen also depends on type of lesions, e.g. in psoriasis, thicker lesions need to be treated with more potent TCS, as also lichenified (LSC) and verrucous lesions.
- *Sites/type of lesion to be treated:*
  - *Thick skin:* Lesions on palms and soles need to be treated with more potent steroids, in ointment base, sometimes under occlusion.
  - *Thin skin sites:* Eyelids and genitalia need to be treated with less potent steroids.
  - *Flexures:* Potent steroids are best avoided in flexures like axilla and groin as these are naturally moist occluded sites.

Table 1.11: Potency of TCS generally employed in different dermatological indications		
Highly responsive dermatoses require mild to moderate potency TCS	Moderately steroid responsive dermatoses require moderately potent to potent TCS	Least responsive dermatoses require potent to very potent TCS
Intertriginous psoriasis Atopic dermatitis (acute flares) Allergic contact dermatitis Irritant contact dermatitis	Atopic dermatitis (chronic/ lichenified) Seborrheic dermatitis Lichen simplex chronicus Pompholyx Papular urticaria Pruritus ani Pruritus vulvae Juvenile plantar dermatosis Chronic actinic dermatitis Vitiligo Lichen planus Chronic plaque psoriasis Parapsoriasis Cutaneous T-cell lymphoma Bullous pemphigoid Alopecia areata	Palmoplantar psoriasis Hand dermatitis Hypertrophic lichen planus Keloids/hypertrophic scars Discoid lupus erythematosus Actinic prurigo Lichen sclerosus Lichen nitidus Morphoea Cutaneous sarcoidosis Granuloma annulare Prurigo nodularis Pyoderma gangrenosum Urticaria pigmentosa Geographic tongue Pruritic urticarial papules and plaques of pregnancy Pretibial myxedema Sweet's syndrome Necrobiosis lipoidica

- *Face:* Potent steroids are best avoided on the face unless the disease warrants it (e.g. lesions of discoid lupus erythematosus on the face can be treated with a very potent steroid because without treatment the lesions will cause more scarring of the face) because of risk of developing topical steroid damaged face.

- *Duration of therapy*: When long term therapy is required, start with mild TCS.

- *Area to be treated*: When large area is to be treated, start with mild TCS.

Choosing Appropriate Vehicle

Vehicles should be chosen considering, the type and site of lesion, the potency of TCS and also occasionally previous history of contact sensitisation (Table 1.12).

Using Appropriate Amount

- Adequate amount must be applied to get the desired therapeutic effect.
- Simple practical guide to quantify the amount of TCS to be used is to ask the patient to use a pea-sized amount (if small area has to be covered; Fig. 1.14a) or the fingertip unit (FTU)[33] if larger area has to be covered. A FTU is quantity of formulation extruded from a tube with a nozzle of 5 mm diameter extending from the distal crease of the forefinger to ventral aspect of the fingertip (Fig. 1.14b).

Table 1.12: Properties of various vehicles used in formulations of TCS

Vehicle	Hydration	Indications	Sites	Cosmesis	Irritation/CD
Ointment	Very good	• Palmoplantar lesions • Lichenified/ thick scaly dermatoses	• Palms and soles • Avoid in naturally occluded areas	Greasy	Generally low
Cream	Moderate	Acute/subacute weeping lesions	Moist skin, intertriginous areas	Elegant	Variable, as contain preservatives
Gel	Drying	Dermatoses in dense hairy areas like scalp. Also mucosal lesions	Naturally occluded areas, scalp, mucosa	Elegant	Higher
Lotion (oil in water)	Drying	Scalp or dermatoses in dense hairy areas	Naturally occluded areas, scalp	Elegant	Higher
Solution (alcohol)	Drying	Scalp or dermatoses in dense hairy areas	Naturally occluded areas, scalp	Elegant	Higher

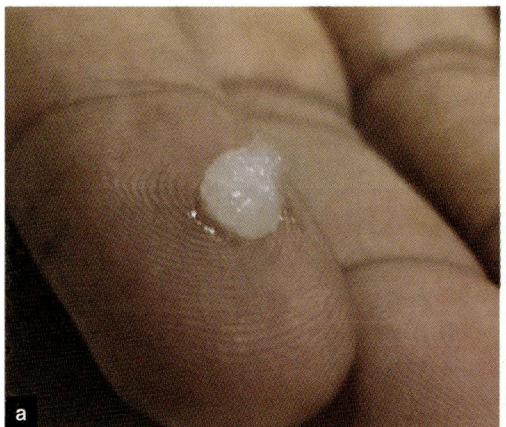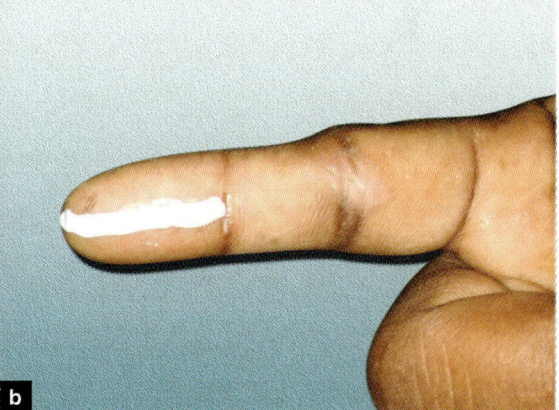

Fig. 1.14. (a) Pea-sized amount. (b) Fingertip unit: Quantity of formulation extruded from a tube with a nozzle of 5 mm diameter extending from the distal crease of index finger to ventral aspect of the fingertip. This unit weighs approximately 0.5 g and covers an area of 300 cm^2.

This unit weighs approximately 0.5 g and covers, on an average, an area of approximately 300 cm^2.

• The requirement to cover different parts of body are shown in Table 1.13 and Fig. 1.15.

• But as a thumb rule no more than 50 g/week of potent and 100 g/week of mild or moderate potent TCS should be applied in an adult.

Frequency and Duration of Treatment

• Once daily application is as efficacious as more than one application of very potent steroid.

Table 1.13: Number of FTUs needed for different body parts	
Anatomical area	Number of FTU/s required
Face and neck	2
Anterior or posterior trunk	7+7
Arm	3
Hands (both sides)	1
Leg	6
Foot	2
Entire body	40

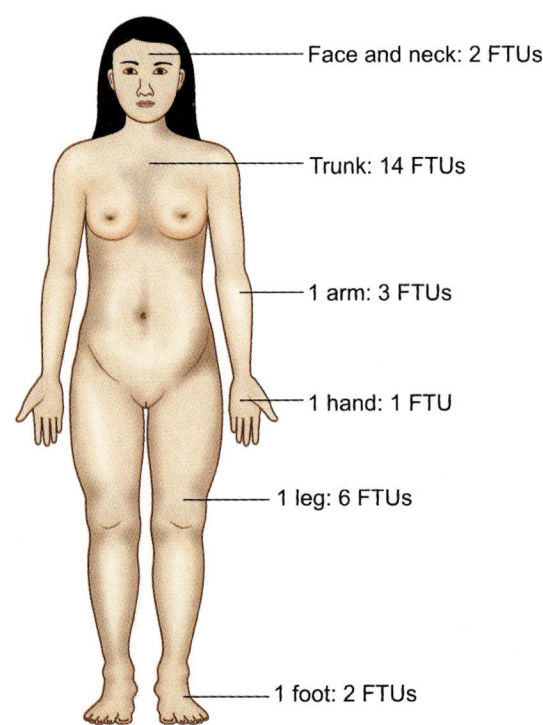

Face and neck: 2 FTUs

Trunk: 14 FTUs

1 arm: 3 FTUs

1 hand: 1 FTU

1 leg: 6 FTUs

1 foot: 2 FTUs

Fig. 1.15: Number of FTUs needed for different body parts.

- High potency formulations should be used for short periods (2–3 weeks) or intermittently and it is prudent to reduce frequency of application to alternate days or week end use) once disease control is partially achieved.
- Sudden discontinuation should be avoided after prolonged use to prevent rebound phenomenon.

Mode of Application

- *As is application*: Patients are most frequently asked to apply appropriate quantity (using pea-sized amount or FTU) after hydration of the skin (after bath or soaks; Fig. 1.16a). When very potent/potent TCS are used, it is advisable

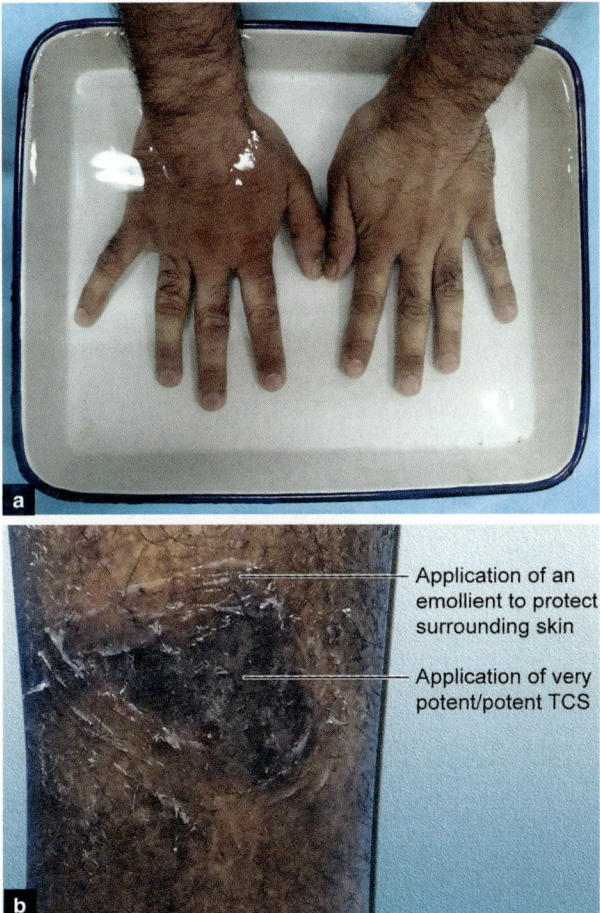

Application of an emollient to protect surrounding skin

Application of very potent/potent TCS

Fig. 1.16: Optimising results with TCS. (a) Hydration of skin: Patients are most frequently asked to apply appropriate quantity (using FTU) after hydration of the skin (bath or soaks). **(b) Protecting surrounding skin.** When very potent/ potent TCS are used, it is advisable to protect the surrounding uninvolved skin with an emollient to avoid side effects.

to protect the surrounding uninvolved skin with an emollient (Fig. 1.16b) to avoid side effects.

- **Under occlusion:** In thick (hyperkeratotic/lichenified) lesions, patient can be asked to use the TCS under occlusion. There are several ways of occluding the lesions:
  - *Bandaging* (Fig. 1.17a)
  - *Gloves and socks* (Fig. 1.17b)
  - *Cling film* (Fig. 1.17c)
- **Wet wraps:** In extensive AD, wet wrap therapy can be particularly helpful to rehydrate and soothe the skin and help TCS work better. Wet wraps are left on skin for several hours or overnight, taking care not to let them dry out. The steps for wet wraps include (Fig. 1.18):

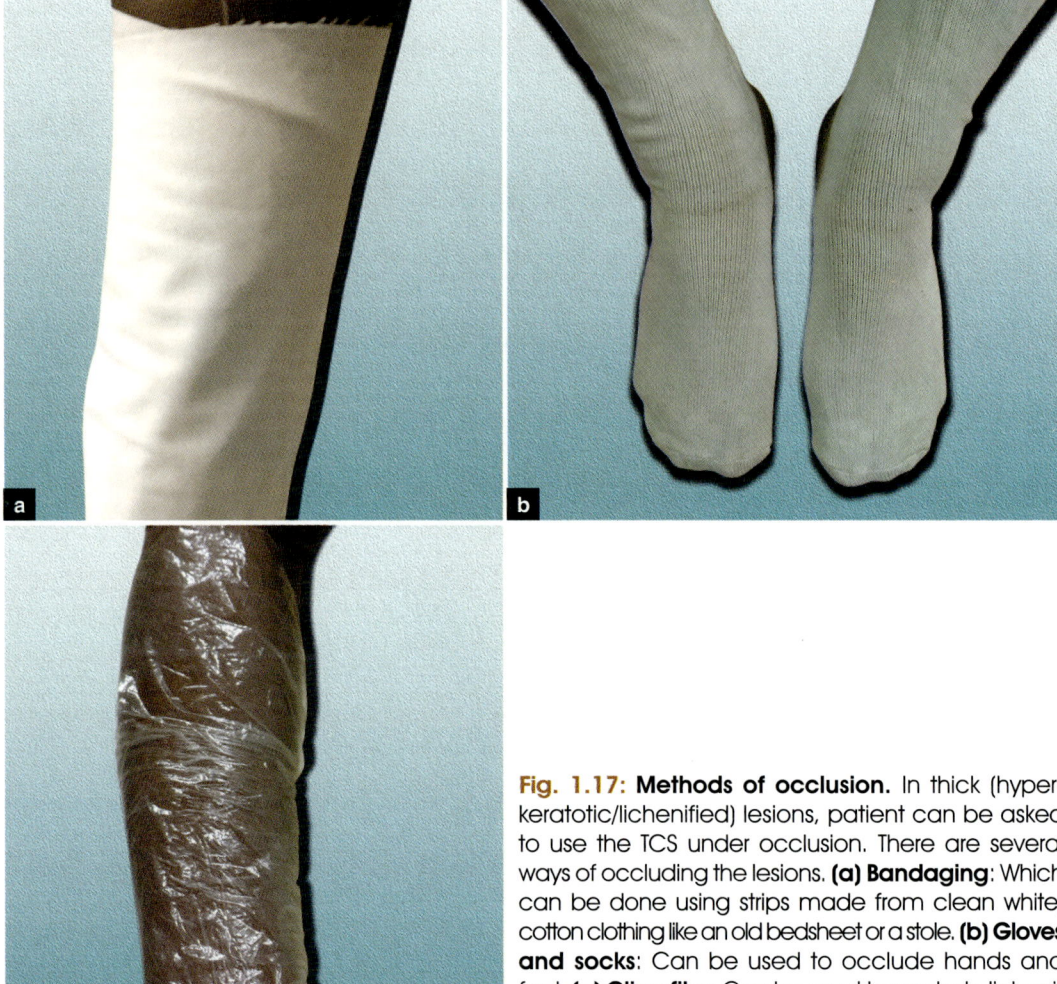

Fig. 1.17: Methods of occlusion. In thick (hyperkeratotic/lichenified) lesions, patient can be asked to use the TCS under occlusion. There are several ways of occluding the lesions. **(a) Bandaging**: Which can be done using strips made from clean white, cotton clothing like an old bedsheet or a stole. **(b) Gloves and socks**: Can be used to occlude hands and feet. **(c) Cling film**: Can be used to occlude lichenified/hyperkeratotic lesions.

- *Step 1*: Bathing/soaking, moisturizing and applying appropriate TCS on the affected area.
- *Step 2*: For the wet layer clean white cotton clothing or gauze from a roll is used. This is first moistened in warm water until slightly damp.
- *Step 3*: This wet dressing is wrapped around the affected area.
- *Step 4*: Then a dry layer is wrapped over the wet one.
- *Step 5*: Lastly, the patient is asked to carefully put on night-time clothing (pajamas or sweat suit) without disturbing the dressing.
- If the eczema is on the feet and hands, cotton gloves or socks are used as the wet layer with vinyl gloves or food-grade plastic wrap as the dry layer.

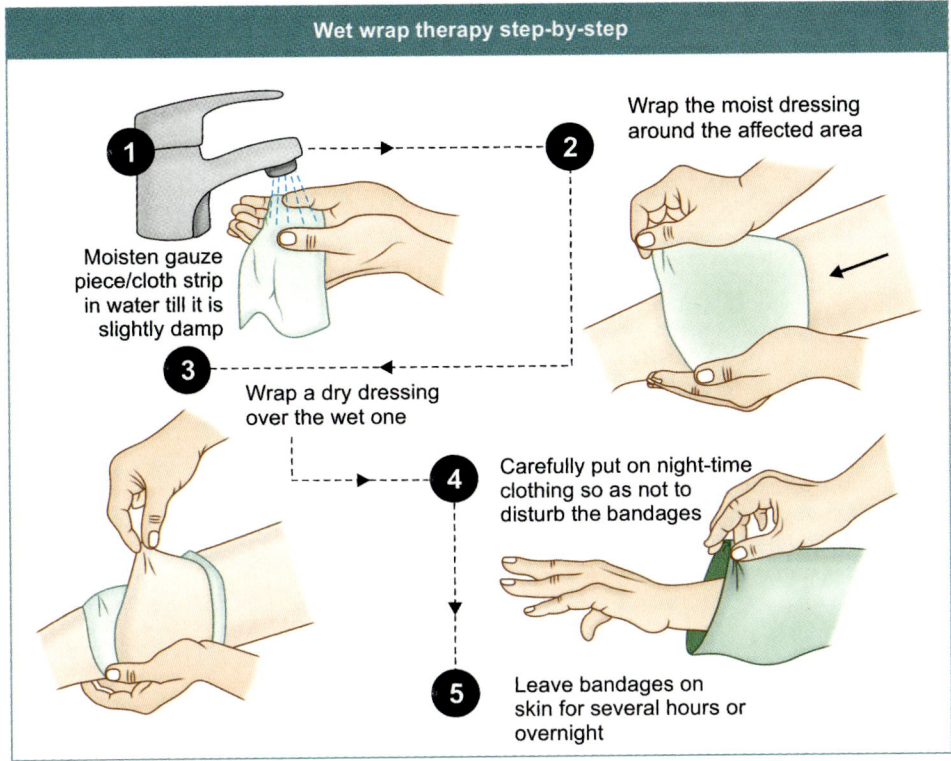

Wet wrap therapy step-by-step

1. Moisten gauze piece/cloth strip in water till it is slightly damp

2. Wrap the moist dressing around the affected area

3. Wrap a dry dressing over the wet one

4. Carefully put on night-time clothing so as not to disturb the bandages

5. Leave bandages on skin for several hours or overnight

Fig. 1.18: Step-by-step of wet wrap therapy.

REFERENCES

1. Mehta AB, Nadkarni NJ, Patil SP, Godse KV, Gautam M, Agarwal S. Topical corticosteroids in dermatology. Indian J Dermatol Venereol Leprol 2016; 82:371–8.

2. Luís Uva, Diana Miguel, Catarina Pinheiro, Joana Antunes, Diogo Cruz, João Ferreira, Paulo Filipe. Mechanisms of action of topical corticosteroids. Int J Endocrinol. 2012; 561018.

3. Abidi A, Ahmad F, Singh SK, Kumar A. Comparison of reservoir effect of topical corticosteroids in an experimental animal model by histamine-induced wheal suppression test. Indian J Pharmacol 2012; 44:722–5.

4. Ashworth J. Potency classification of topical corticosteroids: Modern perspectives. Acta Derm Venereol Suppl 1989;151:20–5.

5. Berth-Jones J. Principles of topical therapy. In: Griffiths CEM, Barker J, Bleiker T, Chabmers R, Creamer D, editors. Rook's Textbook of Dermatology, 9 th ed. WILEY Blackwell; 2016. p. 18.15.

6. Das A, Panda S. Use of topical corticosteroids in dermatology: An evidence-based approach. Indian J Dermatol 2017;62:237–50.

7. Hanifin J, Gupta AK, Rajagopal R. Intermittent dosing of fluticasone propionate cream for reducing the risk of relapse in atopic dermatitis patients. Brit J Dermatol 2002; 147: 528–37.

8. Wolkerstorfer A, Visser RL, De Waard van der Spek FB, Mulder PG, Oranje AP. Efficacy and safety of wet-wrap dressings in children with severe atopic dermatitis: influence of corticosteroid dilution. Br J Dermatol 2000; 143: 999–1004.

9. Green C, Colquitt JL, Kirby J, Davidson P. Topical corticosteroids for atopic eczema: clinical and cost effectiveness of once-daily vs more frequent use. Br J Dermatol 2005; 152:130–41.

10. Callen J, Chamlin S, Eichenfield LF, Ellis C, Girardi M, Goldfarb M, et al. A systematic review of the safety of topical therapies for atopic dermatitis. Br J Dermatol 2007; 156: 203–21.

11. Schlager JG1, Rosumeck S1, Werner RN1, Jacobs A2, Schmitt J3, Schlager C1, Nast A1. Topical treatments for scalp psoriasis: summary of a Cochrane Systematic Review. Br J Dermatol. 2017 Mar;176(3):604–14.

12. Manriquez JJ, Niklitschek SM. Vitiligo. In: Williams HC, Bigby M, Herxheimer A, Naldi L, Rzany B, Dellavalle R. et al., editors. Evidence-Based Dermatology. 3rd ed. Wiley-Blackwell Publishers. 2014. pp.44–9.

13. Bleehen SS. The treatment of vitiligo with topical corticosteroids. Light and electronmicroscopic studies. Br J Dermatol. 1976;94 suppl 12:43–50.

14. Papp KA, Papp A, Dahmer B, Clark CS. Single-blind, randomized controlled trial evaluating the treatment of facial seborrheic dermatitis with hydrocortisone 1% ointment compared with tacrolimus 0.1% ointment in adults. J Am Acad Dermatol 2012;67:e11–5.

15. Chi CC, Kitschig G, Baldo M, Brackenbury F, Lewis F, Wojnarowska F. Topical interventions of genital lichen sclerosus. Cochrane Database Syst Rev 2011; 7: CD008240

16. Neill SM, Lewis FM, Tatnall FM, Cox NH. British Association of Dermatologists' guidelines for the management of lichen sclerosus. Br J Dermatol 2010;163:672–82.

17. Datz J. A double-blind, multicenter trial of 0.05% halobetasol propionate ointment and 0.05% clobetasol 17-propionate ointment in the treatment of patients with chronic, localized atopic dermatitis or lichen simplex chronicus. Am Acad Dermatol 1991; 25: 1157–60.

18. Edgar NR, Saleh D, Miller RA. Recurrent aphthous stomatitis: A review. J Clin Aesthet Dermatol. 2017;10: 26–36.

19. Lenane P, Macarthur C, Parkin PC, Krafchik B, DeGroot J, Khambalia A, et al. Clobetasol propionate, 0.05%, vs. hydrocortisone, 1%, for alopecia areata in children. JAMA Dermatol 2014; 150: 47–50.

20. Trautinger F, Knobler R, Willemze R, Peris K, Stadler R, Laroche L, et al. EORTC consensus recommendations for the treatment of mycosis fungoides/Sézary syndrome. Eur J Cancer 2006;42:1014–30.

21. Hejazi EZ, Werth VP.Cutaneous lupus erythematosus: an update on pathogenesis, diagnosis and treatment. Am J Clin Dermatol 2016; 17: 135–46.

22. Yancey KB, Hall RP, Lawley TJ. Pruritic urticarial papules and plaques of pregnancy. Clinical experience in 25 patients. J Am Acad Dermatol 1984; 10: 473–80.

23. Al-Ghnaniem R, Short K, Pullen A, Fuller LC, Rennie JA, Leather AJ. 1% hydrocortisone ointment is an effective treatment of pruritus ani: a pilot randomized control crossover trial. Int J Colorectal Dis 2007; 22: 1463–7.

24. Weichert GE. An approach to the treatment of anogenital pruritus. Dermatol Ther 2004; 17: 129–33.

25. Lane PR, Moreland AA, Hogan DJ. Treatment of actinic prurigo with intermittent short-course topical 0.05% clobetasol 17-propionate: a preliminary report. Arch Dermatol 1990; 126: 1211–3.

26. Paek SY, Lim HW. Chronic actinic dermatitis. Dermatol Clin 2014; 32: 355–61.

27. Warshaw EM. Therapeutic options for chronic hand dermatitis. Dermatol Ther 2004; 17: 240–50.

28. Menni S, Boccardi D, Crosti C. Painful geographic tongue (benign migratory glossitis) in a child. J Eur Acad Dermatol Venereol 2004;18: 737–8.

29. Burge SM. Hailey-Hailey disease: the clinical features, response to treatment and prognosis. Br J Dermatol 1992; 126: 275–82.

30. Gibbs NF. Juvenile plantar dermatosis. Can sweat cause foot rash and peeling? Postgrad Med 2004; 115: 73–5.

31. Cheng S, Kirtschig G, Cooper S, Thornhill M, Leonardi-Bee J, Murphy R. Interventions for erosive lichen planus affecting mucosal sites. Cochrane Database Syst Rev 2012;2:CD008092.

32. Lodi G, Carrozzo M, Furness S, Thongprasom K. Interventions for treating oral lichen planus: A systematic review. Br J Dermatol 2012;166:938–47.

33. Long CC, Finlay AY. The fingertip unit—a new practical measure. Clin Exp Dermatol 1991; 16:444–7.

ANNEXURE 1: SOME COMMON AVAILABLE BRANDS OF TOPICAL CORTICOSTEROIDS

Generic salt	Brands	Preparation	Potency	Cost (₹)/g or /ml
		High Potent TCS		
Clobetasol 0.05%	Cosvate	Cream	15 g, 30 g	4.6, 3.4
		Ointment		
		Lotion		
	Excel	Cream	15 g	7.6
		Ointment		
		Lotion	15 ml	11.4
	Lobate	Cream	15 g, 30 g	2.5, 2.8
		Ointment		
		Lotion	89 (25 ml)	4.21
	Tenovate	Cream	30 g	3.2
		Ointment	15 g	4.5
		Lotion		
	Topinate	Cream	30 g	2.1
		Ointment	15 g	3.9
		Lotion	15 ml	9.56
	Clop	Cream	30 g	3.8
		Ointment	30 g	1.4
		Lotion	15 ml	3.6
Betamethasone dipropionate 0.05%	Diprobate	Cream	16 g	3.8
		Ointment	15 g	59.0
		Lotion	16 g	2.0
Halobetasol propionate 0.05%	Halovate	Cream	15 g	13.0
		Ointment	30 g	7.8
		Lotion	30 ml	7.4
	Halobet	Cream	15 g	7.6
		Ointment	30 g	7.8
		Lotion	30 ml	7.4
	Halotop	Cream	30 g	6.8
		Ointment	30 g	6.8
		Lotion	50 ml	1.74
	Halox	Cream	15 g, 30 g	10.6, 4.7
		Ointment	20 g	09.2
		Lotion	30 ml	06.6
		Potent TCS		
Betamethasone 0.05%	Diprobate	Lotion	30 ml, 50 ml	1.3, 2.5
Fluocinolone acetonide 0.1%	Flucort H	Cream	20 g	4.38
		Ointment	Unavailable	
		Lotion	30 ml	3.9
Mometasone furoate 0.1%	Momate	Cream	5 g	10.8
		Ointment	15 g	15.3
		Lotion	30 ml	10.9
	Cutizone	Cream	15 g	10
		Ointment	15 g	16
		Lotion	15 ml	7
	Momoz	Cream	30 g	7.4
		Ointment	15 g	9.8
		Lotion		

(Contd.)

(Contd.)

Generic salt	Brands	Preparation	Potency	Cost (₹)/g or /ml
	Momtas	Cream	20 g	8.75
		Ointment	1 g	15.48
		Lotion		
	Elocon	Cream	5 g	18.2
		Ointment	10 g	21.0
		Lotion	5 ml	18.2
Fluticasone proprionate 0.005%	Flutivate	Cream	10 g	13.3
		Ointment	20 g	6.55
		Lotion		
	Flutopic	Cream		
		Ointment	10 g	4.8
		Lotion		
Moderate TCS				
Desonide 0.05%	Desowen	Cream	10 g	16.8
		Ointment		
		Lotion	30 ml	06.1
	Dosetil	Cream	10 g	09.3
		Ointment		
		Lotion	30 ml	04.2
Clobetasone 0.05%	Eumosone	Cream	15 g	04.6
		Ointment		
		Lotion		
Fluocinolone 0.01%	Flucort	Cream	20 g	0.45
		Ointment	15 g	2.13
		Lotion	15 ml	02.7
	Sebowash	Shampoo	100 ml	02.11
Fluocinolone 0.025%	Flucort	Cream	20 g	04.45
		Ointment		
		Lotion	15 ml	06.4
	Flucort forte	Cream		
		Ointment		
		Lotion	15 ml	06.4
Betamethasone valerate 0.1%	Betnovate	Cream	20 g	01
		Ointment		
		Lotion	20 ml	0.7
Mild TCS				
Hydrocortisone acetate 1%	Cutisoft	Cream	10 g	09.00
		Ointment		
		Lotion	50 ml	4.5
	Drocort	Cream	15 g	3.2
		Ointment	15 g	3.3
		Lotion		
Hydrocortisone aceponate, 0.127%	Efficort	Cream	10 g	19.3
		Ointment		
		Lotion		
Triamcinolone acetonide	Kenacort	Oral paste	5 g	13.6
	Cinort	Oral paste	5 g	11.6

Note: This list is not exhaustive. The price is not a reflection on the quality of brands.

2

Complications of Topical Steroids

Abhishek De, Monika Khemka, Aarti Sarda, Savera Gupta, Neena Khanna

SUMMARY

- When used injudiciously, TCS may lead to side effects, but if used as prescribed, they are generally safe and effective and their side effects manageable.
- Factors affecting development of side effects can be drug related, application related or patient related. Drug related factors include the potency and concentration of TCS, used and the vehicle and additives in which TCS are formulated. Application related factors include amount of TCS used, duration and frequency of application, site of application (thickness of skin, whether used in naturally occluded areas), state of hydration of skin, application under occlusion and lack of physician supervision (self medication). Patient related factors include age of patient, condition of skin and underlying dermatological indications.
- Side effects of TCS can be categorized as cutaneous (local) and systemic side effects. The adverse effects of TCS are mostly due to the TCS molecule, though vehicle can potentiate these.
- Cutaneous atrophy, both epidermal and dermal, is the most common local adverse effect of TCS and is generally seen after many weeks of application. It is characterized by wrinkled, shiny skin, hypopigmentation, telangiectasia and prominent deep vessels. TCS-induced cutaneous atrophy can to some extent be prevented by retinoic acid.
- Topical corticosteroid-induced rosacea like dermatitis (CIRD) is characterized by development of small, pink-red papules, pustules and papulovesicles (pseudovesicles), usually with perilesional erythema. The distribution of lesions can be perioral, centrofacial or diffuse. Withdrawal of TCS can be done either as step-down approach or sudden stoppage. Topical steroid dependent (damaged) face (TSDF) is characterized by a plethora of signs and symptoms and psychological dependence on TCS due to unsupervised, prolonged (mis)use of TCS of any potency on the face, resulting in semi-permanent or permanent damage to the skin. It is evident from the Indian data on facial dermatoses that

gross overuse of TCS is quite common in most parts of India. During the last decade dermatologists in India have been regularly campaigning against such misuse.

- TCS promote the growth of vellus hair and long term use of TCS may lead to facial hypertrichosis which usually resolves on discontinuation of TCS, but may persist even months after withdrawal.

- TCS may exacerbate/mask cutaneous infection (bacterial, fungal, viral). TCS are often (mis) used to treat dermatophyte infections, because of their over-the-counter availability and rapid (albeit temporary) response and patients may present with atypical clinical features (tinea incognito, tinea pseudo-imbricata).

- Allergic contact dermatitis (ACD) to TCS is suspected when a TCS responsive dermatitis fails to respond or worsens after TCS therapy and it can be an allergic reaction to the active ingredients (TCS), vehicle or the preservatives. TCS are classified into 4 groups based on cross-reaction patterns. Confirmation of ACD to topical steroids is done by patch testing.

- Tachyphylaxis is a well-known (albeit controversial) problem with chronic TCS use, particularly of higher potency preparations. An intermittent regimen with twice-daily application for 2 weeks followed by 'steroid holiday' for one week may help in preventing tachyphylaxis.

- When TCS are withdrawn after application for a considerable duration of time, there can be a rebound phenomenon of the existing skin lesions.

- Despite rampant often unsupervised use of potent and superpotent TCS, fortunately, systemic side effects are rare, but when seen are more common in infants and elderly patients. HPA axis suppression may be seen with excessive application of TCS. For prevention, recommended weekly dosage of TCS of no more than 50 g of very potent TCS and 100 g of potent TCS be used.

- Every attempt should be made to reduce side effects of TCS. Strategies to do so include using correct potency of TCS for adequate duration and frequency. Once daily application of TCS is as efficacious, more cost effective and safer than twice daily application. Thin sites such as eyelids, scrotum and flexures require special precautions as also when using in children and elderly who are particularly prone to adverse effects.

- Use of TCS should be avoided as monotherapy as far as possible, and depending on the indication, adjuvant therapy should be prescribed to reduce the total amount and duration of TCS used.

- Communication of correct and adequate information about the medication and clear written instructions regarding how to use them is the key to avoid TCS misuse.

FACTORS AFFECTING DEVELOPMENT OF SIDE EFFECTS

Several factors affect development of side effects with use of TCS.

Drug Related Factors

- *Potency of TCS*: TCS molecules have inherent differences in potency based on their structure which determine:
  - *Lipophilicity*: Greater the lipophilicity, higher the percutaneous absorption resulting in better efficacy, but unfortunately more side effects.
  - *Binding affinity to GCR*: Greater the binding to GCR, higher the potency.
  - *Metabolism*: Greater the rate of de-esterification in skin, lower the potency.
- *Concentration TCS used*: The clinical response and side effects to TCS is directly proportional to concentration of TCS used.
- *Vehicle and additives*: The vehicle and additives in which TCS are formulated not only affect the therapeutic effect, but also the adverse effect profile:
  - Occlusive vehicles like ointments enhance a TCS molecule's percutaneous absorption by increasing hydration of stratum corneum.
  - Solvents such as propylene glycol and ethanol (which have high solubility for TCS molecule) enhance local side effects by increasing percutaneous absorption.
  - Emulsifiers help to distribute the drug evenly on the skin surface, thereby reducing uneven concentration, reducing side effects.
  - Addition of keratolytics increases penetration.

Application Related Factors

- *Amount of TCS used*: Adequate amount based on fingertip unit (FTU) must be applied to get the desired therapeutic effect. Inadvertent use of large quantities of TCS leads to side effects.
- *Duration and frequency of application*: Prolonged and frequent unwarranted use of TCS predisposes to development of side effects.
- *Sites of application*: Sites of application also affects penetration:
  - *Thickness of skin*: Percutaneous absorption correlates directly with thinness of stratum corneum.[a] So penetration is maximum through mucous membrane and scrotum and least through palms and soles. Therefore, palms and soles are less prone to developing side effects than adjoining skin, e.g. patient applying very potent or potent TCS on palms and soles sometimes inadvertently apply the medication on adjoining thinner skin which develops side effects (Fig. 2.1). Similarly TCS should not be prescribed (at least nothing more than mild potency) around the eyes and on genitalia, unless strongly warranted.

---

[a]Stratum corneum is the strongest barrier for systemic absorption of TCS, but also serves as a reservoir from which drug absorption continues.

– *Naturally occluded skin*: Naturally occluded areas (flexures) are more prone to developing side effects of TCS due to increased hydration of stratum corneum and higher temperature in these areas (Fig. 2.2).

• *Hydration of skin*: Hydration of stratum corneum (e.g. by soaking the part) results in increased percutaneous absorption.

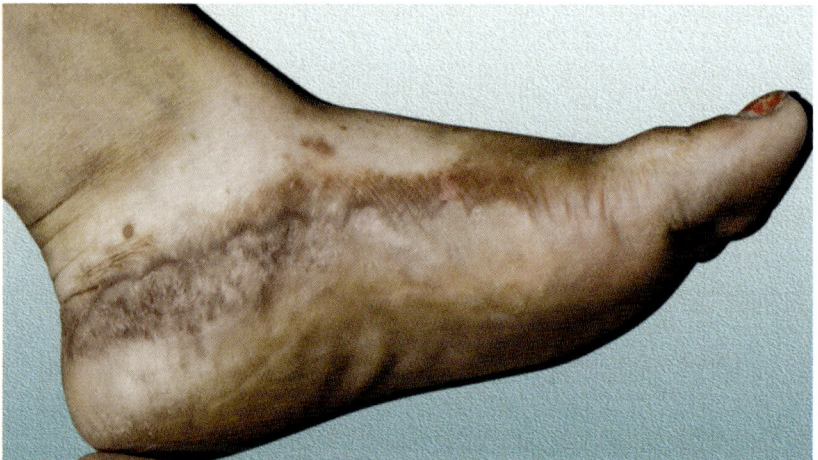

Fig. 2.1: Side effects when TCS are applied to palms and soles: This patient with plantar psoriasis was asked to soak the affected part and immediately apply a combination of clobetasol propionate + 3% salicylic acid. However, he inadvertently applied the medication on adjoining normal skin resulting in hypopigmentation of the area.

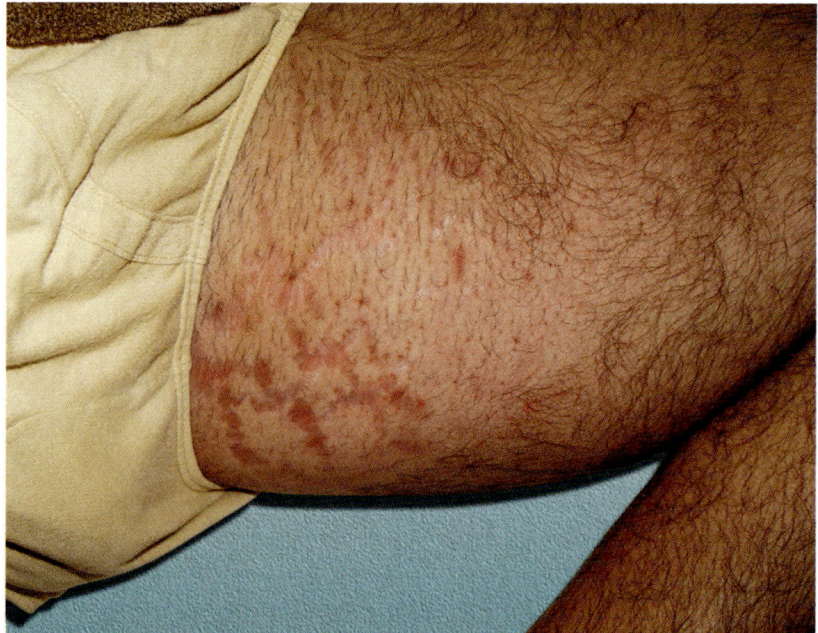

Fig. 2.2: Side effects in flexures: Very potent TCS should not be used in flexures as it may lead to side effects like striae.

- *Occlusion*: Occlusion increases the hydration and temperature of stratum-corneum and thus enhances drug penetration by up to 10 times.
- *Lack of physician supervision*: Patients who self medicate invariably have more side effects than patients whose therapy is physician-supervised.

Patient Related Factors

- *Age of patient*: Children are particularly prone to developing side effects when potent TCS are applied on their skin (Fig. 2.3) because they:
  – Absorb TCS more readily than adults.
  – Have a greater skin surface-to-body volume ratio.
  – Metabolize TCS slowly.
- *Condition of skin*: Absorption of TCS from skin varies from <1 to 7% when applied to intact skin (depending on site of application) to 4–19% in patients with loss of barrier function, e.g. dermatitis, erythroderma, Netherton's syndrome.
- *Underlying dermatological indications*: Stasis dermatitis, leg ulcers, perianal dermatitis, hand and foot eczema, chronic actinic dermatitis and facial dermatitis are some of the conditions particularly prone to developing contact dermatitis to TCS.

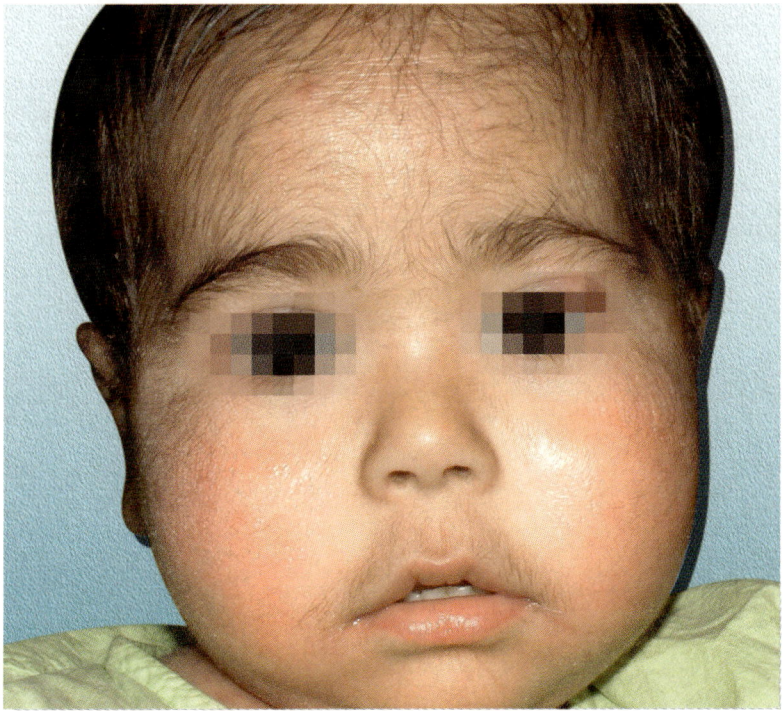

Fig. 2.3: Side effects in infancy: This child had been using very potent TCS for his atopic dermatitis. He developed moon facies. Also note atrophy of skin particularly around eyes, hypertrichosis and a hardoleum.

SIDE EFFECTS OF TCS

The side effects of TCS can be categorized as cutaneous (local) and systemic side effects (Table 2.1).

The adverse effects of TCS are mostly due to the TCS molecule, though vehicle can potentiate these.

CUTANEOUS ADVERSE EFFECTS[1]

Local adverse effects of TCS use are largely due to the antiproliferative effects of these agents.

Cutaneous Atrophy

Cutaneous atrophy, both epidermal and dermal, is the most common local adverse effect of TCS.

- *Mechanism of action*[2]: The mechanism of atrophy following use of TCS remains incompletely understood but may be related to:
  - *Effects of TCS on epidermis*: Which include reduced thickness of stratum corneum and granular layer (which may disappear over time) with reduction in the size of basal keratinocytes which also show reduced mitoses. Synthesis of stratum corneum lipids and keratohyalin granules and formation of corneodesmosomes (required for structural integrity of stratum corneum) are also suppressed by TCS.

Table 2.1: Local and systemic side effects of TCS

Cutaneous
- Skin atrophy
- Barrier function impairment
- Telangiectasia
- Corticosteroid-induced rosacea like dermatitis (CIRD)
- Topical steroid dependent (damaged) face (TSDF)
- Acneiform eruption
- Perilesional depigmentation/ hypopigmentation
- Hypertrichosis
- Infections
- Allergic contact dermatitis
- Vehicle/additive-related adverse effects
- Tachyphylaxis
- TCS rebound syndrome
- Other cutaneous side effects

Systemic
- Ocular
- Suppression of hypothalamic-pituitary-adrenal axis
- Iatrogenic Cushing's syndrome
- Growth retardation in infants and children
- Others

– *Effects of TCS on dermis* include reduction in dermal volume (due to reduction of glycosaminoglycans and water content), reduced activity of fibroblasts with reduced amount and abnormal aggregation of collagen and elastic fibres, starting within 3 days of application but manifesting clinically later (on continued application). This results in dermal vessels becoming visible and fragile due to reduction/loss of fibrous and ground substance support.

- *Risk factors* include potency of TCS, occlusion and site of application and age of patient.
- *Features*: All TCS can cause skin atrophy, albeit to a variable degree. The atrophy is characterized by lax, wrinkled, shiny skin with telangiectasia (Fig. 2.4a), purpura, striae, stellate pseudoscars, hypopigmentation and prominent veins (Fig. 2.4b). Even atrophy of fat and muscle in the diaper area has been reported with fluorinated TCS. Striae develop with initial inflammation and edema of the dermis, followed by the deposition of dermal collagen along the lines of mechanical stress (Fig. 2.5).
- *Time course*: Significant atrophy and striae are generally seen after several weeks of application, though studies have shown that atrophy may occur even within first 7 days of daily application of very potent TCS application under occlusion and within 2 weeks of daily use of potent or very potent TCS without occlusion. Striae have been observed on thighs after 2 weeks of very potent TCS cream.
- *Resolution*: Most signs of superficial cutaneous atrophy and hypopigmentation are said to resolve by 1–4 weeks after discontinuation of the TCS, though in practice it does often take longer. Striae are generally permanent, though they do become less visible with time.
- *Testing for atrophogenic potential of TCS*:
  – The atrophy test is used to determine the atrophogenic/antiproliferative potential of a TCS
  – The test TCS is applied to the same skin area for 3 weeks under occlusion when the resulting atrophy and the extent of telangiectasia are evaluated by means of a defined score.
- *Prevention*: Concurrent use of topical tretinoin 0.1% may reduce incidence of atrophy from chronic steroid applications.[3]

Barrier Function Impairment

- *Pathogenesis*: TCS decrease formation of lipid lamellar bodies delaying recovery of barrier function marginally increasing transepidermal water loss.
- *Clinical implications*: This effect may theoretically worsen already existing barrier function impairment in atopic dermatitis and psoriasis, but in practice the TCS induced substantial reduction in inflammation (and consequent recovery of barrier function) outweighs this marginal direct effect.

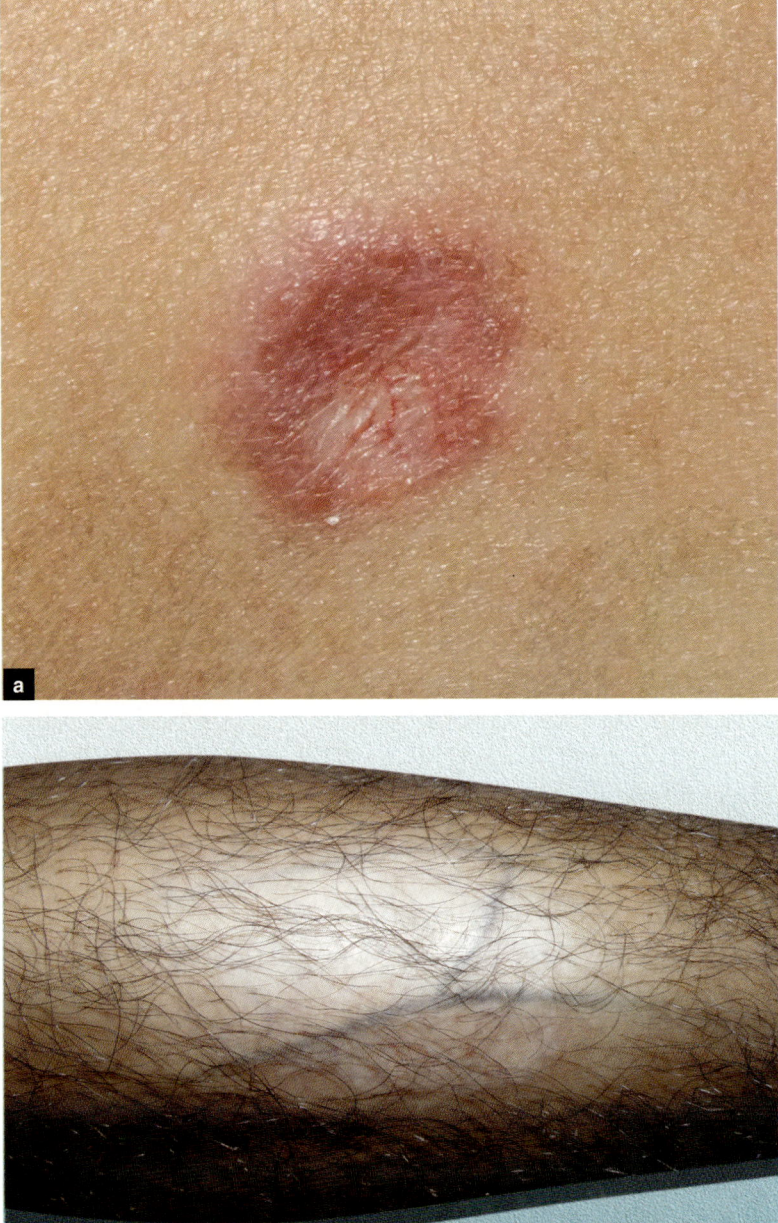

Fig. 2.4: **Atrophogenic potential of TCS. (a) Cutaneous atrophy:** Characterized by lax, wrinkled, shiny skin with telangiectasia. **(b) Prominent veins:** Cutaneous atrophy may manifest as wrinkled, shiny hypopigmented skin with prominent deep vessels.

Telangiectasia

- *Pathogenesis*: Telangiectasia results partly due to loss of support from surrounding tissue and partly due to repeated homeostatic imbalance. Corticosteroids also stimulate microvascular endothelial cells.

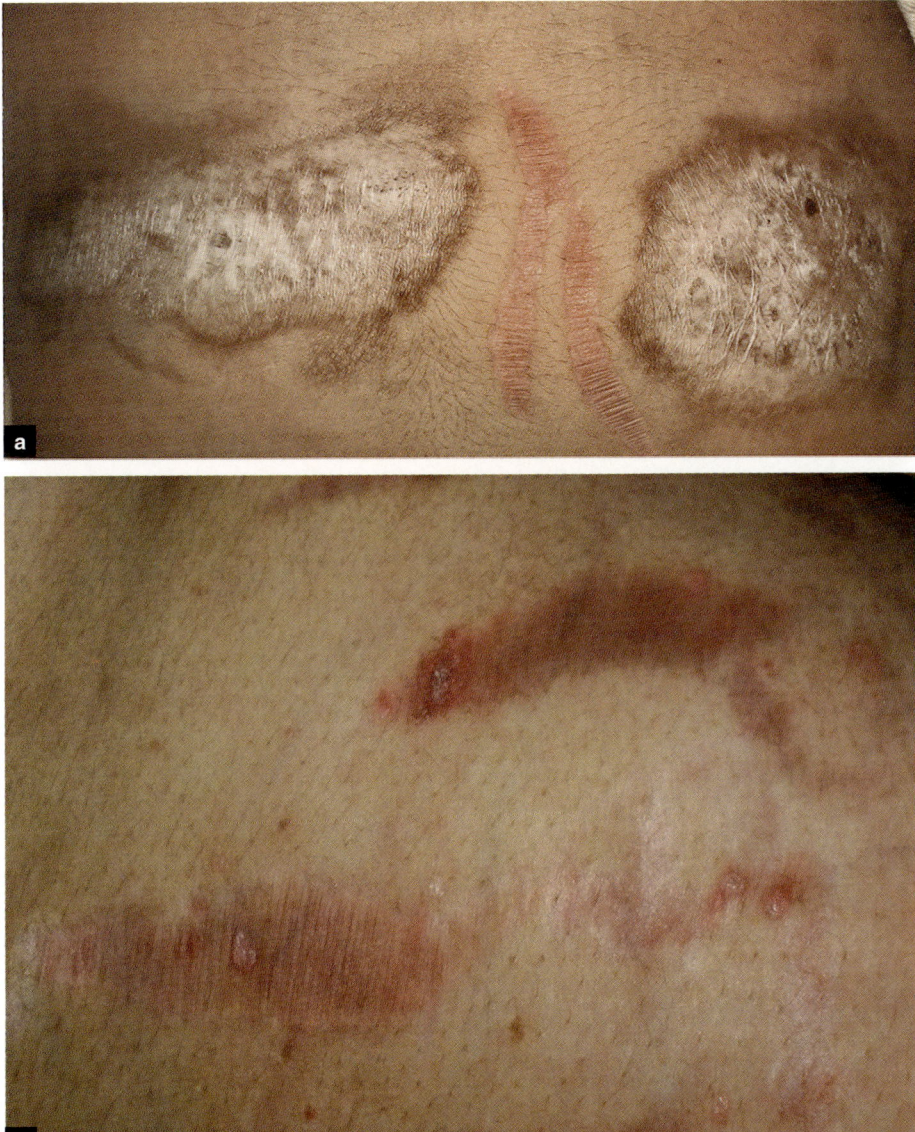

Fig. 2.5: Striae: (a) Striae at site of topical application in a patient with morphea. **(b)** This patient was given potent TCS for his psoriasis. When the TCS were stopped the patient's psoriasis relapsed, with the lesions first appearing in the striae.

- *Risk factors:* Telangiectasias have been reported with prolonged, excessive and occlusive use of TCS, particularly when used in combination with inhaled, intranasal and systemic steroids. Face is a frequently affected site (Fig. 2.6a).
- *Manifestations:* Telangiectasia usually appear with atrophy and hypopigmentation of skin (Fig. 2.6a). Though routine use of TCS in children with eczema does not cause telangiectasia, care should be taken with prolonged, excessive use of very potent TCS (Fig. 2.6b).

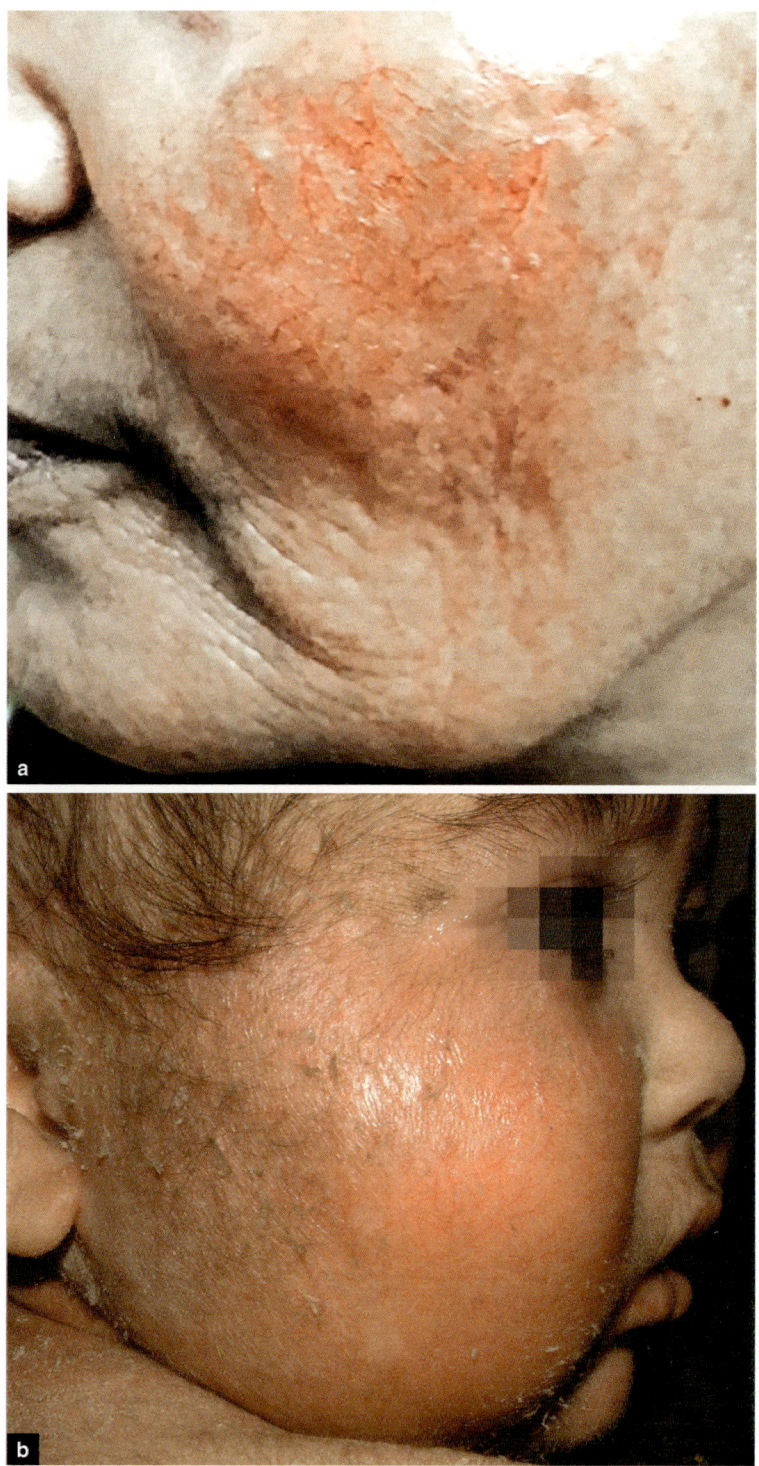

Fig. 2.6: Telangiectasia: (a) Telangiectasia usually appear with atrophy and hypopigmentation of skin (masked by the erythema). **(b)** Telangiectasia in an infant with atopic dermatitis with prolonged and excessive use of very potent TCS.

Topical Corticosteroid Induced Rosacea-like Dermatitis (CIRD)[4]

- *Terminology*: CIRD is an adverse reaction, and is not considered to be a clinical variant of rosacea or perioral dermatitis. Diagnosis of CIRD is often made without knowledge of underlying diagnosis and is sometimes made when TCS application induces CIRD in a patient with pre-existing rosacea/perioral dermatitis.
- *Pathogenesis*: The major mechanism of CIRD development is TCS-induced alteration in normal homeostatic balance of chemical mediators, which modify cutaneous blood flow. There may also be a component of altered permeability.
  - TCS application inhibits release of endothelial nitric oxide[b] (eNO), an endogenous vasodilator, resulting in vasoconstriction.
  - When TCS is discontinued, there is sudden release of the accumulated eNO, resulting in rebound erythema, edema and discomfort (trampoline or neon sign effect).
- *Clinical features*:
  - Patients often complain of sensitive or painful skin with burning, stinging, pruritus, or dryness.
  - CIRD resembles severe papulopustular rosacea, but lesions in CIRD tend to be more diffuse rather than predominantly centrofacial (though other patterns are also described). Primary lesions of CIRD are small, pink–red papules (most common), pustules and papulovesicles (pseudovesicles) usually with perilesional erythema (Fig. 2.7). Lesions often become widespread on the face but perivermilion area is always spared. Papules resolve leaving indurated

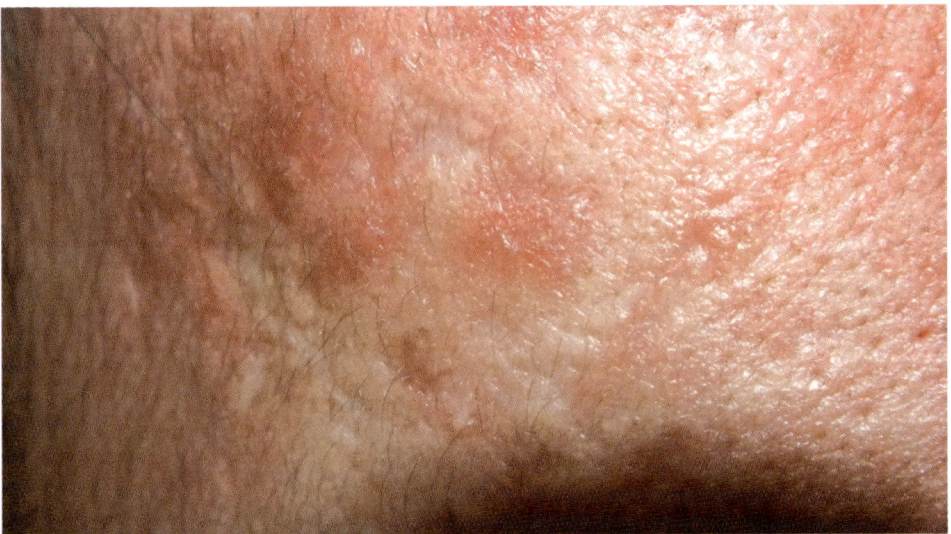

Fig. 2.7: CIRD: Primary lesions of CIRD are small, pink or red papules (most common), pustules and papulovesicles (pseudovesicles) usually with perilesional erythema.

[b]Also referred to as endothelium-derived relaxing factor.

erythema, which is persistent, with a propensity to become more diffuse. Telangiectasias and deeper papules and nodules progressively increase with continued use of TCS.

- The presentation of patients with a red face, often with the headlight sign (large areas of facial erythema with sparing of the nose and upper lip), has been described in adults using potent TCS, mostly for seborrheic dermatitis.

- **Subtypes:** Based on the distribution of lesions, 3 subtypes of CIRD are recognized:
  - *Perioral*: It is the most common manifestation of CIRD, both in adults and children. Patients present with perioral dermatitis (Fig. 2.8a) with a conspicuous perivermilion sparing. There may be associated perinasal and periocular involvement and in children perinasal involvement (often misdiagnosed as seborrheic dermatitis), may be the only site affected.
  - *Centrofacial*: Involves medial aspect of cheeks, lower eyelids, nose, and medial forehead including glabellar region, with absence of perioral involvement (Fig. 2.8b).
  - *Diffuse*: Entire face is involved often with extension onto the neck (Fig. 2.8c).

- **Risk factors:**
  - *Potency of TCS*: Although CIRD may develop with prolonged use of TCS of any potency including hydrocortisone 1%, it is more frequent and severe with very potent TCS.
  - *Duration of use*: CIRD usually develops after 6 months of TCS therapy, but has been reported even as early as 8 weeks of TCS application.
  - *Gender*: CIRD is more common in female patients (72%).
  - *Underlying dermatoses*: History of underlying atopy (67%), rosacea and seborrheic dermatitis is frequently present.

- **Management:**
  - *Counselling*: Depending on duration and severity of CIRD and particularly rebound flares on discontinuation of TCS, patients need continuous support and encouragement.
  - *General measures*: It is strongly recommended to restrict use of any topical applications on the face especially in first few weeks of treatment, to reduce the chances of flares. This includes avoidance of patient-selected skin care products (soaps, astringents, scrubs) as also self-prescribed topical medications. Patient may, however, use a gentle non-medicated cleanser and moisturizer.
  - *Withdrawal of TCS*: Discontinuation of all TCS usually leads to a flare of the eruption but needs to be done. There are 2 approaches to doing this:
    - Step down approach: In which either the frequency of TCS application is reduced (initially to alternate days, then biweekly, then once weekly) or the potency is reduced (substituting a very potent TCS, with potent or moderately potent, again used intermittently) before eventually discontinuing all TCS.
    - Sudden stoppage of TCS use.

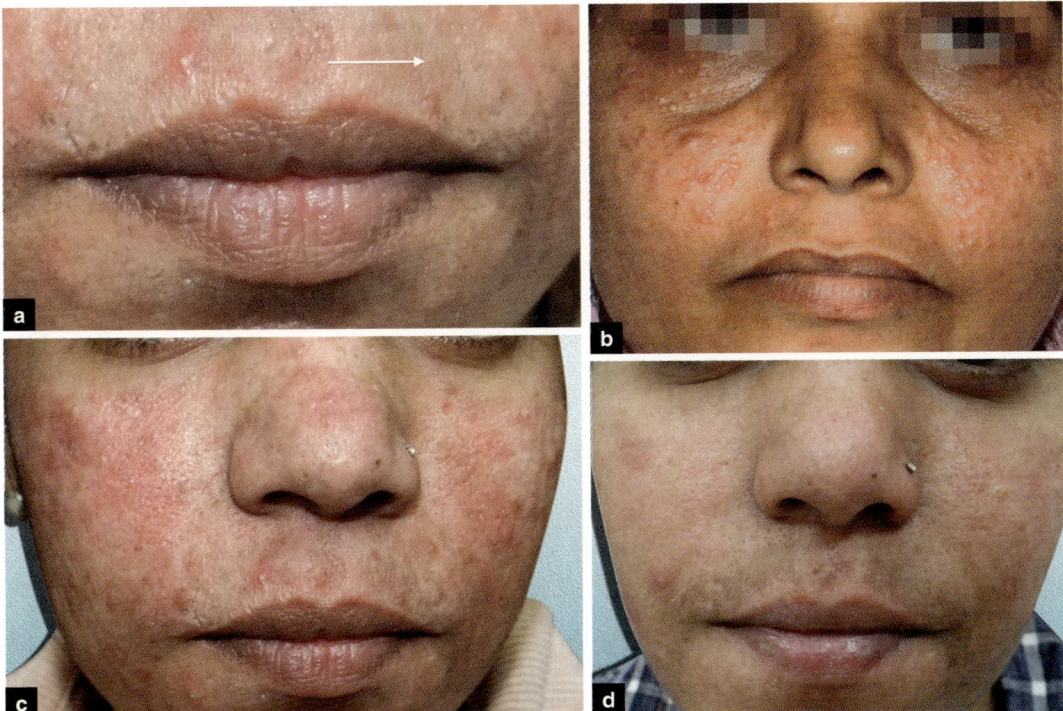

Fig. 2.8: Corticosteroid-induced rosacea-like dermatitis. (a) Perioral CIRD: It is the most common presentation of CIRD, seen in both adults and children. There is a conspicuous perivermilion sparing.Note increased hair in the area due to TCS application. **(b) Centrofacial CIRD:** Involves medial aspect of cheeks, lower eyelids, nose, and central forehead including glabellar region, with absence of perioral involvement. **(c) Diffuse CIRD:** Entire face is involved often with extension onto the neck. **(d) Response to treatment:** Patient was treated with isotretinoin in dose of 10 mg daily for 2 months.

- *Topical therapy*: There are no well-controlled studies to compare the efficacy of the various topical modalities in CIRD.
  - Topical pimecrolimus[5] and tacrolimus[6]: Rapidly reduce the severity of CIRD, may offer quicker initial improvement and more rapid eventual resolution of CIRD.
  - Topical erythromycin: Reduces the time to resolution, but not as quickly as oral medication.
  - Topical metronidazole: Is frequently used to treat perioral dermatitis in children, but evidence for its use in CIRD is relatively weak (case series and a trial showing it to be inferior to oral tetracyclines).
  - Other topical options include azelaic acid and clindamycin (aqueous-based formulations).
- *Oral therapy*:
  - Oral doxycycline or minocycline: Given in dose of 100–200 mg daily for 3–4 months is effective in reducing inflammatory lesions. Doxycycline-MR (modified release) 40 mg once daily has also been used for treatment as the

anti-inflammatory activity is preserved with absence of antibiotic selection pressure.

- Oral tetracycline: Given in initial dose of 500–1000 mg daily followed by a slow taper to 250 mg daily over several weeks, tetracyclines significantly hasten resolution of papules by inhibiting production of NO and also by their anti-inflammatory effects.
- Oral erythromycin: Given in dose of 30 mg/kg daily every 12 hours for 4 weeks is the antibiotic of choice in children as tetracyclines are contra-indicated.
- Oral metronidazole: It is used in patients who are unable to tolerate tetracyclines.
- Isotretinoin: In dose of 2–5 mg daily (often given as a 10 mg dose 2–3 times weekly) for 3 months has been found to be effective, if there is no improvement with a full dose of tetracycline.

Topical Steroid Dependent (Damaged) Face (TSDF)[7]

- *Terminology*: TSDF is a recently described phenomenon characterized by a plethora of signs and symptoms with a psychological dependence to TCS. It occurs due to unsupervised, indiscriminate, irrational, prolonged (mis)use of TCS of any potency on the face, resulting in semi-permanent or permanent damage to the skin.
- *Reason for use*: TCS may be (mis) used on:
  - *Diseased skin*: To treat acne vulgaris, seborrheic dermatitis, photodermatoses.
  - *Normal skin*: As fairness creams without a dermatologist's prescription, often suggested by beauticians, chemists and friends.
- *Manifestations*:
  - Patient complains of burning, stinging, tightness, photosensitivity and diminished tolerance to lubrication.
  - Skin of face appears thin, erythematous, hypo-/hyperpigmented and develops papules, pustules, telangiectasia, desquamation/peeling (Fig. 2.9), acneiform eruption and eventually CIRD. Some patients may also develop an allergic contact dermatitis to components of TCS.
  - Withdrawal of TCS results in erythema (red face) for about 2 weeks followed by desquamation. If the patient does not restart TCS again, the flare resolves but reappears within 2 weeks eventuating into a cycle of relapses and remissions which may continue for some time.
- *Management*: TSDF is difficult and necessitates psychological counseling as well as treatment of CIRD.[7]

Acneiform Eruption/Steroid Folliculitis[8]

- *Pathogenesis*: TCS induce comedone formation by several mechanisms:
  - Increasing the response of follicular epithelium to comedogenesis.

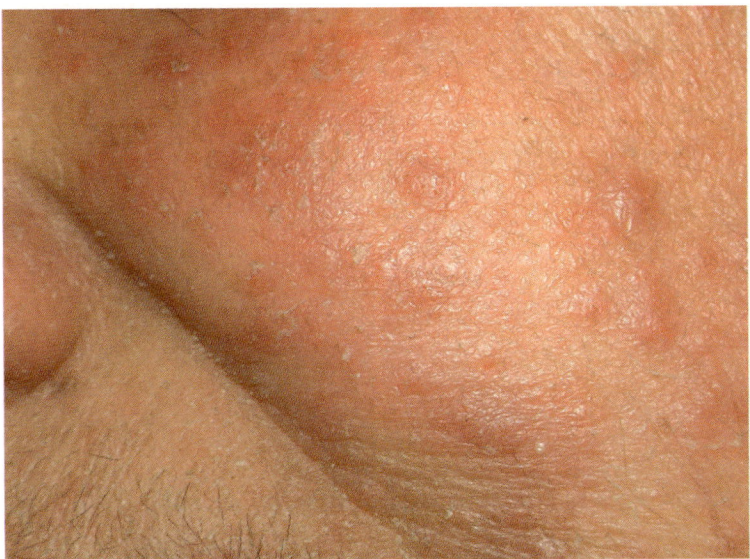

Fig. 2.9: Topical steroid damaged face. On prolonged use of potent TCS on face, the skin of face appears thin, erythematous, and may desquamate. This patient complained of burning, stinging, tightness, photosensitivity and diminished tolerance to topical applications.

- Increasing number of bacteria in the pilosebaceous duct.
- Increasing concentration of free fatty acids in skin surface lipids due to increased lipolysis of sebaceous gland triglycerides.
- Degradation of follicular epithelium, resulting in extrusion of follicular content.

- *Clinical features:* Follows prolonged application of TCS, occurring more on trunk and face and rarely elsewhere. Differs from acne vulgaris in consisting of monomorphic, small, papulopustules (Fig. 2.10a) without comedones, pseudocysts and scars, and are frequently less erythematous. Acneiform lesions due to TCS may be associated with presence of other side effects of steroids like striae (Fig. 2.10b). In psoriasis, use of potent TCS may induce an acneiform eruption surmounted by psoriasiform scales (Fig. 2.10c).
- *Histopathology:* Shows focal folliculitis with a neutrophilic infiltrate in and around the follicle.
- *Treatment:* Stopping TCS use and initiating anti-acne therapy usually with topical retinoids.

Perilesional Depigmentation/Hypopigmentation

- *Mechanism:* The cause of pigment dilution by TCS is incompletely understood but may be due to:
  - Reduced production of melanin by melanocytes.
  - Vasoconstriction due to alteration of normal homeostatic balance of chemical mediators (eNO) and the pallor so produced may be mistaken for hypopigmentation.

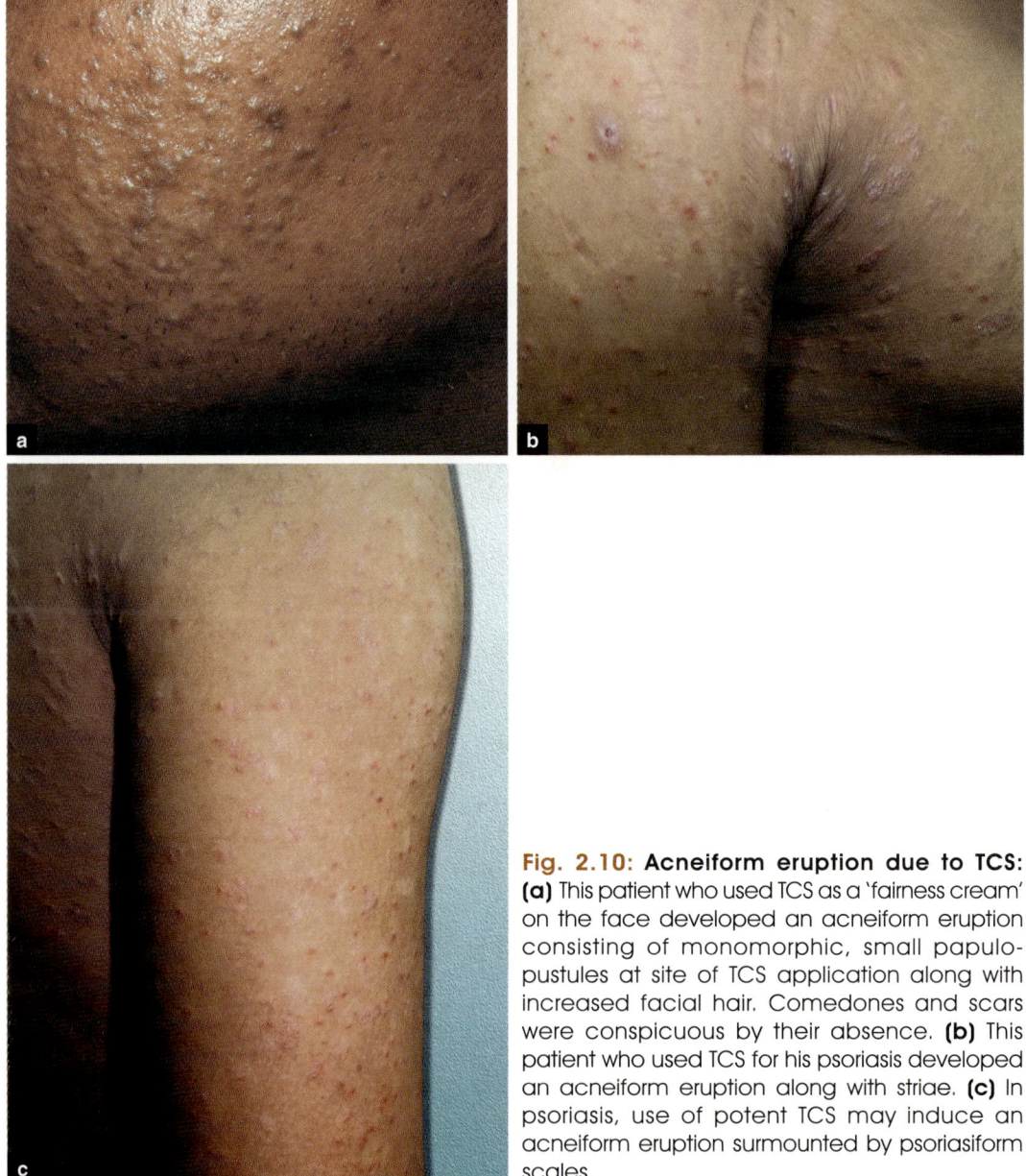

Fig. 2.10: **Acneiform eruption due to TCS:** **(a)** This patient who used TCS as a 'fairness cream' on the face developed an acneiform eruption consisting of monomorphic, small papulopustules at site of TCS application along with increased facial hair. Comedones and scars were conspicuous by their absence. **(b)** This patient who used TCS for his psoriasis developed an acneiform eruption along with striae. **(c)** In psoriasis, use of potent TCS may induce an acneiform eruption surmounted by psoriasiform scales.

- *Manifestations:*
  - Hypopigmentation is frequently seen in perilesional skin when potent and very potent steroids are used especially in ointment formulation to treat thick/lichenified dermatoses (like lichen simplex chronicus and psoriasis; Fig. 2.11a) and to treat keloids (Fig. 2.11b). Hypopigmentation is also commonly seen on dorsal aspects of digits due to inadvertent rubbing of excess ointment of TCS used to treat palmoplantar disease (psoriasis, hyperkeratotic eczema; Fig. 2.11c).

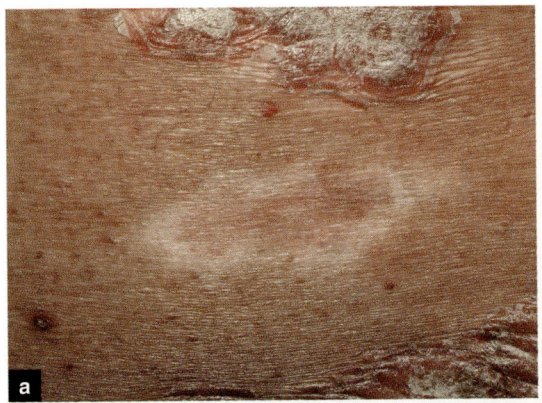
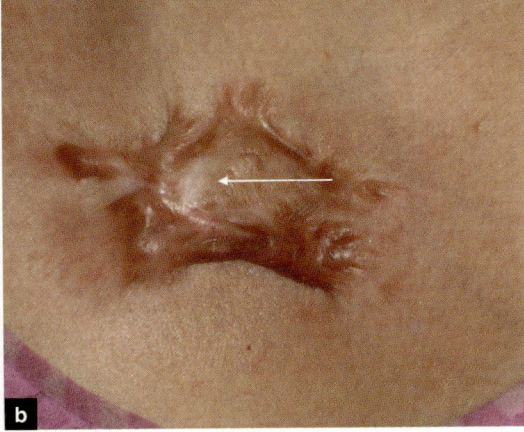
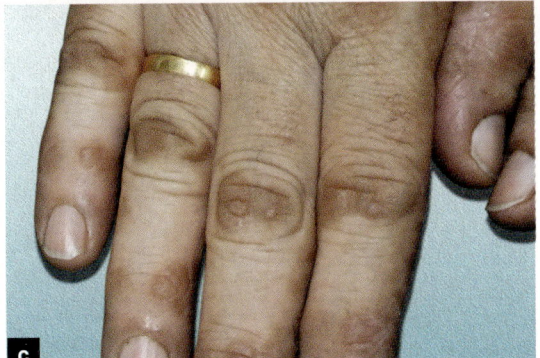

Fig. 2.11a to c: Hypopigmentation due to TCS:
(a) Hypopigmentation is frequently seen in perilesional skin when potent and very potent steroids are used to treat psoriasis. **(b)** Hypopigmentation is seen in flatter normal skin(in this case within the lesion) when very potent steroids in ointment formulation are used to treat keloids. **(c)** Inadvertent rubbing of excess ointment of TCS (here used to treat palmar psoriasis) onto dorsal aspect of hands, resulted in hypopigmentation of dorsal aspects of digits.

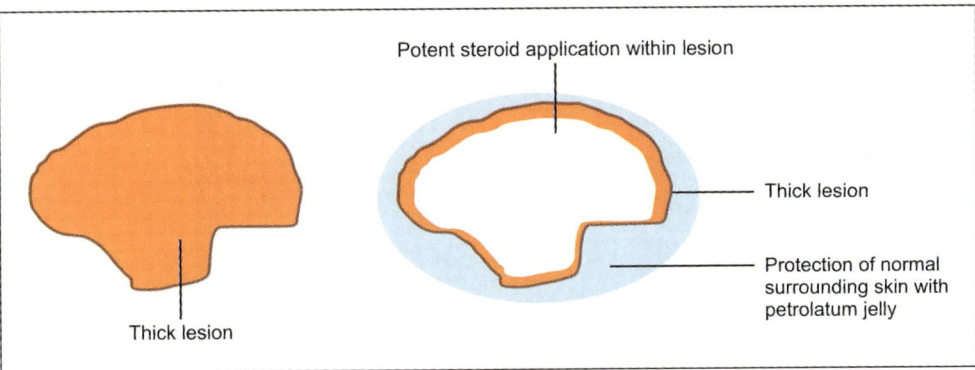

Fig. 2.11d: Carefully applying the TCS within the margin of the skin and protecting the surrounding normal skin with petroleum jelly is a good way to avoid atrophy and hypopigmentation of adjoining skin.

Hypopigmentation of face sometimes occurs along with features of TSDF due to (mis) use of TCS as a fairness cream.

- The hypopigmentation may be associated with atrophy and visibility of deeper vessels (Fig. 2.4b).
- The pigmentary change is temporary and resolves over a period of a few weeks to months following cessation of the TCS use.

Hypertrichosis

- *Mechanism:* TCS promote growth of vellus hair by an unknown mechanism.
- *Manifestations:* Long term use of TCS may lead to facial hypertrichosis. The localised hypertrichosis usually resolves on discontinuation of TCS, but this often takes several months (Fig. 2.12).

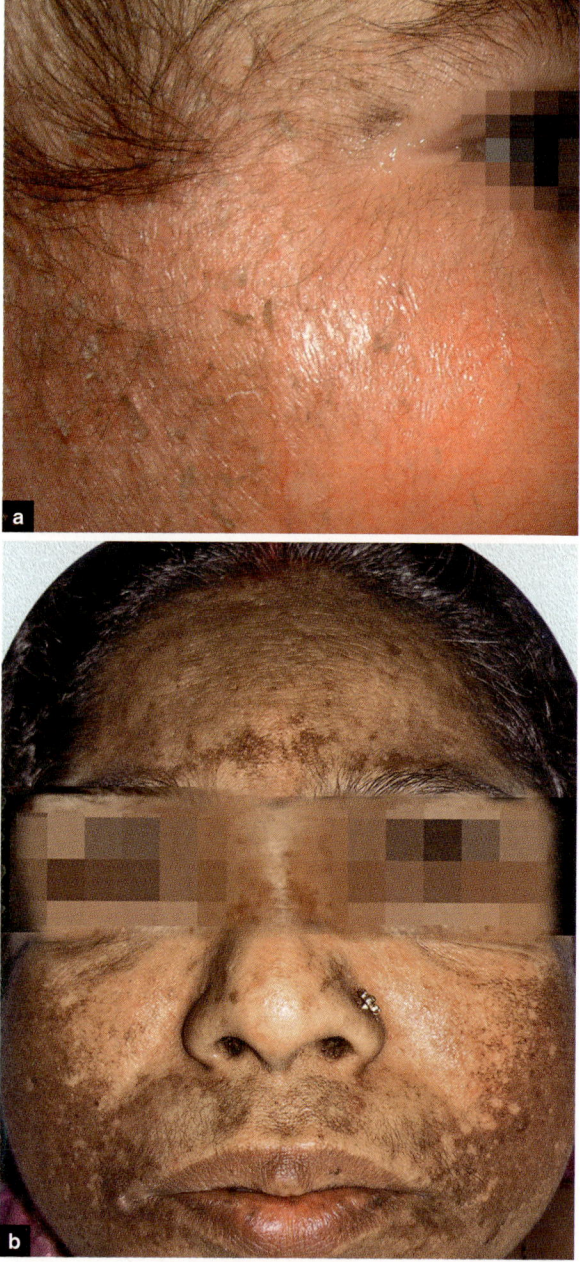

Fig. 2.12: Hypertrichosis due to TCS application: (a) Long term use of TCS often leads to facial hypertrichosis. **(b)** This patient of melasma treated with TCS developed hypertrichosis.

Infections

TCS may exacerbate/mask cutaneous infections with incidence of skin infection varying from 16 to 43%.[9]

- **Bacterial infections:** In case of obviously infected dermatitis, bacterial infection should be treated prior to use of TCS. However, colonization of lesions with bacteria in atopic dermatitis can be reduced by improving the condition of skin by using mild to moderately potent TCS.
- **Dermatophyte infections[10]:** Dermatophyte infections are often self/quack-treated with TCS because they are easily available over the counter, and they improve symptoms rapidly. However, the patient may develop atypical manifestations of tinea:
  - *Tinea incognito*: The classic appearance of tinea is masked due to the anti-inflammatory effect of TCS—lesions lose their active erythematous edge (Fig. 2.13a) develop pustular lesions around the periphery of the existing lesion and often mimic other diseases such as dermatitis (Fig. 2.13b). However, despite clinical masking, lesions continue to be strongly KOH-positive (Fig. 2.13c).
  - *Steroid-modified tinea*:
    - Extensive lesions: TCS-treated tinea lesions are often very large (Fig. 2.14).
    - Tinea pseudoimbricata: Tinea pseudoimbricata refers to usually 2 or rarely 3 complete, but more often incomplete, concentric circles (rings within a ring/double-edged tinea) within a lesion of tinea and is a clue to the application of potent TCS (Fig. 2.14b and c). It is essentially a form of tinea incognito that resembles tinea imbricata, but the latter generally has many more concentric circles. The formation of concentric circles in TCS-treated tinea is probably due to TCS-induced local immunosuppression (allowing dermatophyte to survive in the centre) and its anti-inflammatory effect (masking clinical manifestations). So while TCS is being used, though the dermatophyte survives in the centre (due to inadequate clearance) it does not manifest clinically (due to anti-inflammatory effect of TCS). When the TCS application is discontinued, both the dermatophytes in the centre and at the edge become clinically manifest and if this happens repeatedly, it would lead to multiple active borders and circles leading to tinea pseudoimbricata.
  - *Drug-nonresponsive tinea*: Tinea cruris and corporis is today non-responsive or at best poorly responsive to most anti-fungal agents (both topical and systemic) and this has been attributed at least partly to TCS misuse.
- **Granuloma gluteale infantum:**
  - *Etiology*: Treatment of diaper dermatitis with potent TCS results in impaired immune response to Candida.
  - *Morphology*: Characterized by reddish-purple plaques and nodules in the groin, inner thighs and buttocks.
  - *Histopathology*: Syphilis-like plasma cell infiltrate on light microscopy.
  - *Treatment*: Nodules resolves in a months time on stoppage of TCS.

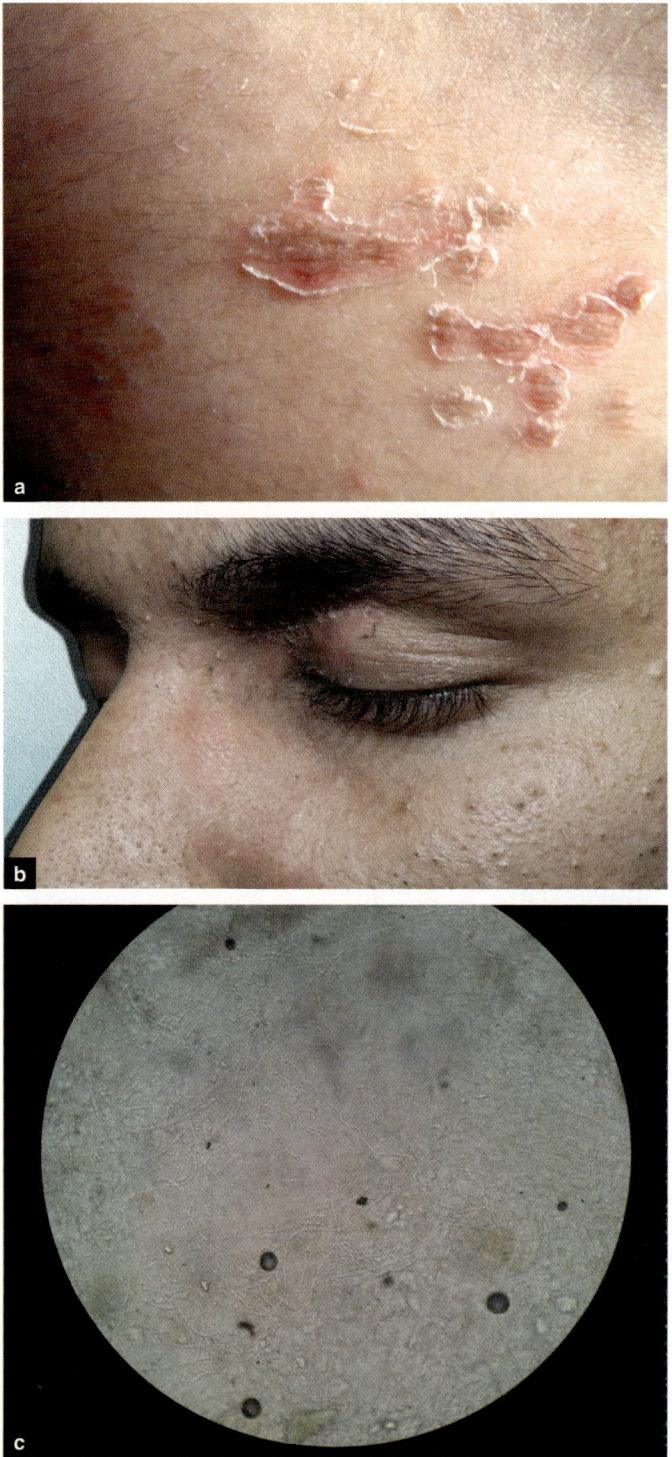

Fig. 2.13: Tinea incognito: When tinea is treated with TCS, its clinical morphology becomes less discernible. **(a)** Lesions lose their active erythematous edge. **(b)** Lesions mimic other diseases such as dermatitis. **(c)** Despite clinical masking, lesions continue to be KOH positive.

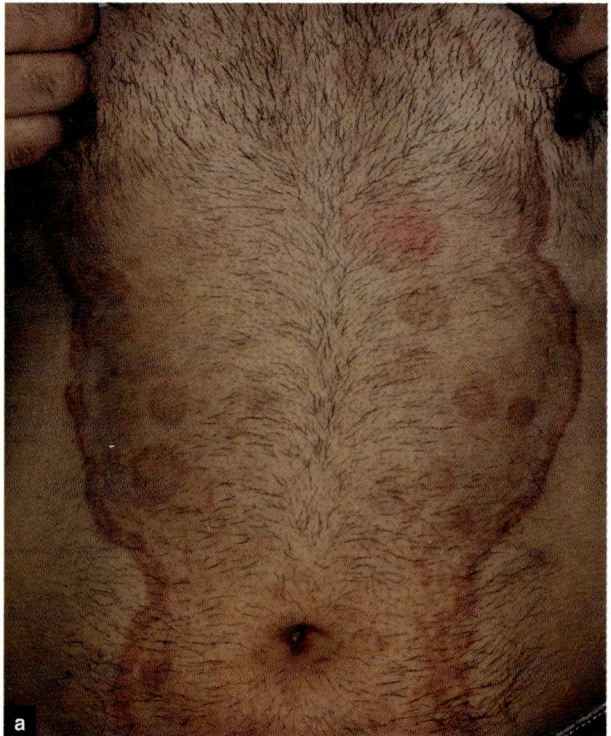

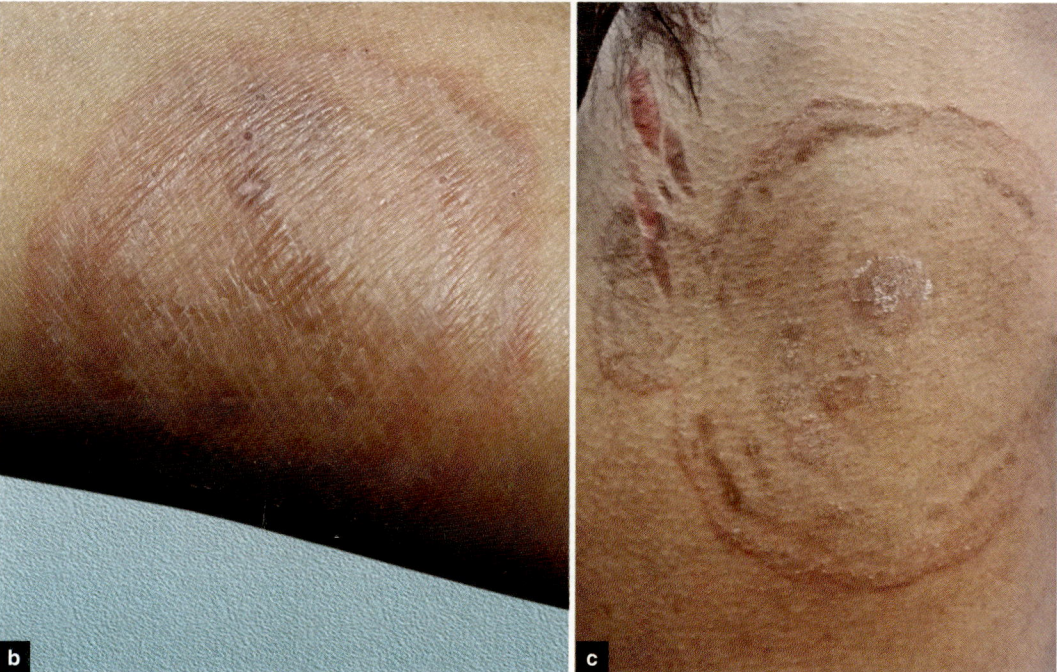

Fig. 2.14: Steroid-modified tinea. (a) Large lesion of tinea corporis: Due to treatment with potent TCS. Note multiple separate rings (rings within a ring) within the giant lesion of tinea. **(b and c) Tinea pseudoimbricata:** Concentric rings (usually only 2–3), some complete others incomplete of tinea corporis.

- *Viral infections*: Application of TCS over active viral infections may disseminate herpes simplex infection (Fig. 2.15), molluscum contagiosum and warts. Complications of use of TCS in genital area include development of anogenital warts and reactivation of genital herpes (GH) and it is recommended that while using TCS on genitals, those with history of GH should be prescribed prophylactic acyclovir.[11]

Allergic Contact Dermatitis (ACD)

- *Prevalence*: ACD to TCS though uncommon, is being increasingly recognized. Prevalence ranges between 0.2 and 6% and TCS were named the American Contact Dermatitis Society's 'allergen of the year' in the year 2005. In a 6-year retrospective study, 127 of 1188 subjects (10.7%) patch tested with TCS showed a positive reaction to at least one agent, with 5% patients reacting to multiple TCS.[12] In a study of 100 Indian patients tested with a commercially available steroid series there was a 2% positive patch test reactivity to tixocortol pivalate, to which the study population had no previous exposure (not commercially available in India).[13] This could be explained by cross reactivity of tixocortol to hydrocortisone acetate, which is marketed in India.

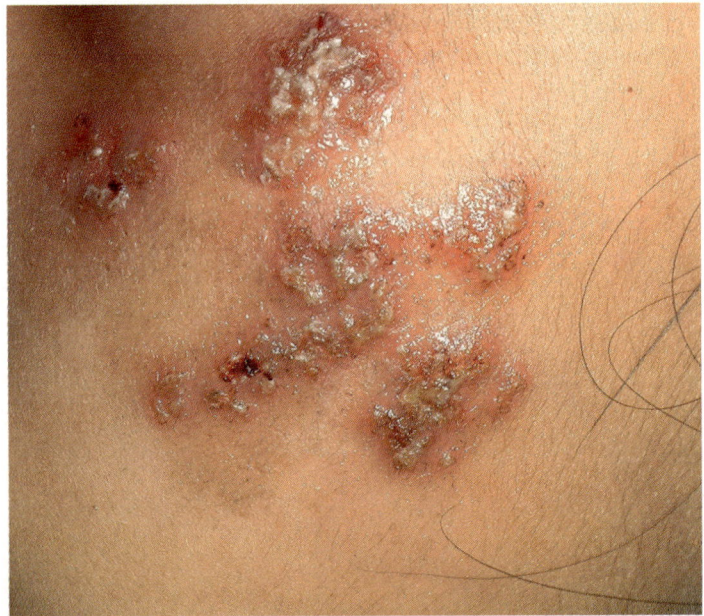

Fig. 2.15: Steroid-modified herpes simplex infection. This child with recurrent HSV infection was treated with very potent TCS, resulting in spread of lesions.

Earlier Dooms-Goossens et al in 1986 had reported several patients who were patch test positive to tixocortol pivalate when that molecule was not even commercially available due to structural similarity to hydrocortisone. Subsequently, it was found that tixocortol pivalate is a sensitive marker for ACD to hydrocortisone (and also to prednisolone, and methylprednisolone. Similarly, budesonide is a sensitive marker for ACD to desonide, and halcinonide and clobetasol propionate is a good proxy for betamethasone dipropionate and fluticasone.

- *Etiology*: Allergic reactions can be due to the active ingredients (TCS), vehicle or the preservatives.
  - *TCS*: Most frequent sensitizers are hydrocortisone, budesonide and hydrocortisone butyrate and sensitivity to more than one TCS is not uncommon. Based on their molecular structure, propensity to cause ACD and their cross reactions, TCS have been classified into 4 groups (Coopman's classification; Table 2.2). Patch test reaction to class A products are most common, whereas patch test reaction to class C are extremely rare.
  - *Vehicle and added products*: Most common allergens are propylene glycol and sorbitan sesquioleate. Others include methylchloroisothiazolinone/methyl isothiazolinone, lanolin, parabens, formaldehyde releasing preservatives and fragrances.[13]
- *Risk factors*:
  - *Underlying skin disorder*: Patients with stasis dermatitis, leg ulcers, perianal dermatitis, hand and foot eczema, chronic actinic dermatitis and facial dermatitis are particularly prone to developing ACD to TCS as also are patients with barrier disruption (like atopic dermatitis).

Table 2.2: TCS classification based on cross-reaction patterns (Coopman's classification)				
Group	*Molecule*	*Screening agent*	*Cross reaction*	*Comment*
A: Hydrocortisone type	Hydrocortisone Tixocortol Methylprednisolone Prednisolone Prednisone	Tixocortol	Cross reacts with group D2	
B: Triamcinolone acetonide type	Triamcinolone Desonide Budesonide Fluocinolone Fluocinonide Halcinonide	Budesonide Triamcinolone acetonide	Budesonide specially cross reacts with group D2	
C: Betamethasone type	Betamethasone Dexamethasone Desoximetasone Fluocortolone Flucortine			Least chance of ACD
D1: Betamethasone dipropionate type	Betamethasone dipropionate Halobetasol Clobetasol Fluticasone Clobetasone	Clobetasol -17- propionate		Halogenated. C16 methylated Less frequent patch test positivity.
D2: Methylpredni-solone acepponate type	Methylprednisolone acepponate Prednicarbate Hydrocortisone butyrate Hydrocortisone acepponate	Hydrocortisone-17-butyrate	Cross react with group B and group A	Non-halogenated. Not C16 methylated More frequent patch test positivity.

- *Prolonged exposure*: Risk of ACD increases with prolonged use of TCS.
- *Steroid structure*: Nonfluorinated TCS (e.g. hydrocortisone, hydrocortisone-17-butyrate and budesonide) cause more ACD than fluorinated compounds because of greater binding to amino acid arginine which is a prerequisite for development of allergic reaction to TCS.
- *Formulations*: Solutions and ointments are least allergenic.
- **Clinical features**: Because it is uncommon and TCS themselves are used for treating allergic dermatoses, ACD to TCS is often not suspected. To avoid missing ACD to TCS, it is important to suspect it when:
  - A normally TCS-responsive dermatitis fails to respond to or worsens after TCS use (Fig. 2.16a and b).
  - A steroid-responsive dermatosis develops a dermatitis.
- *Management*:
  - *Patch test*: When an allergy to TCS is suspected, a patch test using patient's own TCS and a corticosteroid series (Table 2.3, Figs 2.17 and 2.18a and b) is done to confirm the diagnosis and TCS from another group is prescribed (Table 2.3).
  - *Patch test facility not available*: If patch testing facility is not available, and patient needs to use a TCS, then a class C steroid with a vehicle that contains no allergens (like propylene glycol and lanolin), preferably in ointment formulation (because of fewer additives) may be prescribed.

Vehicle/Additive-related Adverse Effects

The vehicle/additives used in a TCS preparation can either increase the adverse effects of the TCS or may cause local adverse effects of their own.

- Occlusive vehicles can cause folliculitis, miliaria, and exacerbation of acne and rosacea.
- The vehicle and various additives used can cause symptoms like pruritus and burning, contact urticaria and contact dermatitis (Table 2.4).

Tachyphylaxis

- **Definition**: Tachyphylaxis is development of acute tolerance (loss of clinical effect) to action of a drug after repeated doses and is a well-known (albeit controversial) problem with prolonged use particularly of very potent TCS.
- **Occurs to**: Both vasoconstrictive effects on human skin and to antiproliferative effects in hairless mouse skin.
- **Measured by histamine-induced wheal suppression**: At baseline, volume of wheal induced by pricking with histamine acid phosphate solution on the flexor of forearms is calculated. The TCS being tested is applied daily under occlusion for 14 days at the same site. The histamine test is repeated on the same site on day 14.[16]

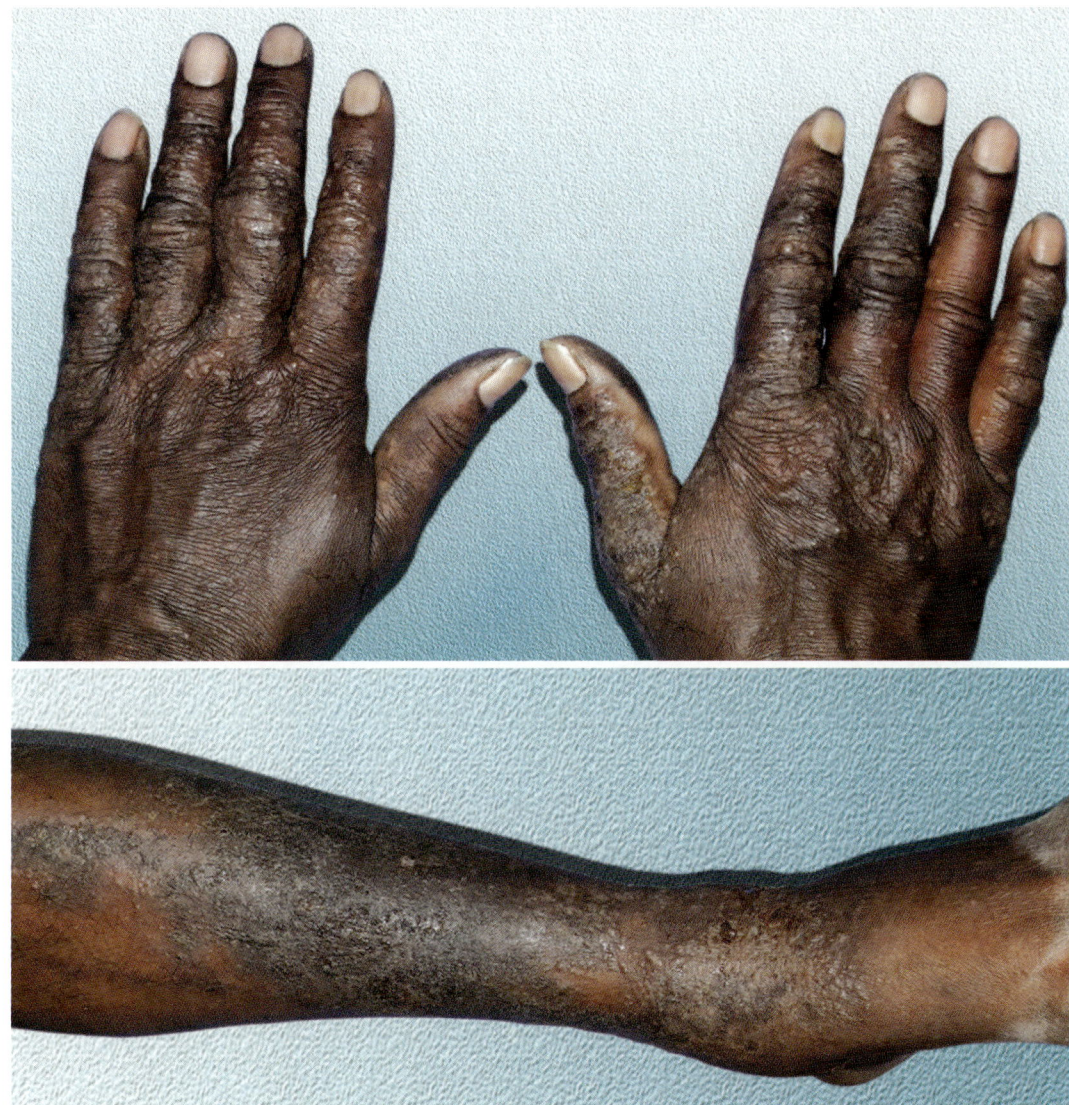

Fig. 2.16: Allergic contact dermatitis to TCS. This patient's normally TCS-responsive endogenous dermatitis failed to respond to TCS.

- **Clinical implications** are debatable as clinical studies in patients with psoriasis have failed to demonstrate any tachyphylaxis.
- **Prevention:** The most effective way to prevent tachyphylaxis is also debatable. An intermittent regimen with twice-daily application for 2 weeks followed by 'steroid holiday' for one week may help in preventing tachyphylaxis.

Note: Subjects with plaque psoriasis applied TCS twice daily × 12 weeks to their plaques, with 1 plaque left untreated. Plaques were evaluated 2 weekly using a 9-point scale. Clinical detection of tachyphylaxis was defined as an increase in plaque elevation of at least 2 occurring after a detectable decrease in plaque elevation. At 12 weeks, none of 32 patients exhibited detectable signs of tachyphylaxis.

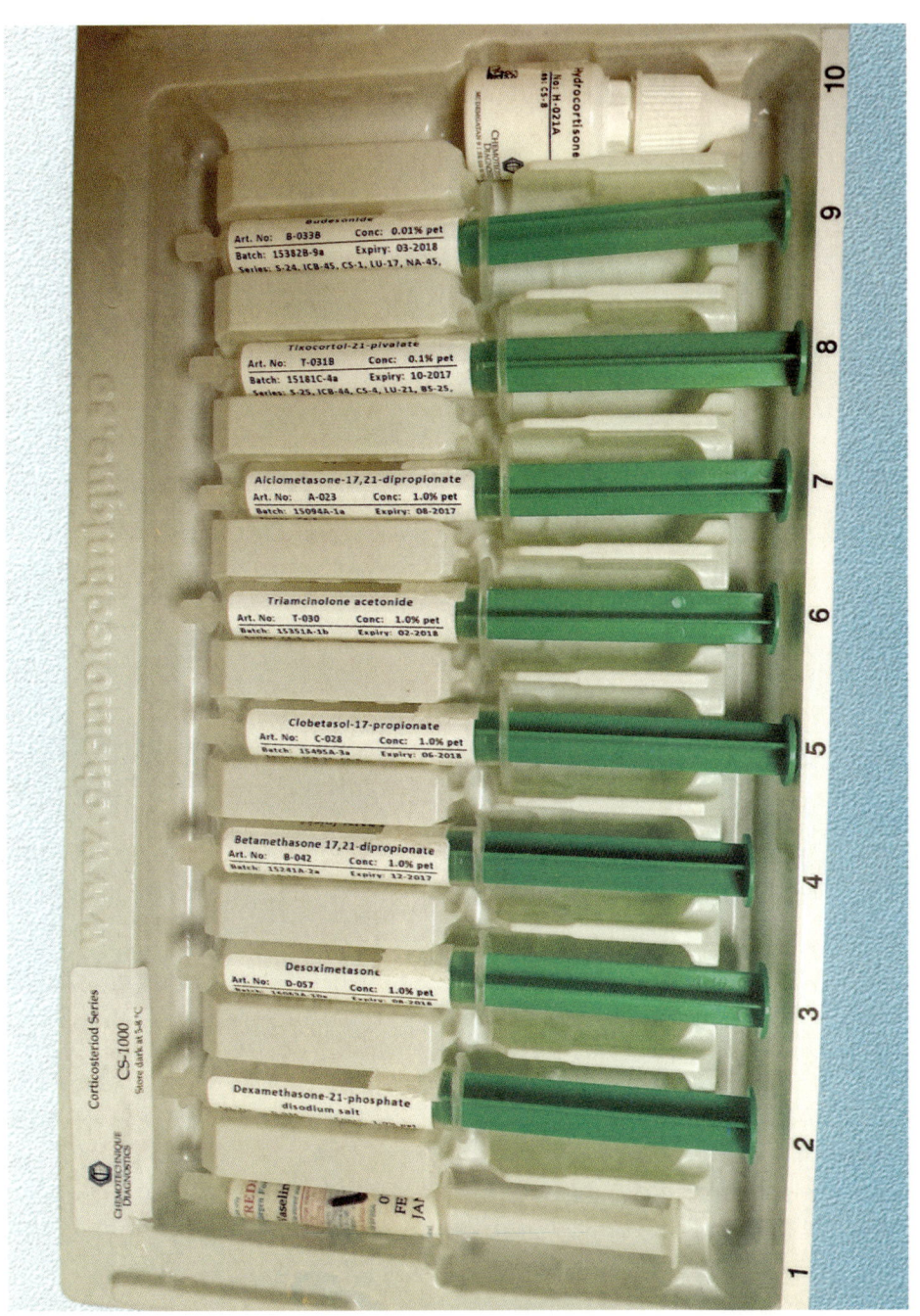

Fig. 2.17: TCS patch test series for testing allergic contact dermatitis to TCS. Contains **(1)** petrolatum (as control) **(2)** dexamethasone-21-phosphate disodium salt 1%, **(3)** desoximetasone 1%, **(4)** betamethasone-17-21 dipropionate 1%, **(5)** clobetasol-17-propionate 1% **(6)** triamcinolone acetonide 1%, **(7)** alclometasone-17-21 dipropionate 1% **(8)** tixocortol-21-pivalate 0.1%, **(9)** budesonide 0.01%, **(10)** hydrocortisone-17-butyrate.

Table 2.3: List of allergens in TCS patch test series

S. No.	Allergen	Group
1.	Vaseline	
2.	Dexamethasone-21-phosphate disodium salt	C
3.	Desoximetasone	C
4.	Betamethasone-17-21 dipropionate	D1
5.	Clobetasol-17-propionate	D1
6.	Triamcinolone acetonide	B
7.	Aclometasone17-21 dipropionate	D
8.	Tixocortol -21-pivalate	A
9.	Budesonide	B
10.	Hydrocortisone-17-butyrate	D2

Table 2.4: Reactions to different components of TCS

Type of reaction	Vehicles responsible
Stinging	Benzoic acid, cinnamic acid compound, lactic acid, urea, emulsifiers, formaldehyde and sorbic acid
Irritant contact dermatitis	Propylene glycol, alcohol and acetone
Allergic contact dermatitis	Propylene glycol and sorbitan sesquioleate
Non-immunologic contact urticarial	Acetic acid, alcohols, balsam of Peru, benzoic acid, cinnamic acid, formaldehyde, sodium benzoate and sorbic acid
Immunologic contact urticaria	Acrylic monomer, alcohols, ammonia, benzoic acid, benzophenone, diethyltoluamide, formaldehyde, menthol, parabens, polyethylene glycol, polysorbate, salicylic acid and sodium sulphide

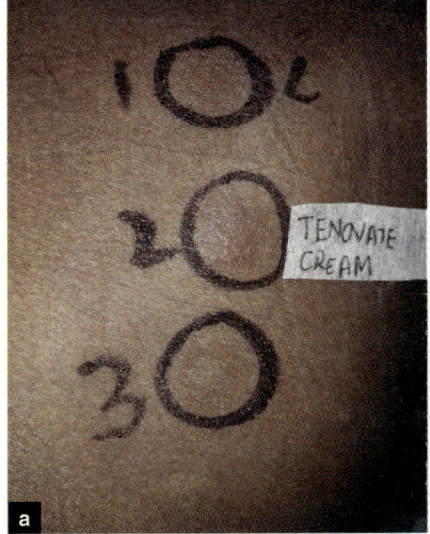 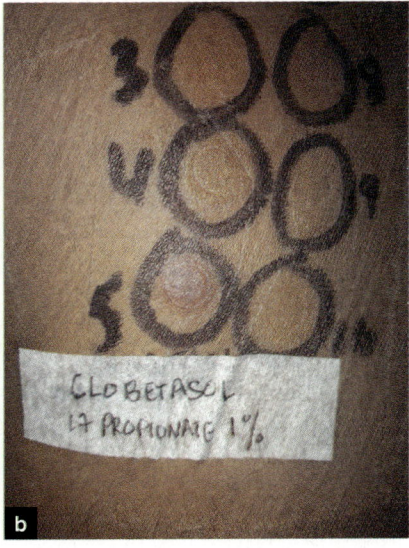

Fig. 2.18: TCS patch test reading. (a) Showing positive (2+) to patient's own medication. **(b)** Showing positive (2+) to clobetasol propionate in the TCS patch test series.

TCS Rebound Syndrome

When TCS are withdrawn after prolonged use, there can be a rebound phenomenon of the existing skin lesions.

- When potent TCS is used for the treatment of widespread lesions of plaque of psoriasis, the withdrawal may lead to pustular psoriasis (Figs 2.19a and b).
- In patients who have developed striae to TCS application, often the psoriasis relapses in the striae.

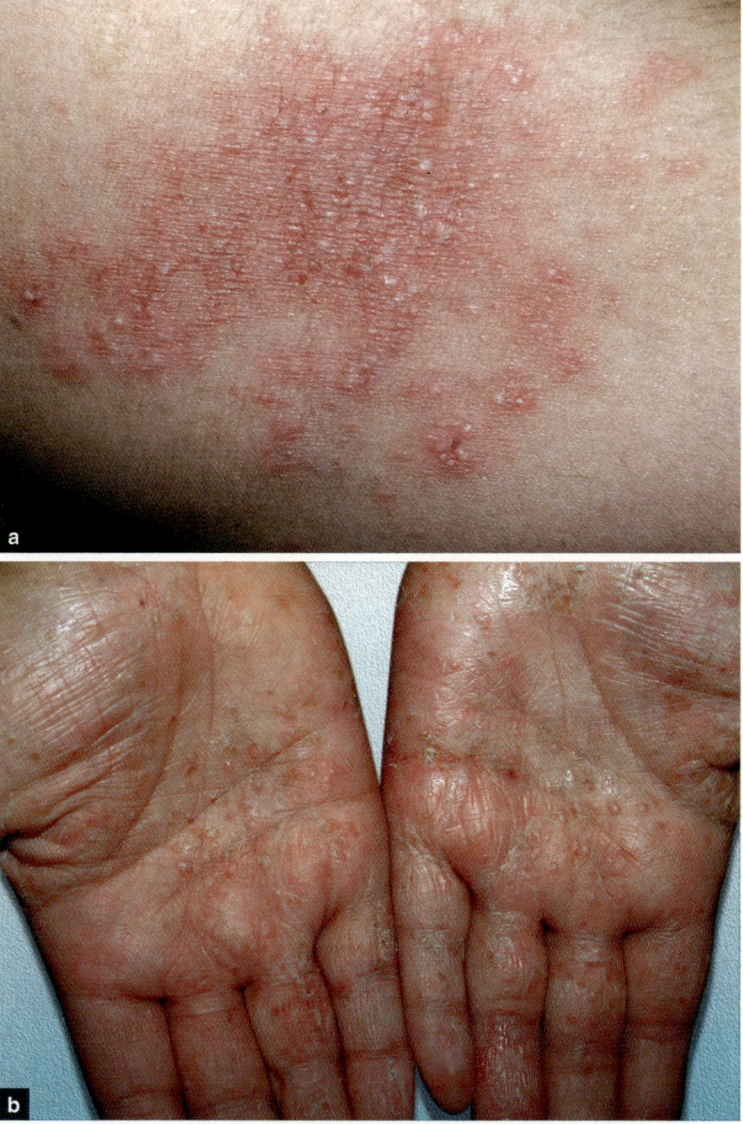

Fig. 2.19: TCS rebound syndrome: (a) Pustular psoriasis: This patient's chronic plaque psoriasis was treated with very potent TCS. On stopping the treatment, lesion relapsed with pustular lesions. **(b) Palmoplantar pustulosis:** This patient's palmoplatar psoriasis was treated with very potent TCS. On stopping the treatment, lesions relapsed as palmoplantar pustulosis.

Other Cutaneous Side Effects

- *Delayed wound healing*:
  - *Due to*:
    - Reduced mitoses of keratinocytes resulting in delayed reepithelialisation.
    - Reduced activity of fibroblasts.
    - Impaired angiogenesis resulting in delayed formation of granulation tissue formation).
  - Other local effects of TCS include folliculitis, miliaria, genital ulceration.

SYSTEMIC SIDE EFFECTS OF TCS

Despite rampant, often unsupervised use of potent and very potent TCS, fortunately, systemic side effects are rare, but when seen, they are more common in infants and elderly patients.

Ocular Effects[17]

- *Why the concern?* There is concern about potential ocular side effects to TCS because:
  - Use of systemic corticosteroids is associated with ocular side effects like glaucoma and cataract.
  - Rate of absorption of TCS is 50–300-fold higher from eyelids than from other sites and can increase further (by 2–10-fold) in diseased skin (like atopic dermatitis) due to a defective epidermal barrier.
- *Clinical relevance*: Only anecdotal reports are available for ocular side effects of TCS:
  - Prolonged use of TCS in eyes can lead to glaucoma, cataract, slower healing of traumatic ulcers, exacerbation of herpetic ulcers and increased susceptibility to fungal and bacterial infections.
  - Prolonged, inappropriate use of potent TCS in periorbital areas can lead to decreased vision due to glaucoma.
  - There is no evidence to suggest that application of mild TCS to the face or potent TCS to areas other than the eyes results in ocular complications.

Effects on HPA Axis[18]

- *Basis*: Exogenous glucocorticoids suppress effects of hypothalamic cortisol releasing hormone and pituitary adrenocorticotropic hormone (ACTH). With prolonged use, suppression of HPA axis and adrenal insufficiency with adrenal gland atrophy may occur and it takes a long period to recover after treatment discontinuation.
- *Evidence*: TCS have been found to induce some degree of cortisol suppression in 38% of patients using them with there being a linear decrease in cortisol levels with an increase in potency of TCS. However, even though biochemical

alterations are seen, clinical manifestations are rare and are seen only with gross misuse of TCS.

- **Risk factors:**
  - *Drug related factors:*
    - Potency of TCS: Though all TCS possess the potential to suppress the HPA axis, very potent TCS such as clobetasol propionate, betamethasone dipropionate, and diflorasone diacetate have an increased ability to suppress adrenal function. As little as 14 g/week of clobetasol propionate 0.05% may induce suppression in children, while 49 g/week of betamethasone dipropionate is required to significantly reduce plasma cortisol levels.
    - Formulation: Risk is greatest with occlusive formulations like ointments
  - *Application related factors:*
    - Quantity of TCS: HPA axis suppression may be seen with excessive application of moderately potent TCS or by relatively modest use of very potent TCS and has been documented even with hydrocortisone in children, if large quantity is applied over large areas.
    - Occlusion: Increases risk.
  - *Patient related factors:*
    - Age of patient: Children are at a greater risk and even hydrocortisone, if applied over large areas can cause HPA suppression in children with atopic dermatitis.
    - Condition of skin: Patients with atopic dermatitis are most prone.
- **Course:** Fortunately, recovery within 4 months of discontinuation of TCS application is the rule.
- **Diagnosis:** HPA suppression is diagnosed by:
  - *Determining morning cortisol level*: Finding of decreased fasting cortisol level is the most cost-effective means of diagnosing clinically significant suppression.
  - *1 µg ACTH test*: Finding of blunted cortisol response to ACTH is a more sensitive means of assessing the HPA axis.
  - *Metyrapone test*: Confirmed by stimulation studies with overnight metyrapone test.
- **Treatment:** Treatment of TCS-induced HPA axis suppression involves:
  - *Reducing potency and amount of TCS*: There are no formal practice guidelines for this and duration and rate of TCS taper depends on degree of adrenal suppression and potency, amount and duration of TCS treatment.
  - *Supplementation with an oral corticosteroid*: A physiologic dose of oral cortico-steroid is given to prevent an adrenal crisis for 3–4 months and is discontinued when HPA axis recovery is confirmed by normal morning cortisol levels.
- **Prevention:** For prevention, recommended weekly dosage of TCS is:
  - <50 g of very potent TCS, e.g. clobetasol, halobetasol.

– <100 g of potent TCS, e.g. betamethasone, mometasone, fluticasone.
– Even at this level, prolonged usage is best avoided in high-risk patients.

Steroid-induced Cushing's Syndrome[19]

• There are anecdotal reports of iatrogenic Cushing syndrome developing after indiscriminate use of very potent TCS (clobetasol) use, both in children and adults.
• Most of these reports are from developing countries where sale of these drugs is unrestricted and mostly in infants with diaper dermatitis and sometimes in adults with psoriasis.

Others

• *Hyperglycemia*: Significant percutaneous absorption of TCS may result in hyperglycemia and unmasking of latent diabetes mellitus especially in patients with pre-existing hepatic disease. However, this is decidedly rare.
• *Effect on growth*: Glucocorticoids excess leads to short stature both due to decreased release of growth hormone releasing hormone (GHRH) and growth hormone (GH) from the hypothalamus and pituitary respectively. Growth impairment has been reported in child treated with 30 gram/week of betamethasone valerate (0.1%) ointment for three years.[19]
• *Epiphyseal closure*: Long-term treatment with TCS should also be avoided in adolescents because of chance of premature epiphyseal closure before catch-up growth can occur.[20]
• *Decrease in bone mineral density*: Osteoporosis is a serious side effect of systemic and inhaled corticosteroid therapy, but has also been reported with the use of TCS.[21] The bone loss caused by glucocorticoids is trabecular in nature affecting vertebrae and ribs of the axial skeleton.
• *Avascular necrosis of femoral head*: Osteonecrosis of femoral head following application of clobetasol propionate has been described in a case of atopic dermatitis.[22]

STRATEGIES TO REDUCE SIDE EFFECTS OF TCS

Every attempt should be made to reduce side effects of TCS, and some of the strategies to prevent/counter these have already been discussed under the relevant side effect. However, there are general principles which help to curtail side effects of TCS include:

• *Using correct potency*: The potency of TCS to be used depends on several factors including the dermatological indication and site of use. Nevertheless, therapy should always be started with least potent TCS likely to control the disease followed by titrating down with the response.

- *Optimum duration*: Once disease control is achieved, alternate day application or weekend therapy is recommended. Prolonged use (especially unmonitored) of TCS may lead to side effects.
- *Frequency*: Once daily application of TCS is as efficacious and more cost effective as compared to twice daily application. More frequent applications do not offer additional benefits, but increase the risk of side effects.[23]
- *Site specific precautions*: Thin sites such as eyelids, scrotum and flexures such as groin and axilla have higher absorption of topical medications and, therefore, lower potency TCS should be used at these sites for a minimum duration of time.
- *Age related precautions*: Caution must be exercised while prescribing TCS in:
  - *Children*: Who are particularly prone to adverse effects due to their higher body surface area to weight ratio and immature skin barrier function.
  - *Elderly*: Skin of elderly is thin and fragile, increasing risk of adverse effects including atrophy, purpura, delayed wound healing and susceptibility to infections.
- *Use of adjuvant therapy*: Monotherapy with TCS is best avoided and adjuvants added depending on the indication, so as to reduce both the total amount of TCS used and the duration of therapy:
  - *Atopic dermatitis*:
    - Emollients should be used liberally, so as to wean the patient of TCS.
    - Topical calcineurin inhibitors should be used as alternatives to TCS whenever possible.
  - *Psoriasis*: Coal tar, anthralin, salicylic acid can be used initially along with TCS.
  - *Seborrheic dermatitis*: Topical azoles are used in seborrheic dermatitis as anti-inflammatory agents.
- *Patient education*:
  - Communication of correct and adequate information about the medication and clear written instructions regarding how to use them is the key to avoiding steroid misuse.
  - Patients can be provided with an information leaflet (Annexure 2) with details on how to apply the TCS in adequate amount based on FTU and ensuring regular follow up to avoid prolonged, inadvertent use of TCS.
  - Patients must be educated to strictly avoid prescription sharing and using old prescriptions indefinitely.

REFERENCES

1. Hengge UR, Ruzicka T, Schwartz RA, Cork MJ. Adverse effects of topical glucocorticosteroids. J Amer Acad Dermatol 2006;54:1–15.

2. Lehmann P, Zheng P, Lavker RM, et al. Corticosteroid atrophy in human skin. A study by light, scanning, and transmission electron microscopy. J Invest. Dermatol. 1983; 81: 169–76.

3. McMicheal AJ, Griffiths CE, Talwar HS, et al. Concurrent application of tretinoin (retinoic acid) partially protects against corticosteroid-induced epidermal atrophy. Brit J Dermatol. 1996;135: 60–64.

4. Rathi SK, Kumrah L. Topical corticosteroid-induced rosacea-like dermatitis: A clinical study of 110 cases. Indian J Dermatol VenereolLeprol 2011;77:42–6.

5. Chu CY. An open-label pilot study to evaluate the safety and the efficacy of topically applied pimecrolimus cream for the treatment of steroid-induced rosacea-like eruption. J Eur Acad Dermatol Venereol 2007;21:484–90.

6. Goldman D. Tacrolimus ointment for the treatment of steroid-induced rosacea: A preliminary report. J Amer Acad Dermatol 2001;44:995–8.

7. LahiriK, Coondoo A. Topical steroid damaged/dependent face (TSDF): An entity of cutaneous pharmacodependence. Indian J Dermatol 2016;61:265–72.

8. Condoo A, Phiska M, Verma S, Lahiri K. Side effects of topical steroids: A long overdue revisit. Indian Dermatol Online J 2014;5:416–25.

9. Aucott JN. Glucocorticoids and infection. Endocrinol Metab Clin North Am 1994;23:655–70.

10. Verma S, Madhu R. The great Indian epidemic of superficial dermatophytosis: An appraisal. Indian J Dermatol 2017;62:227–3.

11. Neill SM, Lewis FM, Tatnall FM, Cox NH. British Association of Dermatologists' guidelines for the management of lichen sclerosus. Br J Dermatol 2010;163:672–82.

12. Davis MD, el-Azhary RA, Farmer SA. Results of patch testing to a corticosteroids series: a retrospective review of 1188 patients during 6 years at Mayo clinic. J Am Acad Dermatol 2007;56:921–7.

13. Sahu U, Handa S, De D. Contact sensitivity to topical corticosteroids in India. Indian Journal of Dermatol Venereol Leprol 2016; 82:184–86.

14. Coopman S, DeGreef H, Dooms-Goossens A. Identification of cross-reaction patterns in allergic contact dermatitis from topical corticosteroids. Br J Dermatol 1989;121:27–34.

15. Dooms-Goossens A, Verschaeve H, DeGreef H, van Berendoncks J. Contact allergy to hydrocortisone and tixocortol pivalate: Problems in the detection of corticosteroid sensitivity. Contact Dermatitis 1986;14:94–102.

16. Singh G, Singh PK. Tachyphylaxis to topical steroids measured by histamine-induced wheal suppression. Int J Dermatol 1986; 25:324–6.

17. Cubey RB. Glaucoma following application of corticosteroid to the skin of the eyelids. Br it J Dermatol 1976;95:207–8.

18. Gilbertson EO, Spellman MC, Piacquadio DJ, Mulford MI. Super potent topical corticosteroid use associated with adrenal suppression: clinical considerations. J Amer Acad Dermatol 1998;38:318–21.

19. Keipert JA, Kelly R. Temporary Cushing's syndrome from percutaneous absorption of betamethasone 17-valerate. Med J Aust 1971;1:542–4.

20. Takahashi H, Bando H, Zhang C, Yamasaki R, Saito S. Mechanism of impaired growth hormone secretion in patients with Cushing's disease. Acta Endocrinol (Copenh) 1992;127:13–7.

21. Nymann P, Kollerup G, Jemec GB, Grossmann E. Decreased bone mineral density in patients with pustulosis palmaris et plantaris. Dermatology. 1996;192:307–11.

22. Millard TP, Antoniades L, Evans AV, Smith HR, Spector TD, Barker JN. Bone mineral density of patients with chronic plaque psoriasis. ClinExp Dermatol. 2001;26:446–8.

23. Green C, Colquitt JL, Kirby J, Davidson P. Topical corticosteroids for atopic eczema: Clinical and cost effectiveness of once-daily vs. more frequent use. Br J Dermatol 2005;152:130–41.

ANNEXURE 2: INSTRUCTIONS TO PATIENTS PRESCRIBED TOPICAL STEROIDS

What are topical steroids?

Topical steroids are medicines applied directly to skin to reduce inflammation and irritation.

Are all topical steroids equally effective?

- No. There are many topical steroids, and they can be broadly categorized as:
  - Mild
  - Moderately potent
  - Potent
  - Very potent.
- Do not substitute the steroid prescribed by your doctor by another, as they may have different potencies.

What are the formulations in which topical steroids are available?

- Topical steroids are available in several formulations and the doctor prescribes a formulation which is most suited for the site of disease and type of disease.
- The formulation may also change the potency of the medicine. Do not substitute the formulation of steroid prescribed by your doctor by another, as they may have different potencies.
- Formulations in which topical steroids are available include:
  - *Creams*: The most frequently used formulation.
  - *Ointments*: These are greasy and used in very scaly diseases.
  - *Lotions and solutions*: Used in hairy areas.
  - *Gels and foams*: Cosmetically elegant.
  - *Paste*: Used in mouth.

What are the conditions for which a topical steroid is prescribed?

Several skin diseases (especially several itchy skin diseases) are treated with topical steroids, but they generally do not cure these conditions, but help relieve the symptoms. They are used in:

- *Psoriasis*: Which causes scaly patches.
- *Vitiligo*: Which causes white spots.
- *Eczema*: Such as atopic eczema, hand eczema
- *Seborrheic dermatitis*: Which causes dandruff and scaly patches on the skin
- *Nappy rash*
- *Lichen planus*: Which causes an itchy, blue-black rash
- *Skin irritation*: Caused by insect bites or stings, allergic rashes to chemicals like hair dyes and metals.

When should topical steroids be avoided?

Most adults can use topical steroids safely, but there are situations when they are not recommended or need to be used with caution.They should not be used:

- If there is a skin infection like ringworm. Though there is an initial improvement (infection may even get masked), over period of time the infection spreads (large lesion, several rings) and often becomes resistant to standard antifungal therapy.
- In skin conditions like rosacea (red, sensitive face), acne and open sores.

Can I use topical steroids prescribed to some one else?

No, never. Because different skin diseases and different sites need to be treated with steroids of different potency and formulation and treatment is often individualised.

When should topical steroids be used with caution?

- Most topical steroids are considered safe to use during pregnancy, but it is best to avoid very potent topical steroids during pregnancy, though exceptions are sometimes made under the supervision of a skin specialist.
- Most topical steroids (best to avoid very potent ones) are considered safe to use during breastfeeding. However, you should wash off any steroid cream applied to your breasts before feeding your baby.
- It is best to avoid use of very potent and potent steroids in children, because there is an increased risk of absorption.

How to use topical steroids?

- Use this medication exactly as directed on the label or as it has been prescribed by your doctor. Do not use the medication in larger amounts or for longer than recommended.
- Most people only need to use the medication once or twice a day for a week or two, although occasionally your doctor may suggest using it less frequently over a longer period of time.
- The medication should only be applied to affected areas of skin. Gently smooth it into your skin in the direction the hair grows.
- If the lesion is thick, your doctor may prescribe a potent steroid. In that case it is a good idea to protect the surrounding skin with petroleum jelly before applying the steroid on the diseased skin to avoid side effects developing in adjacent area.
- If the disease is on palms and soles, your doctor may ask you to soak these parts in water (or salt water). Apply the medicine on the affected part only, after pat drying the skin. Do not rub excess amount of medicine on unaffected areas as this may lead to side effects.

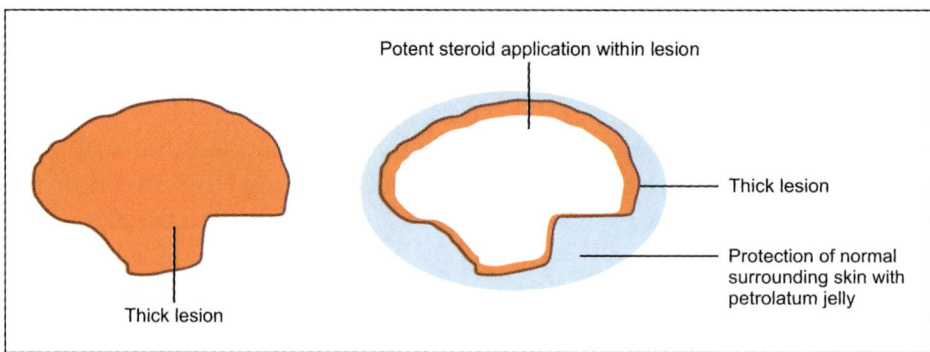

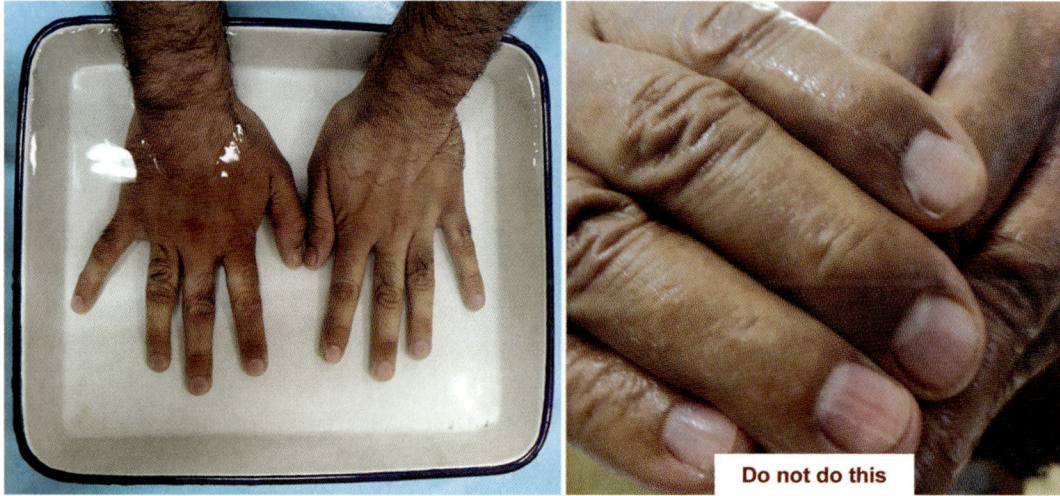

Do not do this

- Do not cover treated skin areas with a bandage or other covering unless your doctor has advised you to do so. If you are treating the diaper area of a baby, do not use plastic or tight-fitting diapers. Covering the skin that is treated with topical steroid can increase the amount of the drug your skin absorbs, which may lead to unwanted side effects.

- Avoid using this medication on your face, near your eyes, or on body areas where you have skin folds or thin skin, unless advised by the doctor.

- If you are using both topical steroids and emollients, you should apply the emollient first. Then wait about 30 minutes before applying the topical steroid.

How much to use?

- If the area on which the steroid is to be applied is small, then the doctor will probably tell you to apply a pea-sized amount to the lesion.

- If the area on which the steroid is to be applied is large, then the doctor will probably indicate the amount of medication needed using fingertip units (FTUs).

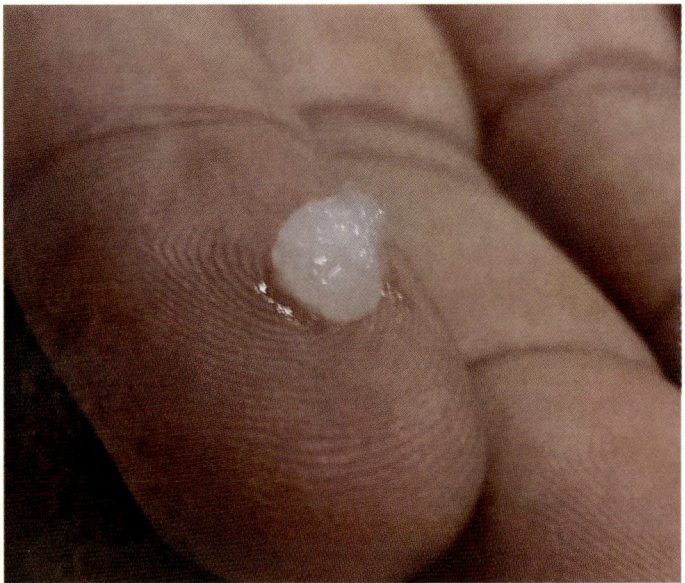

Pea-sized amount

- A FTU (about 0.5 g) is the amount of medication needed to squeeze a line from the tip of an adult finger to the first crease of the finger. It should be enough to treat an area of skin double the size your palm with your fingers together.

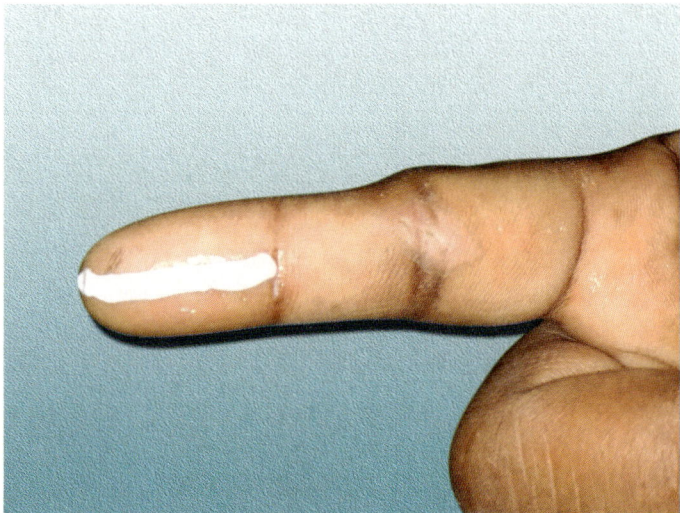

Fingertip unit

- The recommended dosage will depend on area of the part of body being treated. For adults, the recommended FTUs to be applied in one single dose are:
  - Scalp: 3 FTUs
  - Face and neck: 2 FTUs

- Trunk: 14 FTUs
- Arm (1): 3 FTUs
- Hand (2): 1 FTU
- Leg (1): 6 FTUs
- Foot: 2 FTUs
- Hand + elbows + knee: 1 FTU
- Hand+ arm together: 4 FTUs
- Buttocks: 4 FTUs
- Legs+ chest: 8 FTUs
- Legs + back: 8 FTUs
- Genitals: 0.5 FTU

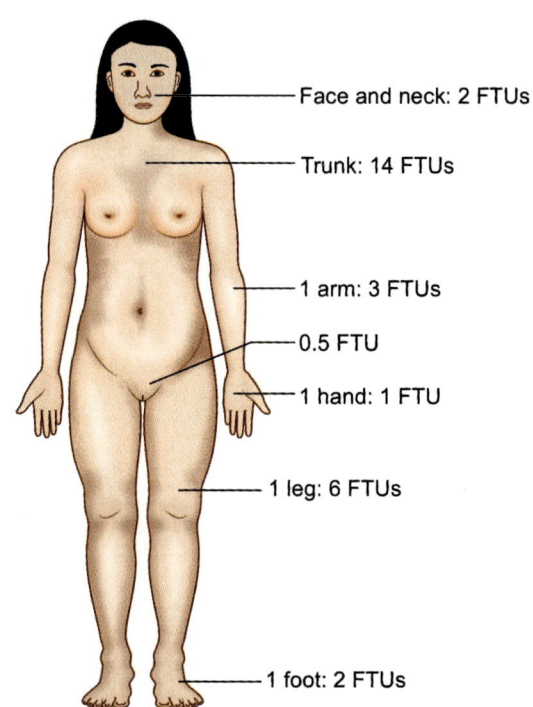

Face and neck: 2 FTUs
Trunk: 14 FTUs
1 arm: 3 FTUs
0.5 FTU
1 hand: 1 FTU
1 leg: 6 FTUs
1 foot: 2 FTUs

- For children, the recommended FTUs will depend on their age. Your doctor can advise you on this.

Side Effects of Topical Steroids

This is not a full list of all the possible side effects. For more information on side effects, see the leaflet that comes with your medication.

- Common side effects of topical steroids include:
  - Worsening of a pre-existing skin infection: This being especially true for ring worm infection.

- Whitening of skin: Never use topical steroids as whitening agent for face as it is likely to cause intense redness of the face and permanent damage to the skin of the face.
- Thinning of the skin: This can make the affected skin more vulnerable to damage; for example, you may bruise more easily.
- Stretch marks: Which are likely to be permanent, although they do become less visible over time.
- Folliculitis and acne: Inflammation around the hair and worsening of existing acne.
- Rosacea: A disease that makes the face red and sensitive to sun and to anything you apply to it.
- Excessive hair growth on area of application.
- Allergy: Skin irritation caused by a allergic reaction to the substances in a particular topical steroid
- If potent or very potent topical steroids are used for a long time or over a large area, there's a risk of the medication being absorbed into the bloodstream and causing internal side effects, such as:
  - Decreasedgrowth in children
  - Cushing's syndrome
- Side effects are more likely:
  - If you use a more potent steroid.
  - If you use it for a very long time.
  - If you use it over a large area.
  - In elderly and very young.
  - If you occlude the area, e.g. with bandage or using it at sites which are naturally occluded like armpits and groins.

3

Intralesional Steroids

Abhishek De, Sujata Sinha, Aarti Sarda, Savera Gupta, Neena Khanna

SUMMARY

- Intralesional steroid (ILS) injection is a mode of drug delivery commonly used to treat localized disease, often circumventing the need of topical (sometimes even systemic) steroid therapy.
- It has advantages of being a targeted therapy where the drug is deposited directly at the site of disease activity, with faster onset of action, sustained effect for longer duration and minimal side effects.
- ILS are used in situations where TCS are either not effective or have a limited role and as adjunct to TCS.
- ILS can be used as monotherapy or in combination with other intralesional drugs.
- ILS are used in various dermatological conditions in different concentrations. Keloid, hypertrophic scar, nodulocystic acne, alopecia areata, hypertrophic lichen planus are some of the common indications.
- Triamcinolone acetonide (TAC) is the most frequently used preparation of ILS, available as 10 mg/ml and 40 mg/ml suspension.
- TAC can be diluted with normal saline or 2% lignocaine (without adrenaline) to make the desired concentration.
- TAC is injected into the skin lesion using a 0.5-inch long, 26 to 30-gauge fine needle, with the needle being positioned at an angle of about 15–30° with bevelled tip up.
- Drug should be injected deep in the dermis as this is the site of pathology in most inflammatory conditions and also minimizes side effects.
- The end point of amount injected is when the injected skin becomes raised and blanches.
- Dose per session of TAC is generally 0.1 ml/cm^2 of involved skin given at distance of 1 cm^2, not to exceed 40 mg/session and injections are generally given at an interval of 3 to 6 weeks.

- The required number of injections depends on the disease, sites of lesions, age of patient and response to previous injections.
- International advisory panel on scar management has recommended the use of ILS for the treatment of keloids and hypertrophic scars. ILS have shown efficacy when used either alone or in combination with other modalities like verapamil, 5-fluorouracil, bleomycin, silicone gel sheet, cryotherapy and lasers.
- ILS in nail apparatus includes intramatricial injection, nail bed injection and hyponychial injection.
- Side effects of ILS can be early and delayed effects. Early effects include pain, bleeding, bruising, infections, contact allergic dermatitis, impaired wound healing, skin necrosis, ulcerations and inadvertent intravascular injection. The avoidance of intravascular injection is especially important when injecting lesions around the forehead where accidental intra-arterial injection and retrograde flow of a bolus of particles may result in retinal artery occlusion and blindness. Delayed adverse effects include cutaneous and subcutaneous atrophy, hypo- or hyperpigmentation, telangiectasia, striae, localized hypertrichosis, steroid induced acne, suppression of HPA axis, Cushing's syndrome.
- Face, genitalia, lips, buccal mucosa, etc. are particularly prone to development of atrophy and hence ILS should be avoided over these sites or only minute quantities and very dilute concentrations of ILS should be used if need be.

INTRODUCTION

- Intralesional steroid (ILS) injection is a mode of drug delivery which allows introduction of high concentration of medications into the lesion.
- Commonly used to treat localized disease, often circumventing the need to use topical (sometimes even systemic) steroid therapy.
- They may be used as monotherapy, in combination with other intralesional drugs or as an adjunct to topical and systemic steroid therapy.

Rationale of Using ILS[1]

- *Targeted therapy*: ILS injection helps to deposit the drug directly to the site of disease activity, bypassing the superficial barrier zone, which is an important obstacle to percutaneous absorption of topical corticosteroids (TCS).
- *Sustained effect*: Since the most frequently used preparation of steroid for ILS is triamcinolone acetonide (TAC) suspension, which is a depot preparation (acts as a reservoir for the medication in the dermis) releasing the drug slowly thereby prolonging its local effect.
- *Minimal systemic effects*: With ILS, a high concentration of drug is achieved in skin lesion without long term use (and side effects) of TCS and systemic corticosteroids.

Advantages of ILS Therapy

- Drug administered directly at the site it is required, overcoming physiological barriers in the way. ILS in nail unit allows delivery of drug to anatomically unreachable sites in least invasive way.
- Eliminates the need for long-term topical therapy and side effects of systemic treatment.
- Faster onset of action and prolonged action due to depot/reservoir effect.
- Reduced dependence on patient compliance.
- Can be combined with other modalities for synergistic action. For example, ILTAC with cryotherapy or 5-fluorouracil for the treatment of keloids.

Mechanism of Action

- The mechanism of action is essentially similar to that of TCS, being mediated by classical genomic and non-genomic pathways.
- ILS have anti-inflammatory, antiproliferative and potent atrophogenic effects.

Indications[2]

ILS are used in the following situations, where (Table 3.1):

- *TCS are not effective or have a limited role*: Some conditions are treated with ILS because topical agents are either not potent enough or because they cannot be delivered at the disease site with the topical route, e.g. in nodulocystic acne, nail lichen planus, nail psoriasis, myxoid cyst. ILS have a definite role where TCS have only limited utility (due to limited percutaneous absorption), e.g. in thick/hypertrophic/lichenified lesions in conditions such as hypertrophic lichen planus, lichen simplex, keloid/hypertrophic scar.
- *As an adjunct to TCS*: In conditions such as psoriasis, alopecia areata, lichen planus, mycosis fungoides, though TCS are effective, ILS may be used as an adjunct in single/few lesions which are thick or recalcitrant to treatment.
- *TCS use is associated with adverse effects*: In conditions such as discoid lupus erythematosus or necrobiosis lipoidica diabeticorum, in which epidermal atrophy is a recognized component of the disorder, monthly ILS can be used in place of daily potent TCS to reduce the risk of steroid-induced atrophy.

Contraindications

- Infection at or around the site of injection
- Previous history of hypersensitivity
- Dermal or subcutaneous atrophy as a sequelae of repeated ILS injections
- Peripheral vascular compromise should be ruled out before injecting in nail unit.

Table 3.1: Diseases and specific indications where ILS can be useful	
Conditions	Comments
Acne vulgaris	Few persistent nodulocystic lesions, poorly responsive to conventional treatment
Psoriasis	Few recalcitrant thick plaques, poorly responsive to conventional treatment Nail psoriasis
Localized dermatitis	Prurigo nodularis Lichen simplex chronicus
Lichen planus	Hypertrophic lichen planus Nail lichen planus Oral lichen planus
Pemphigus	Resistant oral lesions Resistant scalp lesions
Alopecia areata	Few patches Shorter duration, presence of exclamation hair, positive hair pull test, indicating disease activity and better response to ILS
Hidradenitis suppurativa	Inflammatory solitary/few nodules
Granuloma annulare	Solitary/few lesions
Granuloma faciale	Solitary/few lesions
Cutaneous sarcoidosis	Small papular/localized lesions
Pretibial myxedema	As adjunct to TCS and compression bandage
Pyoderma gangrenosum	Intralesional/perilesional injection into skin around active margins of lesion
Keloids/hypertrophic scars	Mainstay of treatment
Nodular scabies	Use ILS cautiously as scrotal skin is prone to atrophy.
Necrobiosis lipoidica diabeticorum	Progression of new lesions may be halted by ILS into margin of lesion
Lymphocytoma cutis	For localized disease
Pyogenic granuloma	May be used when lesion is at an unfavourable location for excision or other destructive modalities.
Myxoid cyst	Simple drainage/evacuation followed by ILS to prevent recurrence.
Angiolymphoid hyperplasia with eosinophilia	Complete surgical excision is preferred for persistent lesions. ILS is an alternate option.
Other localised inflammatory skin diseases	

FORMULATIONS OF ILS

- *Preparations available*:
  - *Most frequently used*: Triamcinolone acetonide (TAC) suspension (10 and 40 mg/ml).
  - *Others*: Triamcinolone hexacetonide, triamcinolone diacetate, betamethasone sodium phosphate/acetate, dexamethasone acetate, dexamethasone sodium phosphate, hydrocortisone acetate, methyl-prednisolone acetate.

- ***Preparation of choice***: Out of the various preparations of ILS available, triamcinolone acetonide is most frequently used, because of:
  - *Ease of injection*:
    - Small particle size: Resuspends easily with shaking.
    - Relatively painless, whereas betamethasone can frequently be irritating.
  - *More effective*: Because of small crystals it is more efficiently delivered to treatment site, thereby decreasing the total administered dose of the drug (and so reducing the risk of systemic side effects and skin atrophy).
  - *Less side effects*:
    - Less atrophogenic than triamcinolone hexacetonide.[3]
    - Less chance of small vessel occlusion or embolic phenomenon, due to smaller particle size. Triamcinolone hexacetonide is relatively insoluble and so more likely to cause small vessel occlusion.
  - *Longer duration of action*: Because it is better depot preparation, than triamcinolone diacetate, betamethasone and prednisolone.
  - *Character of molecule*:
    - Tends not to form crystals.
    - Stable at room temperature, for at least 1 week.

METHOD OF ADMINISTRATION

What is needed?

ILS injection does not need any expensive equipment (Fig. 3.1).

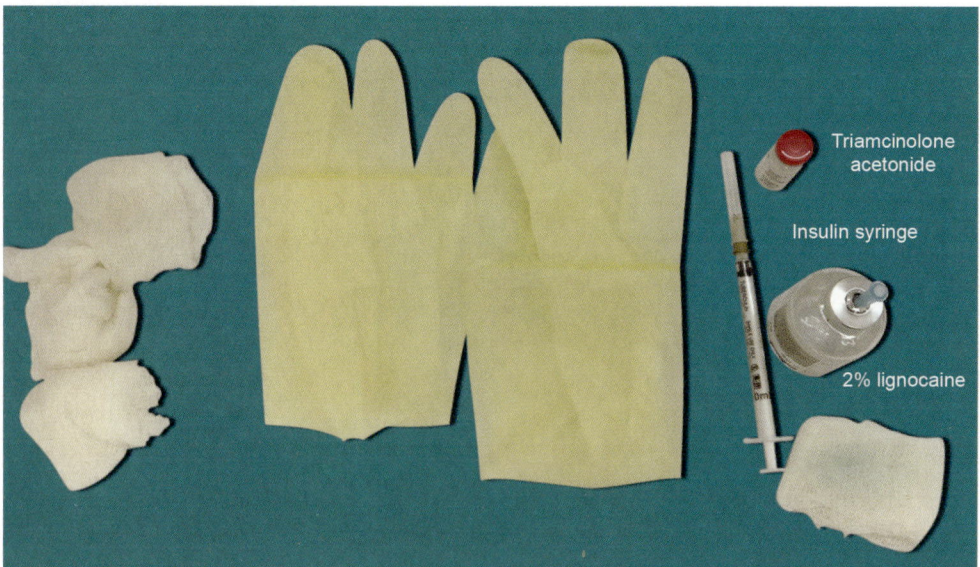

Fig. 3.1: What is needed for ILS injection: 1 ml syringe (usually insulin) with 26–30 G needle, triamcinolone acetonide (10 mg/ml or 40 mg/ml), 2% lignocaine/ normal saline (to dilute), alcohol swabs, gauze pieces and gloves.

Mixing the Solution

- Gently shake TAC vial and take the required amount of drug in 1 ml insulin syringe.[a]
- Dilute[b] with normal saline or 2% lignocaine (without adrenaline) to make the desired concentration. Sterile saline is preferred over lignocaineas a diluent, as the latter stings more (due to acidic pH[4]) and do not dilute TAC with bupivacaine (causes precipitation).
- Gently shake/roll syringe before injection to ensure even suspension of the drug in the diluent.

Injection Technique

- Topical anaesthetic may be applied 30–60 minutes before injection, to minimize pain, especially if multiple injections have to be given.
- Using aseptic precautions (cleaning the site to be injected, with alcohol or antiseptic solution) TAC is injected into the skin lesion using a 0.5-inch long, 26 to 30-gauge fine needle, with the needle being positioned at an angle of about 15–30° with bevelled tip up (Fig. 3.2).
- Drug should be injected deep in the dermis when possible, as this is the site of pathology in most inflammatory conditions. Injection in dermis also minimizes the risk of atrophy.

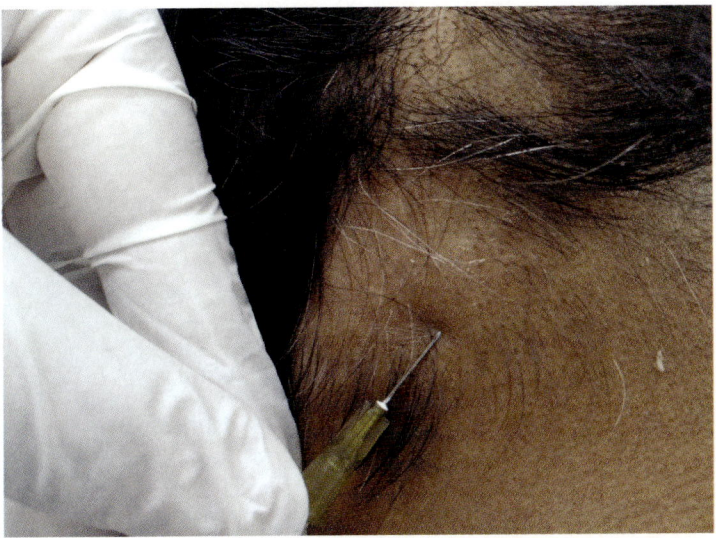

Fig. 3.2: ILS injection in alopecia areata: Inserting the needle at 15 to 30° with bevelled tip up.

---

[a]**Insulin syringe:** Though any syringe can be used, insulin (1 ml) syringe is preferred, because there is hardly any leak (which may occur with other syringes) if injecting into 'tough' tissue like keloids, due to good fit of syringe and needle.
[b]**Dilute:** Example to get 20 mg/ml strength of TAC, draw 0.5 ml of 40 mg/ml TA and 0.5 ml of normal saline in the insulin syringe.

- The end point of amount injected is when the injected skin becomes raised and blanches (Fig. 3.3).
- Single injection may be sufficient for small lesions. For a larger or multiple lesions, withdraw the needle and inject additional areas as described above, either by threading technique or multiple puncture technique (Fig. 3.4).

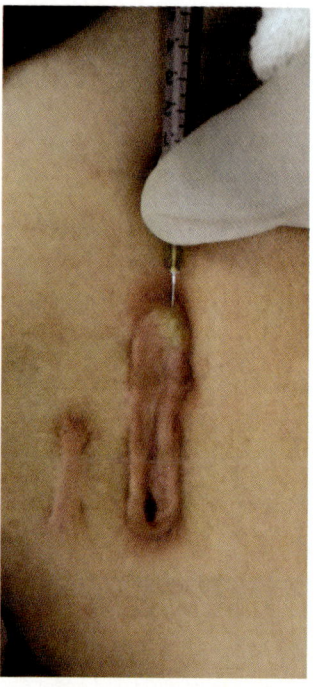

Fig. 3.3: ILS in keloid over chest: The blanching of the lesion is noticeable.

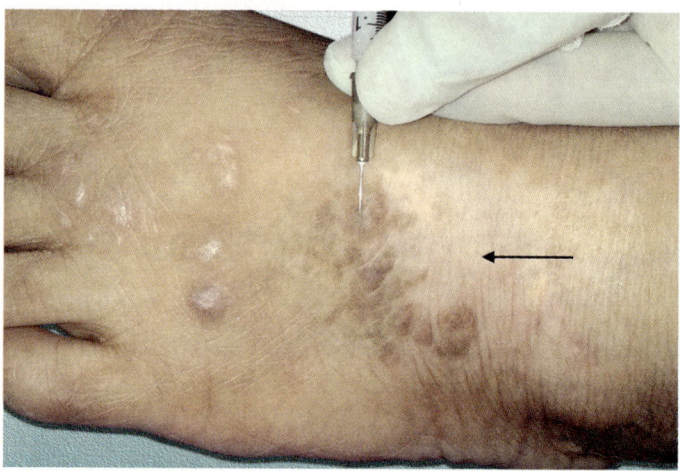

Fig. 3.4: Lichen simplex chronicus: On dorsum of foot treated with topical corticosteroids (TCS) for several months and lesion partly resolved with TCS induced hypopigmentation. The residual multiple smaller lesions are being treated with ILS by multiple puncture technique to avoid TCS adverse effects.

- When injecting into thick keloids or hypertrophic scars, there is a risk of 'splashing' the drug. One can use an insulin syringe, a luer lock syringe or steady the junction of needle and syringe with hand while injecting.
- Care must be taken to avoid injecting into the subcutaneous tissue.
    - Unlike intradermal injection where some resistance is felt, injection into the subcutaneous tissue is easier because of lack of resistance offered by loose fatty tissue.
    - To avoid adverse effects due to deeper injections, a simple device prepared from a needle cap for better control of the depth of intralesional injections is suggested.[5] The desired depth of ILS is measured by placing the needle close to the lesion and marked on the needle with a surgical marker pen. Then the needle cap is put and the cap is marked parallel to the needle mark. Then the cap is cut at that level using a surgical blade (#22). This cut piece of cap on the needle works as a guard and controls the depth of placement of intralesional injection (Fig. 3.5).

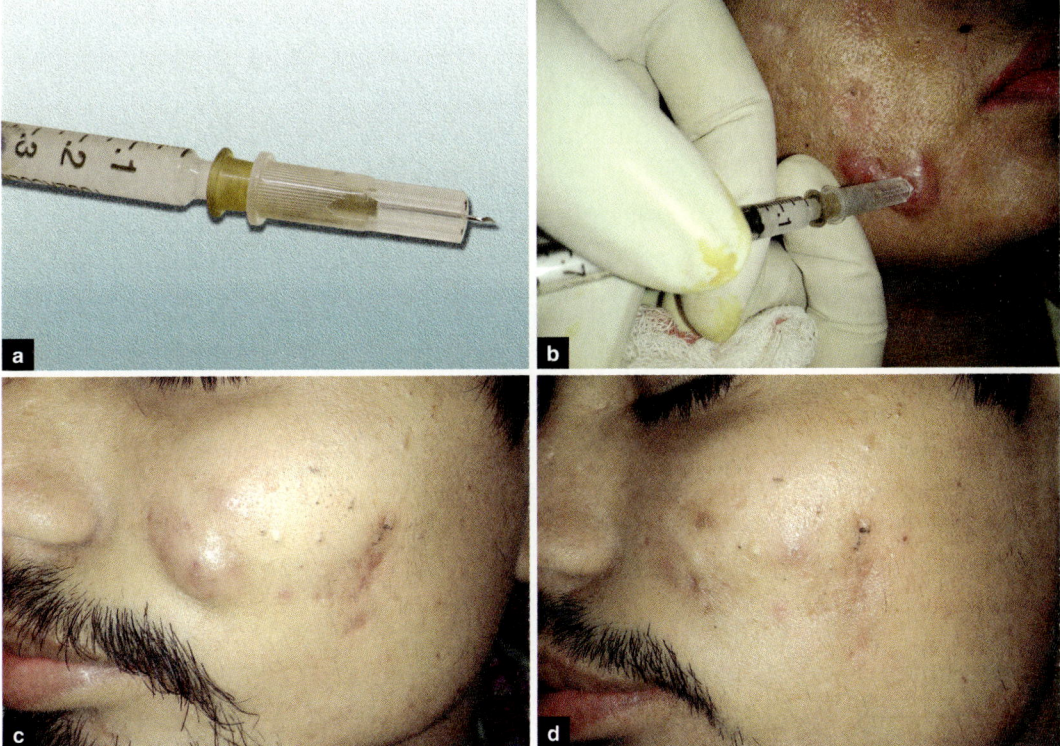

Fig. 3.5: (a) Needle with the cut cap at marked site based on the desired depth of the acne cyst; **(b)** ILS being given with the needle cap acting as the guard to control depth of injection; **(c)** Nodulocystic acne before ILS; **(d)** The lesion settled after 2 weeks of single session of ILS (2 mg/ml).

Dosage

- *Dose per session*: Of TAC is generally 0.1 ml/cm² of involved skin given at distance of 1 cm.[6] The recommended dose of TAC for various indications is shown in Table 3.2.
- *Maximum dose*: Not to exceed 40 mg/session.
- *Frequency*: Injections are generally given at an interval of 3 to 6 weeks.
- *Number of sessions*: The required number of injections depends on the disease, sites of lesions, age of patient and response to previous injections.

SPECIAL SITUATIONS

ILS Injections in Keloids

- *Indication*: International advisory panel on scar management has recommended the use of ILS for the treatment of keloids and hypertrophic scars.[7]
- *Mechanism of action*: ILS (steroids in general) induce keloid regression through several mechanisms:
  - Reduce fibroblast proliferation (and so new collagen formation) and increase fibroblast degeneration.
  - Reduce plasma protease inhibitors, allowing collagenase to degrade collagen.
  - Reduce alpha-1-antitrypsin and alpha-2-macroglobulin levels, which are natural inhibitors of collagenase in human skin.
  - Suppress inflammation by inhibiting leukocyte and monocyte migration and phagocytosis.
  - Vasoconstriction, reducing delivery of oxygen and nutrients to wound bed.

Table 3.2: Recommended strength of ILTAC in various indications	
Indication	Dosage/session (mg/ml)
Keloids • Thick • Moderate/hypertrophic scar	40 10
Discoid lupus erythematosus/sarcoidosis/localized psoriasis/ hypertrophic lichen planus/nail lichen planus	5–10
Granuloma annulare	3–10
Alopecia areata • Scalp • Face/eyebrows	2.5–10 5–10 2.5
Nodulocystic acne • Face • Extra facial	1–2 2–5
Hidradenitis suppurativa	2–5
Trachyonychia/twenty-nail dystrophy, nail lichen planus or nail psoriasis	2.5 to 10

- *Response*: Clinically, the response to ILS alone is variable with 50–100% regression and a recurrence rate of 33% and 50% at 1 and 5 years, respectively. Five-year recurrence rates for surgical excision followed by TAC administration were reported to be between 8% and 50%.
- *Factors determining response*:
  - *Trigger*: Better response in lesions caused by a trauma or a surgical scar rather than in those resulting from varicella or vaccination.
  - *Site*: Earlobe keloids had a worse response than those on other locations.
  - *Age of keloid*: Had no effect on response to treatment.
- There is considerable difference among practitioners in the dose, frequency and duration of treatment (Table 3.3) as also in combinations in which ILS are used with other treatments (Table 3.4).

ILS Injection in Nail Apparatus[8]

Intramatricial Nail Injections

- *Indications*: Nail lichen planus, nail matrix psoriasis (manifesting as pitting or nail dystrophy), trachyonychia/20 nail dystrophy.
- *Strength of TAC used*: 2.5–10 mg/ml.
- *Technique*:
  - Patient is made to lie prone with hand/foot to be injected extended towards the operator.

Table 3.3: Response of keloids to intralesional steroids		
Study	*Treatment given*	*Result*
Rahban and Garner, 2003	2–3 injections of 10 mg/mL TAC 4–8 weeks apart	
Darzi et al, 1992	Dose of TAC 10 mg/mL based surface area of keloid, given in 4 injections: • 1–2 cm²: Total dose of 20–40 mg • 2–6 cm²: 60–80 mg • 6–12 cm²: 80–120 mg	At 10-year follow-up: • 71% full flattening • 29% partial flattening • 71% symptom relief
Robbles et al, 2007	Trunk/extremities: 40 mg/mL and then titrated accordingly at subsequent visits	
Acosta et al, 2016	TAC, 40 mg/mL injected monthly till lesion was not palpable. Volume change measured using ultrasound	Assessment 82.7% reduction in size, with median number of injections needed/keloid being 2 mg (range 1–5), median dose/session being 16 mg (range 4–40 mg) and median dose to complete treatment being 32 mg (range 4–80 mg).

Table 3.4: Response of keloids to intralesional steroids and other treatments

Study, year	Methodology	Result
	TAC and verapamil[c]	
Ahuja and Chatterjee, 2014	• TAC (40 mg/mL) *vs* verapamil (2.5 mg/mL) IL given every 3 wk until complete flattening of keloid (upto 8 sessions). • Scar pliability, vascularity, height and pigmentation assessed by Vancouver Scar Scale (VSS) score.	• Response faster and better with TAC • More complications (skin atrophy and telangiectasia) in TAC group *vs* verapamil group (only injection-related pain)
Danielsen *et al* 2016	In paired split-scar design, 14 patients with surgically excised keloids were randomly allocated to receive postoperatively and every 4 wk thereafter for 3 m: • Triamcinolone 1–2 mg/cm (max total dose 10 mg) in ½ of suture line • Verapamil 0.5 mg/cm (maximum total dose 2.5 mg) in other ½ of suture line	At 12-month follow-up, TAC was more effective in preventing keloid recurrence after surgical excision
Kant *et al*, 2018	• In a retrospective study of 58 patients treated with a 1:1 mixture of TAC 40 mg/mL and verapamil[1] 2.5 mg/mL given at wk 0, 1 and 5 • Improvement in scar surface area and pliability, assessment scale (POSAS) scores done at 1–3, 3–4, 4–6, 6–12 and >12 ms)	Combined therapy is effective and offers long-term stable results
	TAC and 5FU[d]	

Saha and Mukhopadhyay, 2012	Patients randomized into 2 groups receiving injections at wkly intervals up to 6 injections up to 2 mL:
	• 1st gp: IL 5-FU, 50 mg/mL
	• 2nd gp: TAC, 40 mg/mL
		• Reduction in keloid volume and itching and recurrence at 6 m comparable in 2 groups
		• Side effects significantly higher in 5-FU group *vs* TAC gp:
		  – Pain (95 *vs* 4%)
		  – Hyperpigmentation (90 *vs* 12.5%)
		  – Superficial ulceration (65 *vs* 0%)

(Contd.)

[c]**Verapamil:** Calcium antagonist used for treating hypertension and cardiac arrhythmias increases synthesis of procollagenase leading to an increase in collagen degradation.

TAC acts by decreasing proteinase inhibitors and verapamil by increasing procollagenase secretion, so both have synergistic effect.

[d]**5-FU:** Is a pyrimidine analog which blocks collagen synthesis *in vitro* by reducing fibroblast activity and also inhibits TGF-β-induced expression of type I collagen gene in human fibroblasts.

Table 3.4: Response of keloids to intralesional steroids and other treatments (Contd.)

Study, year	Methodology	Result
Sadeghinia and Sadeghinia, 2012	Patient randomised into 2 gp treated 4 wkly: • IL TAC (40 mg/mL) • 5-FU (50 mg/mL) administered by tattooing keloid with 27 G needle followed by occlusion	• Better response in 5-FU gp (decrease in height and surface of lesions, erythema, induration and pruritus) • At week 44, no side effects noted in both groups
Fitzpatrick, 1999	1 mg TAC + 45 mg of 5-FU/mL administered 5–10 times.	Better efficacy with reduction of injection-related pain
Khan et al, 2014	Compared wkly injections × 8 wks: • IL TAC alone vs • 4 mg of TAC (0.1 mL of 40 mg/ 1 mL) + 45 mg 5-FU (0.9 mL of 250 mg/5 mL)	Combination superior: • Faster and greater reduction in keloid • Fewer side effects (skin atrophy and telangiectasias)
TAC and bleomycin		
Payapvipapong et al, 2015	26 patients randomised to once every 4 wk × 3 injections of: • IL bleomycin injections (1 IU/mL) • IL TAC (10 mg/mL) injections Results assessed objectively (photography and ultrasonography), and subjectively (POSAS and patient satisfaction score)	• Response comparable in 2 groups • High rate of hyperpigmentation (71.4%) in darker skin suggesting TAC is recommended over bleomycin in darker skin
TAC and silicone gel sheet		
Tan et al 1999	Compared: • Silicone gel sheet used daily vs • IL TAC (40 mg/mL) 4 wkly	IL TAC significantly superior to silicone sheet in treatment of keloids
TAC and lasers		
Kassab and El Kharbotly, 2012	Ear lobule keloids treated with 980 nm diode laser (single mode, 4-sec duration, 5 W power, 20 J/cm² fluence, 5–9 passes). followed by IL TAC (1 mL of 40 mg/mL), 2–5 sitting	• 75% keloid reduced by at least 75% • Skin erythema seen immediately in all patients, and persistent hyperpigmentation in 4
Rossi A et al 2013	Comparison: • 300 µs 1064 nm Nd: YAG laser + IL TAC • IL TAC	Combination superior
Behera et al 2016	Comparison • ILTAC with carbon dioxide laser • ILTAC with cryotherapy	Both were found to be equally effective in treatment of keloids
TAC and Cryotherapy		
Yosipovitch et al, 2001	Comparison • ILS plus cryotherapy • ILS alone • Cryotherapy alone	Combined ILS + Cryotherapy better than ILS or cryotherapy alone in terms of reducing thickness ($p < 0.001$) Itch responded only to combined treatment or ILS alone.

(Contd.)

Table 3.4: Response of keloids to intralesional steroids and other treatments (Contd.)

Study, year	Methodology	Result
Sharma S et al, 2007	Compared • Cryospray • Cryospray + ILS monthly × 6	Combination treatment better than cryospray alone Less recurrence in the combination group at 18 months (3.3% vs 16.7%, p <0.01)
Weshahy AH et al, 2015	Keloids treated with single intralesional cryosurgery followed by 3 monthly ILS × 4 sessions, then 6 monthly × 4 sessions (n = 22)	Significant reduction in the volume, hardness, redness scores and symptoms
TAC and interferon alpha 2b		
Lee et al, 2008	Comparison • TAC plus interferon alpha 2b • TAC alone	Statistical significant decrease in depth and volume in combination group. The main side effects were fever, flu-like symptoms, mild pain and inflammation at the site of injection.
TAC and onion extract gel		
Koc et al, 2008	Comparison • TAC plus onion extract gel • TAC alone	Both treatment groups had statistically significant improvement at week 20. The combination group was better in terms of pain sensitiveness, itching and elevation.
TAC and Botulinum toxin A		
Shaarawy et al, 2015	Comparison • Intralesional TAC • Intralesional botulinum toxin A	Statistically significant reduction in volume of lesions from baseline was seen in both groups without statistically significant difference between the two.

- A 1 ml insulin syringe[e] with a built in[f] 30–31 G needle with 6–8 mm length is used for the injection.
- Point of entry of needle is 2 mm below and lateral to junction between the lateral and proximal nail folds (Fig. 3.6), the needle being kept almost parallel to skin surface till there is a feeling of give up to middle of proximal nail fold. Drug is slowly infused[g] to raise a semilunar blanch in the lunula, which is the endpoint of injection and no more than 0.1–0.2 ml of TAC can usually be administered in an average sized nail.

---

[e]**Insulin syringe:** Preferred to a tuberculin syringe as it has a longer needle for subcutaneous administration compared to tuberculin syringe which is intradermal administration.
[f]**Built in:** Needle should be built-in syringe to enable injection under pressure and avoid any needle dislodgement and backsplash.
[g]**Infused:** After trying to aspirate, to ensure that needle is not in a vessel.

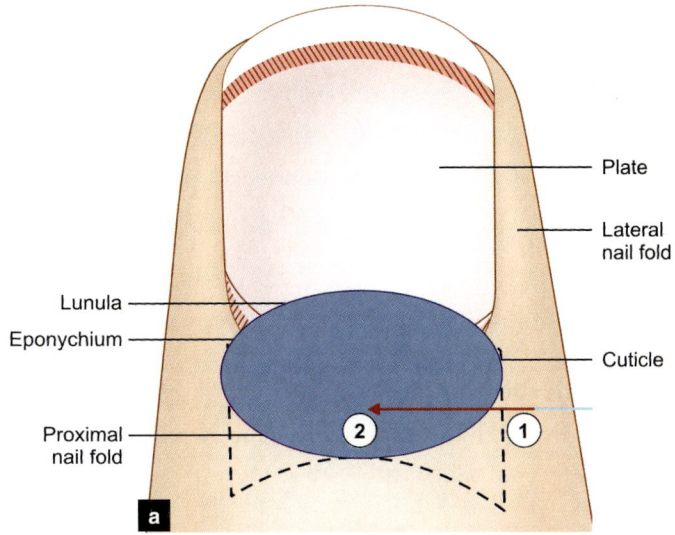

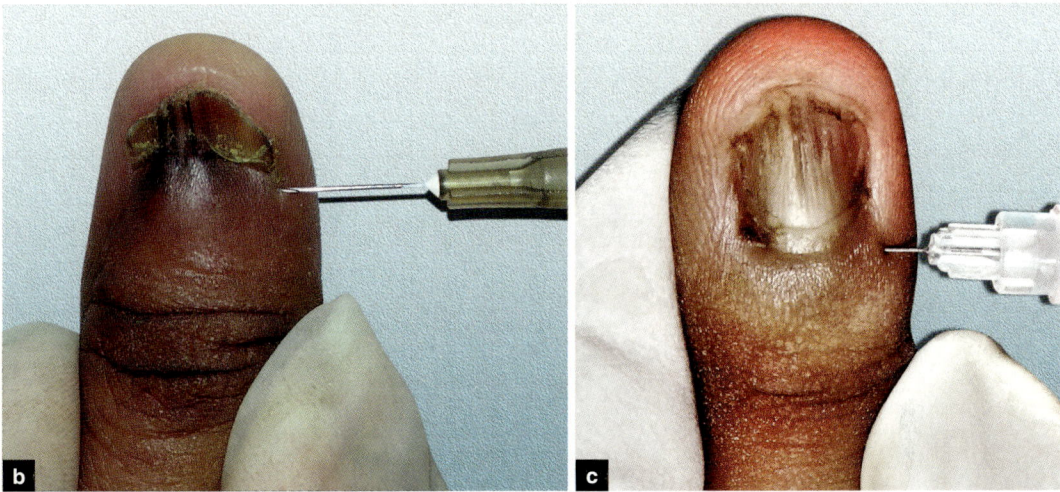

Fig. 3.6: Intramatricial injection. (a) Schematic diagram of intramatricial injections. Needle, with bevelled tip up, is inserted into skin at a point (marked 1) which is 2 mm below and lateral to junction between proximal and lateral nail folds, keeping the needle almost parallel to skin surface (as shown by direction of arrow) till there is a feeling of give at middle of proximal nail fold (head of arrow, marked 2). TA is slowly infused (usually 0.1–0.2 ml) to raise a semilunar blanch (blue area) in the lunula and proximal nail fold, this being the endpoint of injection. **(b) Intramatricial injection in nail lichen planus.** Needle, with bevelled tip up, being inserted into skin at a point (marked 1) which is 2 mm below and lateral to junction between proximal and lateral nail folds, keeping the needle almost parallel to skin surface. **(c)** TA is slowly infused (usually 0.1–0.2 ml) to raise a semilunar blanch in lunula and proximal nail fold (Fig. 3.6c, *Courtesy*: Prof Chander Grover).

- After with drawing the needle, sustained pressure is maintained at the injection site for 1–2 minutes to ensure adequate hemostasis to prevent subungual hematoma formation.
- Injections are repeated at 4 weekly intervals initially, till a desired improvement is seen and 6–8 weeks thereafter to maintain response and prevent relapses.

- *Side effects and complications*: Complications are largely preventable and fortunately reversible:
  - Proximal nail fold hypopigmentation and atrophy is not uncommon.
  - Matrix injections may occasionally cause disturbed nail growth.
  - Rarely hypersensitivity reactions and vasovagal attack, hence injections should be administered in a proper OT setup, with adequate positioning of the patient as well as readiness to handle dermatosurgical emergencies.
  - Nicolau syndrome following intramatricial triamcinolone has been reported as a rare complication.

Nail Bed Injection of Steroids

- *Indications*: For disorders like nail bed psoriasis (prominent distal onycholysis and subungual hyperkeratosis), nail bed injection of TAC is effective.
- *Technique*:
  - Point of entry of needle is slightly more medial than entry point in intramatricial injection, the needle being kept almost parallel to skin surface (Fig. 3.7a). The needle is directed towards the digital tip (as shown by direction of arrow) and advanced towards the centre of the nail bed carefully.
  - TAC is slowly infused to raise a more distal blanch in the nail bed area (Fig. 3.7b), which is the endpoint of injection and no more than 0.1–0.2 ml of TAC can usually be administered.

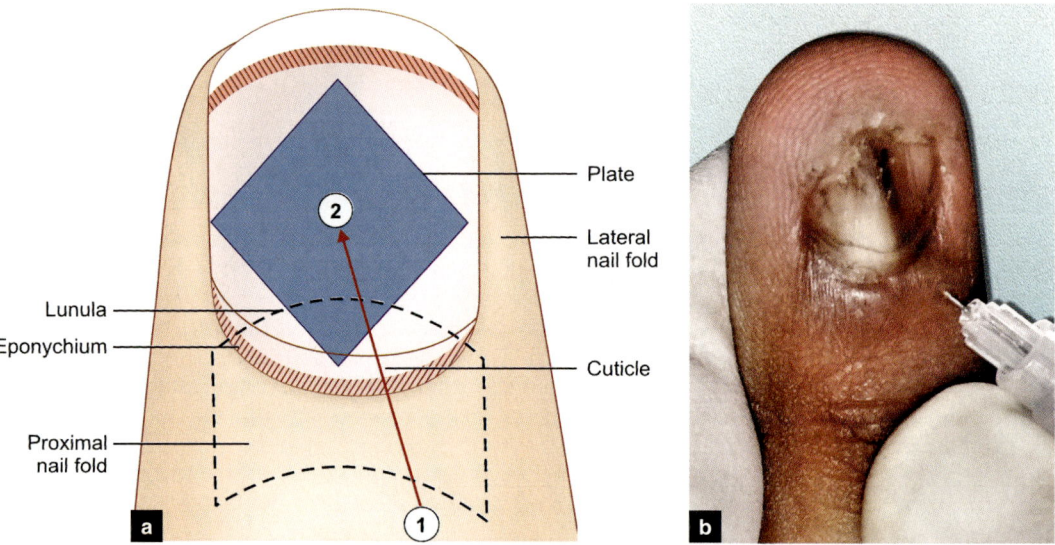

Fig. 3.7: Schematic diagram of intrabed injections. (a) Needle, with bevelled tip up, is inserted into skin at a point (marked 1) which is slightly medial to entry in intramatricial injection. Keeping the needle almost parallel to skin surface (as shown by direction of arrow), the needle is directed towards the digital tip and advanced towards the centre of the nail bed (head of arrow, marked 2). TA is slowly infused (usually 0.1–0.2 ml) to raise a blanch in centre of nail bed (blue area). **(b)** Blanch in centre of nail bed (Fig. 3.7b, *Courtesy*: Prof Chander Grover).

- Injections are repeated at 4 weekly intervals initially, till desired improvement is seen and 6–8 weeks thereafter to maintain response and prevent relapses.
- *Side effects*:
  - Nail bed injections are more painful than nail matrix injections as it is a closed compartment hence more sensitive to volume infiltration.
  - Hematoma formation.

Hyponychial Injections

- This approach is even more painful and is not routinely recommended.

Jaipur Block

- Consists of local subcutaneous infiltration of 2% xylocaine (30 ml), 0.5% bupivacaine (20 ml) and 4 mg/ml dexamethasone (1 ml) solution
- Used in patients of refractory post-herpetic neuralgia, resulted in pain relief in most cases.[9]

SIDE EFFECTS[10]

Side effects can be early and delayed effects.

Early Side Effects

- *Pain*: ILS is associated with significant injection pain, often requiring the administration of local anaesthetic. The pain is greater when ILS is being given into a closed compartment (nail bed, nail matrix) and into dense fibrotic tissue (keloids). The injection itself may be physically challenging due to the density of the lesion and the physician must be able to comfortably generate enough injection pressure to overcome this resistance. Vo *et al*[11] investigated the effects of different syringe and needle combinations and found that a 1 mL polycarbonate syringe with a 25 G, 16 mm needle was the most ergonomic combination for injecting into keloids requiring the lowest injection force.
- *Bleeding and bruising*: Tend to be self limiting.
- *Infections*
- *Contact allergic dermatitis*: May be due to the drug itself or due to preservative, benzyl alcohol.
- *Impaired wound healing*
- *Skin necrosis and ulcerations*
- *Inadvertent intravascular injection*: The avoidance of intravascular injection is especially important when injecting lesions around the forehead where accidental intra-arterial injection and retrograde flow of a bolus of particles may result in retinal artery occlusion and blindness. In this location, counter pressure should be applied around the injection site at the time of injection to avoid this disastrous complication.[12]

Delayed Adverse Effects

- *Cutaneous and subcutaneous atrophy:*
  - Appear as depression of skin at sites of injection and is often associated with hypopigmentation and telangiectasia. Atrophy usually becomes clinically visible a few weeks after treatment and is usually permanent (Fig. 3.8).
  - Face, genitalia, lips, buccal mucosa, etc. are particularly prone to development of atrophy and hence ILS should be avoided over these sites or only minute quantities and very dilute concentrations of ILS should be used if need be.
  - Can be prevented by optimizing depth of injection of steroid (too superficial results in epidermal atrophy and hypopigmentation and too deep leads to subcutaneous atrophy; Fig 3.8a) and avoiding too frequent injections or injecting high concentrations or large volumes of injections per site.
- *Hypo- or hyperpigmentation:* Can occur at the site of injection (Fig. 3.8b) or spread from the site of injection along lymphatics resulting in linear hypopigmented/depigmented and atrophic streaks. These may resolve or persist for long time.

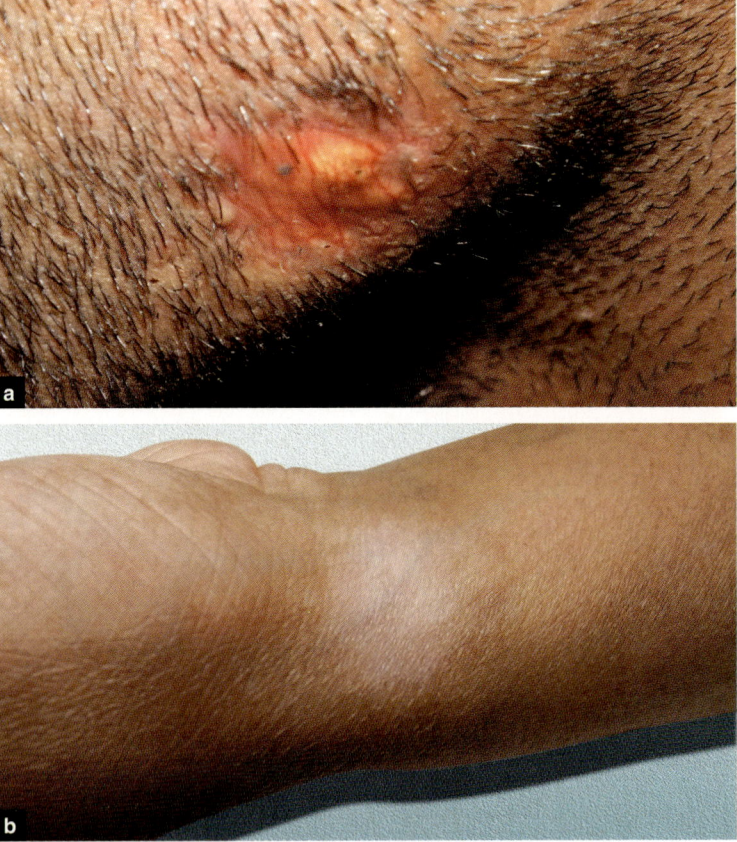

Fig. 3.8: **Side effects to IL TAC: (a)** Atrophy of dermis and telangiectasia with subcutaneous tissue becoming visible. **(b)** Hypopigmentation at site of IL TAC given to treat ganglion cyst.

- *Telangiectasia*:
  - Usually associated with atrophy (Fig. 3.8a).
  - Can be treated if necessary by laser or intense pulsed light (IPL).
- *Striae*
- *Localised hypertrichosis*: Increased hair growth at the site of injection, which usually resolves with time.
- *Localised or distant steroid acne*
- *Systemic effects*: Repeated use of ILS injections in adults can result in systemic effects but in children these have been reported even after a single dose of ILS with 40 mg of triamcinolone given in very large lesions. These systemic effects include:
  - *Suppression of HPA axis*
  - *Cushing syndrome*: Cushing's syndrome associated with ILS is a rare but possible complication, usually reported in children, although a few cases have been described in adults as well.

REFERENCES

1. Savant S, editor. Intralesional therapy. In: Textbook of Dermatosurgery and Cosmetology. 2nd ed. Mumbai, India: ASCAD; 2005. pp 100–106.
2. Callen JP. Intralesional corticosteroids. J Am Acad Dermatol 1981;4:149–51.
3. Shapiro J. Alopecia Areata: Update on therapy. Dermatol Clin 1993;11:35–46.
4. Shapiro J, Price VH. Hair regrowth: Therapeutic agents. Dermatol Clin. 1998;16:341–56.
5. Gupta S, Jangra RS, Gupta S, Mahendra A, Gupta S. Creating a guard with a needle cover to control the depth of intralesional injections. J Am Acad Dermatol 2016;75:e67–8.
6. Alkhalifah A, Alsantali A, Wang E, McElwee KJ, Shapiro J. Alopecia Areata update: Part II: Treatment. J Am Acad Dermatol. 2010;62:191–202.
7. Mustoe TA, Cooter RD, Gold MH, et al. International Advisory Panel on Scar Management. International clinical recommendations on scar management. Plast Reconstr Surg 2002;110:560–571.
8. Grover C, Bansal S. A compendium of intralesional therapies in nail disorders. Indian Dermatol Online J 2018;9:373–82.
9. Bhargava R, Bhargava S, Haldia KN, Bhargava P. Jaipur block in post herpetic neuralgia. Int J Dermatol. 1998;37:465–8.
10. Verbov J. The place of intralesional steroid therapy in dermatology. Br J Dermatol 1976;94:51–8.
11. Vo A, Doumit M, Rockwell G. The Biomechanics and Optimization of the Needle-Syringe System for Injecting Triamcinolone Acetonide into Keloids. J Med Eng. 2016;2016:5162394.
12. S. Walayat Hussain, Richard J. Motley, Timothy S. Wang. Principles of skin surgery. In: Burns T, Breathnach S, Cox N, Griffiths C, (editors). Rook's Textbook of Dermatology, 9th ed. Singapore: Wiley Blackwell; 2016. p. 20.44.

Systemic Corticosteroids in Dermatology

Manik Aggarwal, Savera Gupta, Neetu Bhari

SUMMARY

- Corticosteroids are one of the most effective and frequently used therapeutic agents in dermatology. However, their strong therapeutic profile is offset by serious and potentially life-threatening side effects.
- Their prudent use and monitoring will minimize, although not obviate, adverse effects.
- Corticosteroids are broadly classified into glucocorticoids and mineralocorticoids based on their predominant mechanism of action. Glucocorticoids are further classified based on duration of action and relative anti-inflammatory properties.
- Administered orally, corticosteroids are almost completely and quickly absorbed with maximum absorption occurring in jejunum.
- Approximately 90% of cortisol is bound to corticosteroid binding globulin and only 5–10% is free which is responsible for tissue action.
- They are metabolized predominantly in the liver and the metabolites are then conjugated with sulphate or glucuronic acid to make them water soluble, before being excreted in the urine.
- Oral absorption of corticosteroids is almost complete and it is the most commonly used mode of administration.
- Through investigation before starting corticosteroid therapy to identify absolute and relative contraindications decreases the risks of adverse effects.
- The pretreatment screening depends on the expected duration of therapy with corticosteroids.
- Prior to initiating corticosteroid therapy, the patient should receive appropriate education regarding the potential adverse effects. A steroid treatment card should be provided and the information on it should be kept uptodate.
- Traditionally, prednisolone (the biologically active metabolite of prednisone) is the most commonly used oral corticosteroid in dermatological practice.

- The daily basal production of corticosteroid by the body is prednisone equivalent: 5–7.5 mg daily (physiological dose).
- The pharmacological dose of prednisolone depends on the clinical diagnosis, its severity and the presence or otherwise of cautionary factors. In most situations, it is reasonable to consider commencing prednisolone at a starting dose of up to 1 mg/kg body weight daily.
- A single daily dose is less likely to cause adverse effects than a divided dose, and a morning dose less likely to result in HPA axis suppression than when given at other times of day.
- Based on dose, systemic steroid therapy is classified as high doses (>60 mg daily of prednisone equivalent), intermediate doses (40–60 mg daily of prednisone equivalent), low doses (<40 mg daily of prednisone equivalent).
- Based on duration, systemic steroid therapy is classified as brief duration of therapy (lasting <4 weeks), intermediate duration of therapy (for 4 to 12 weeks) and chronic therapy (for >12 weeks of therapy).
- As a general rule, once adequate disease control is achieved, consideration should be given to tapering long-term corticosteroid to the minimal effective dose in order to minimize the risk of side effects. The rate of dose reduction is determined by disease activity and duration of therapy.
- If supraphysiological doses of corticosteroids are required in the long term, adjusting to an alternating day regimen may ultimately allow recovery of the HPA axis and cause less metabolic disruption than daily administration.
- While on corticosteroid therapy, regular clinical and laboratory monitoring is required to identify adverse effects at an early stage and intervene accordingly. This includes specific history, blood pressure and weight (and height in children) recording, serum electrolytes, fasting glucose and lipids profile, ophthalmic examination and bone mineral density scan.
- There are a large number of potential interactions between systemic corticosteroid and other drugs, although only a small number are potentially serious.
- Various indications for systemic corticosteroid include bullous dermatoses, autoimmune connective tissue disorders, vasculitis, neutrophilic dermatoses, dermatitis, papulosquamous dermatoses and leprosy reactions.
- The first-line therapy for all forms of pemphigus is systemic corticosteroids. Mortality in this group of disorders has come down drastically since the introduction of corticosteroids. There is clinical evidence that early intervention with definitive treatment leads to a better long-term outcome. Prednisone (equivalents) of 1–1.5 mg/kg/day (lean body weight) as the starting dose is the most commonly used regimen. Patients must be monitored for corticosteroid-induced osteopenia and those without a history of renal calculi may be given prophylactic supplemental calcium 1500 mg daily and vitamin D 400 to 800 IU daily.

- In bullous pemphigoid, patients with generalized disease in which topical therapy is not feasible can be treated with systemic steroids. Prednisone at an initial dose of 0.5 to 0.75 mg/kg/day (depending on disease severity and overall health of the patient) is started and continued till active inflammation, blistering and pruritus have stopped which mostly happens in about 6–8 weeks. The steroids are then tapered gradually and are usually stopped completely in 3–6 months.
- Systemic corticosteroids are not commonly used in the milder forms of lupus, however, severe cutaneous disease or internal organ involvement necessitate their use. They may also be used to bridge the gap between the initiation and the achievement of peak levels of antimalarials which form the mainstay of management of cutaneous lupus.
- Corticosteroids are the mainstay therapy for acute as well as long-term management of patients with dermatomyositis. High dose therapy (1 mg/kg) for the first 4–6 weeks to achieve control the disease and then gradual tapering till the lowest effective dose is reached by the next 6–9 months is the preferred therapy.
- Systemic corticosteroids have been found extremely effective in neutrophilic dermatoses (Sweet's syndrome, pyoderma gangrenosum) with response being so dramatic that it is included in the diagnostic criteria for these conditions.
- Idiopathic cutaneous small vessel vasculitis is often self-limited and requires only supportive care. However, patients developing cutaneous necrosis, ulceration or hemorrhagic blisters require systemic corticosteroids.
- In urticarial vasculitis, systemic corticosteroids are indicated in moderately severe disease and in combination with other immunomodulatory drugs for severe disabling disease.
- Systemic corticosteroids are the mainstay therapy for leprosy reactions (both type 1 and type 2). In type 1 reaction, corticosteroids are vital in preventing permanent nerve damage. The duration of steroid therapy is an important determinant of success of therapy and should be long enough to cover the period during which the antigen load is high enough to mount an immune response.

INTRODUCTION

- Corticosteroids are a family of steroid hormones that have vital immuno-modulatory and metabolic functions and are one of the most effective groups of therapeutic agents due their dramatic and consistent efficacy in various inflammatory and autoimmune conditions.[1–3]
- They are an indispensable part of dermatologists' therapeutic armamentarium; however, their prolonged use can lead to numerous side effects. Therefore, dermatologists should follow certain principles and exercise caution while penning down a prescription of steroids.
- Their prudent use and monitoring will minimize, although not obviate, adverse effects.

CLASSIFICATION

- Corticosteroids are broadly classified (based on their predominant action) into:
  - *Glucocorticoids*: Which have varying degrees of anti-inflammatory action and
  - *Mineralocorticoids*: Which do not have clinically significant anti-inflammatory action.
- In practice, the term glucocorticoid is often used synonymously with corticosteroid, although, strictly, the latter includes both GCs and mineralocorticoids, both produced within the adrenal cortex.
- Glucocorticoids are further classified based on duration of action and relative anti-inflammatory properties (Table 4.1).

Table 4.1: Classification of systemic corticosteroids based on the duration of action			
	Equivalent doses (mg)	*Relative anti-inflammatory activity*	*Duration of action (hours)*
Short acting			
Hydrocortisone (cortisol)	20	1	8 to 12
Cortisone acetate	25	0.8	8 to 12
Intermediate acting			
Prednisone	5	4	12 to 36
Prednisolone	5	4	12 to 36
Methylprednisolone	4	5	12 to 36
Triamcinolone	4	5	12 to 36
Long acting			
Dexamethasone	0.75	30	36 to 72
Betamethasone	0.6	30	36 to 72

BASIC PHARMACOLOGY OF CORTICOSTEROIDS

- Cortisol is synthesized from cholesterol in a multiple-enzymes catalyzed pathway. Cortisol, the naturally occurring active form, is formed by hydroxylation in the liver by 11β-hydroxysteroid dehydrogenase at the 11-ketone of cortisone. This naturally occurring corticosteroid has modest glucocorticoid activity.
- Addition of Δ1–2 bond of the A ring forms prednisone and 11-hydroxylation forms the active molecule prednisolone. The unsaturation leads to increased glucocorticoid activity and decreases degeneration.
- Methylation of prednisolone at 6th carbon results in formation of methylprednisolone which has increased glucocorticoid activity with little mineralocorticoid activity.[5]
- Fluorination of cortisol at the 9-α position yields 9-α fluorohydrocortisone (fludrocortisone) which has increased mineralocorticoid and less, glucocorticoid

activity and is the building block for topical steroids. Addition of ester links to side chains such as acetonide, valerate and propionate decreases the mineralocorticoid activity of topical preparations.

- Fluorination and desaturation at Δ1–2 bond of the A ring of cortisol with hydroxylation and methylation forms triamcinolone, dexamethasone and betamethasone, respectively. These are biologically active compounds with high glucocorticoid and low mineralocorticoid activity with long duration of actions.[6]
- Cortisol secretion from the adrenal glands is under the control of pulsatile adreno-corticotrophic hormone (ACTH) secretion which follows a circadian rhythm. It peaks early in the morning hours after waking up and also increases after meals. Normal stress free secretion is 10–20 mg/day.

PHARMACOKINETICS

Absorption

- Administered orally, corticosteroids are almost completely and quickly absorbed with maximum absorption occurring in jejunum.
- Peak plasma levels are achieved 30–100 minutes after drug intake.
- Food delays but does not decrease its absorption.

Circulation and Distribution

- In plasma, 90% of cortisol is bound to corticosteroid binding globulin (CBG)[a] and this is metabolically inactive, acting as a reservoir. CBG synthesis increases in hyperestrogenic states (pregnancy, exogenous estrogen administration and hyperthyroidism) and decreases in protein deficiency states and hypothyroidism.
- Approximately 5% of cortisol is loosely bound to corticosteroid-binding albumin and can exert its effect on target tissues.

Metabolism

- Liver plays the major role in cortisol metabolism by conjugating it with glucuronic acid or sulfate at C3 and C21 hydroxyls, respectively. This makes the metabolites water soluble before being excreted in the urine.
- Tissues with mineralocorticoid receptor and 11-hydroxysteroid dehydrogenase convert about 20% cortisol into corticosterone.
- $T_{1/2}$ of cortisol is 60–90 minutes and is increased during times of stress, hypothyroidism or liver disease. However, it is a poor measure of duration of action which correlates more with the duration of ACTH suppression after giving a compound.[7,8]

---

[a]**CBG:** An globulin synthesized by the liver. CBG is saturated at plasma cortisol levels of 20–30 µg/dl and after that there is an exponential increase in free cortisol levels leading to toxicity.

Excretion

- Approximately, 1% of cortisol is excreted unchanged in the urine.
- One-third is excreted as dihydroxy ketone metabolites and measured as 17-hydroxysteroids.
- Rest is excreted as conjugated metabolites synthesized in liver.

Modification in Presence of Systemic Diseases and Altered Physiologic States

- End-stage renal disease: Does not require a dose adjustment.[9]
- Inflammatory bowel disease: Does not affect the pharmacokinetic profile of systemic corticosteroids.[10]
- Nephrotic syndrome: Non-renal clearance is higher whereas renal clearance is lower in these patients.[11]
- Obesity: Obesity can affect the uptake, storage, and metabolism of glucocorticoids, although results are somewhat contradictory. Ideal body weight rather than total body weight should be used for dosing of glucocorticoids in the obese.[12]
- Severe liver disease: Activation of prednisone to 6β-hydroxyl compounds is impaired which potentially affect the efficacy of glucocorticoid therapy.[13] Prednisone is the prodrug, which is converted by the liver into active prednisolone and the latter is therefore the glucocorticoid of choice in patients with liver disease.

MECHANISM OF ACTION OF SYSTEMIC CORTICOSTEROIDS

Receptors

Glucocorticoids after diffusion across cell membrane bind to intracytoplasmic receptors[b] of which there are 2 types:

- *Glucocorticoid receptor (GR)*: After binding to cortisol, the GR is released from HSP90 and after homodimerization translocates to the nucleus, where it causes direct activation of transcription of multiple genes (transactivation). The glucocorticoid receptor also binds to multiple proinflammatory molecules such as nuclear factor-B (NF-B) and represses the transcription of genes regulated by these molecules (transrepression).[14]
- *Mineralocorticoid receptor (MR)*: This is also known as aldosterone receptor. Activation of MR upon the binding of its ligand results in its translocation to the cell nucleus, homodimerization and binding to hormone response elements present in the promoter of some genes. This results in transcription regulation of inflammatory cascade.[15–20]

Corticosteroids act through classical genomic pathway and non-genomic pathway.[20,21]

---

[b]**Cytoplasmic receptors:** Which are primarily in oligomeric complexes with heat shock protein-90 (HSP 90) and other molecules.

PRINCIPLES OF SYSTEMIC CORTICOSTEROID THERAPY

- Always be sure of the indication for systemic corticosteroid use.
- Investigate thoroughly before starting corticosteroid therapy to identify absolute and relative contraindications (Table 4.2).

Table 4.2: Contraindications of systemic corticosteroid	
Absolute contraindications	*Relative contraindications*
Active systemic fungal infection	Cardiovascular: Hypertension, Congestive heart failure
Herpes simplex keratitis	Central nervous system: Prior psychosis, severe depression
Hypersensitivity to corticosteroid molecule	Gastrointestinal: Active peptic ulcer disease, recent surgery (anastomosis)
	Infections: Active tuberculosis
	Metabolic: Diabetes mellitus
	Musculoskeletal: Osteoporosis
	Ocular: Cataract, Glaucoma
	Pregnancy (Category C)

Pre-treatment Screening[23]

The pre-treatment screening depends on the expected duration of therapy with corticosteroids.

- Short course therapy: If a short course (up to 3 weeks) of corticosteroids therapy is anticipated, history of the following coexisting conditions must be taken:
  - Diabetes
  - Psychosis
  - Glaucoma
  - History and examination to rule out any infective focus
  - Peptic ulcer disease
  - Active diverticulitis
  - Recent surgery
  - Drug history for potential drug interactions
- Extended therapy (more than 3 weeks): In addition, following evaluations are recommended:
  - Blood pressure, weight, height and body mass index
  - Anthropometry in case of children
  - Baseline ophthalmic examination for cataracts and ocular hypertension
  - Chest X-ray to screen for active or latent tuberculosis and other infections
  - Fasting glucose, fasting lipid profile and serum electrolytes

- – Assessment of fracture risk
- – Some practitioners commonly perform bone mineral density scan when initiating long term systemic steroid therapy.
- Prior to initiating corticosteroid therapy, the patient and family members should receive appropriate education, in particular about the potential adverse effects and the monitoring details. A steroid treatment card should be provided and the information on it should be kept uptodate.

Administration

Oral Administration

- Oral absorption of corticosteroids is almost complete and thus is the most commonly used mode of administration.
- Oral corticosteroids are ideally given in the early morning to conform to the natural circadian rhythm of endogenous glucocorticoid production.
- Traditionally, prednisolone (the biologically active metabolite of prednisone) is the most commonly used oral corticosteroid in dermatological practice, although betamethasone, deflazacort, dexamethasone and methylprednisolone can be given orally.

Intramuscular Administration

- Intramuscular administration of corticosteroid has the advantage of guaranteeing that a possibly unreliable patient receives treatment and also avoids the gastrointestinal side effects.
- The disadvantages are:
  - – Absorption is highly variable from patient to patient
  - – A constant plasma levels are achieved without the natural diurnal variation
  - – Precise tapering is not possible
- Complications of intramuscular corticosteroids include:
  - – Subcutaneous fat atrophy
  - – Abscess formation at the injection site
  - – Menstrual irregularities in women: Intramuscular route is more likely to induce menstrual irregularities as compared to oral route. This is possibly because the intramuscular route results in constant levels of circulating corticosteroid without the diurnal variation, thereby suppressing gonadotropin release.
- Triamcinolone acetonide is the favored corticosteroid for intramuscular use.
- A typical regimen for intramuscular triamcinolone is 80 mg two or three times a year.

Intravenous Administration

- It is generally only used in situations where it is desirable to bring very serious steroid-responsive conditions under rapid control.
- It is usually given in 'pulses' on an inpatient basis.

Dosing and Tapering

Physiological Dosing

- Basal production of cortisol: 20–30 mg daily
- Prednisone equivalent: 5–7.5 mg daily.

Pharmacological (Supra-physiological) Dosing

- Depending on the clinical diagnosis, its severity and the presence or otherwise of cautionary factors, it is reasonable to consider commencing prednisolone at a starting dose of up to 1 mg/kg body weight daily, ideally given as a single dose in the morning.
- A single daily dose is less likely to cause adverse effects than a divided dose, and a morning dose less likely to result in HPA axis suppression than when given at other times of day.

Tapering

- As a general rule, once adequate disease control is achieved, consideration should be given to tapering long-term corticosteroid to the minimal effective dose in order to minimize the risk of side effects, although, despite their use over many decades, the optimal regimen has yet to be determined.
- The rate of dose reduction is determined by disease activity and duration of therapy.
  Brief duration of therapy: Minimal to no risk of HPA axis suppression, so tapering is not required unless warranted by disease process.
  Intermediate duration and chronic therapy:
  - Supra-physiological doses for >4 weeks requires tapering to circumvent HPA axis suppression, as abrupt cessation or too rapid a withdrawal may precipitate acute adrenal crisis.
  - Recommended to decrease the dose by 20–30% every 1–2 weeks[c] and achieve alternate day doses to maintain disease control. However, some dermatoses such as pemphigus require even slower tapering at intervals of 3–4 weeks to prevent a flare up.
- When withdrawing corticosteroids, it is reasonable to attempt to reduce the dose rapidly to a physiological level (7.5 mg prednisolone daily or equivalent), followed thereafter by a more gradual reduction.

Alternate Day Dosing

- If supra-physiological doses of corticosteroids are required in the long term, adjusting to an alternating day regimen may ultimately allow recovery of the HPA axis and cause less metabolic disruption than daily administration.

---

[c]**Tapering for long term, high dose therapy:** 20 mg decrements till daily dose of 60 mg, 10 mg decrements till daily dose of 20–30 mg, 5 mg decrements till daily dose of 10 mg and 2.5 mg decrements till cessation of therapy.

- It is based on principle that the anti-inflammatory effects of steroids last longer than HPA axis suppression. So alternate day regimes allow HPA axis to recover while still maintaining reasonable anti-inflammatory activity. This strategy is particularly useful for patients who require maintenance of achieved disease control.
- Three strategies are available to switch from daily to alternate day steroid therapy:
  - Double dose on 'on' day and drop dose on 'off' day
  - Increase dose on 'on' day and decrease equally on 'off' day
  - Decrease doses on 'off' day while maintaining dose on 'on' day
- If the patient has slight flare up on 'off' day, then:
  - A physiological dose of prednisone or other non-steroidal agent may be prescribed on 'off' day
  - Or 'on' day dose maybe increased by ~25%
- Once an 'on' day dose of 10–15 mg is reached, further continuation provides little advantage. The patient can then be shifted to 5 mg daily and tapered off slowly or maintained if required.

Monitoring

- Regular clinical and laboratory monitoring is required to identify adverse effects at an early stage and intervene accordingly.
- A reasonable follow-up frequency for patients on oral corticosteroid treatment is at first month and then every 2–3 months. At each visit, the following should be done:
  - History and examination to rule out any infective focus and look for evidence of adverse effects
  - Blood pressure, weight, and height measurement in adults
  - Anthropometry in case of children
  - Fasting glucose, lipid profile and electrolytes
  - Bone mineral density scan (DEXA scan) one-year post initiation and then every 2–3 years if stable
  - Ophthalmological examination every 6–12 months for cataracts and glaucoma. More frequent evaluation is necessary for patients at higher risk.
  - A neutrophilia frequently occurs with corticosteroid therapy. This should not be assumed to be necessarily the result of infection as it is often innocent, resulting from a shift of neutrophils from the marginated to the circulating pool, with a minor contribution from an increased release from bone marrow.

DRUG INTERACTIONS

- Absorption of oral glucocorticoids is decreased when taken with antacids such containing aluminum or magnesium.[24,25]

- CYP 3A4 family of enzymes is involved in metabolism of steroids in the liver. Inducers of this enzyme like carbamazepine, phenobarbital, phenytoin and rifampicin decrease bioavailability of oral glucocorticoids.[26–30]
- Enzyme inhibitors such as oral contraceptives, azole antifungals, protease inhibitors and antibiotics such as clarithromycin increase the chances of adverse effects. P-glycoprotein efflux pumps are involved in the movement of dexamethasone, methylprednisolone and prednisolone across cells and inhibitors of this efflux pump increases glucocorticoids activity.
- The risk of gastrointestinal bleeding is increased when given corticosteroids are taken synchronously with NSAIDs.
- Corticosteroids antagonize the hypotensive effects of angiotensin converting enzyme inhibitors, β-blockers, angiotensin-II receptor antagonists, calcium-channel blockers and clonidine.
- Corticosteroids antagonize the oral hypoglycaemics.
- Corticosteroids antagonize diuretics and increase risk of hypokalemia.
- Corticosteroids have a variable effect on the anticoagulant action of coumarins.
- Oestrogen-containing oral contraceptives increases plasma concentrations of corticosteroids.
- Corticosteroids may impair immune response to vaccines.

INDICATIONS

Various dermatologic indications for systemic steroids are as follows (Table 4.3).

Pemphigus Vulgaris

- Pemphigus is an autoimmune blistering disease of the skin with an established immunologic basis but unknown etiology (Figs 4.1 and 4.2).
- The primary goal of treatment in all forms of pemphigus is to reduce the synthesis of autoantibodies by the immune system.
- The first-line therapy for all forms of pemphigus is systemic corticosteroids.[31,32] Mortality in this group of disorders has come down drastically since the introduction of corticosteroids.
- Tapering should be initiated once complete disease control is attained and the goal is to take the patient off steroids completely. Adjuvant steroid-sparing immunosuppressive drugs should be introduced at the start of tapering.[33–35]
- Corticosteroids work relatively quickly and are relatively safe when used in appropriate doses for limited periods. The average time to cessation of blistering is around 2–3 weeks and complete disease control within 6–8 weeks. A good clinical response, defined as a resolution of the majority of existing lesions and absence of newly developing lesions, should be evident within 2 to 3 months.

Table 4.3: Dermatologic indications for use of systemic corticosteroids*	
Bullous dermatoses	Pemphigus group Bullous pemphigoid Cicatricial pemphigoid Herpes gestationis Epidermolysis bullosa acquisita Linear IgA bullous dermatosis Stevens-Johnson syndrome/TEN Erythema multiforme minor
Autoimmune connective tissue diseases	Lupus erythematosus Dermatomyositis
Vasculitis	Cutaneous Systemic
Neutrophilic dermatoses	Pyoderma gangrenosum Behçet's disease Aphthous ulcers Sweet's syndrome
Dermatitis/Papulosquamous dermatoses	Contact dermatitis Atopic dermatitis Exfoliative dermatitis Lichen planus
Leprosy	Type 1 reaction Type 2 reaction
Miscellaneous	Sarcoidosis Urticaria and angioedema

*Wolvertan SE. In: Wolvertan SE, editor. Comprehensive dermatologic drug therapy, 3rd ed. Elsevier Saunders, Edinburgh; 2013. p 143–67.

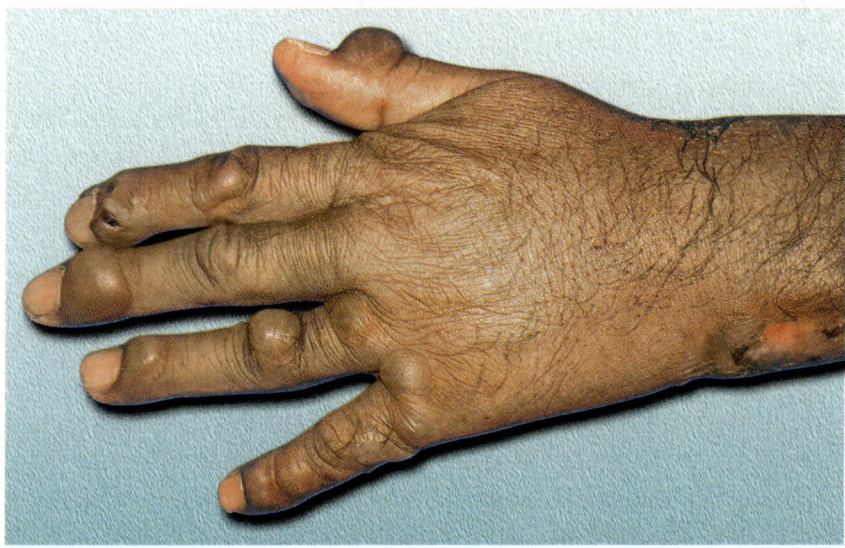

Fig. 4.1: Flaccid blisters in pemphigus vulgaris.

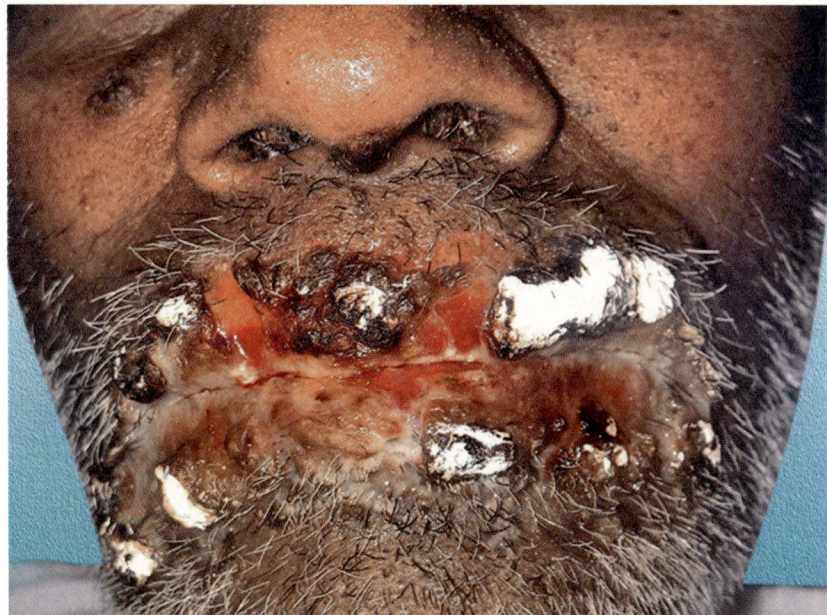

Fig. 4.2: Mucosal erosions and crusting in pemphigus vulgaris.

- Prednisone (equivalents) of 1–1.5 mg/kg/day (lean body weight) as the starting dose is the most commonly used regimen.[36] Higher doses (2–2.5 mg/kg/day) have not been found to hasten the response.[37,38] If disease progression is rapid on 1–1.5 mg/kg/day, hiking the dose up to 2 mg/kg/day can be done. Intravenous or oral pulsed glucocorticoids have been successfully utilized for the treatment of pemphigus vulgaris.[31,39,40]
- In recent years, there is more evidence that the addition of rituximab early in the course of the disease provides a safe and extremely effective treatment that allows an accelerated tapering of systemic corticosteroids, minimizing their devastating side effects.
- The use of a second-line therapy is certainly indicated if significant corticosteroid side effects develop or are expected to develop during the ideal prednisone taper, if the disease does not improve sufficiently to allow continuous tapering, or the disease flares.
- Patients must be monitored for corticosteroid-induced osteopenia by bone mineral density studies (DEXA scan) at the institution of therapy and annually thereafter.
- Patients without a history of renal calculi may be given prophylactic supplemental calcium 1500 mg daily and vitamin D 400 to 800 IU daily.
- In patients with osteopenia or osteoporosis, additional therapies may include hormonal replacement in women (estrogen/progesterone or raloxifene in those with a contraindication for estrogens, such as a history of breast carcinoma) or exogenous testosterone in men with low serum testosterone levels or a bisphosphonate such as alendronate or intranasal calcitonin.

Bullous Pemphigoid

- The Cochrane Skin Group[d] updated its review on the treatment of bullous pemphigoid and concluded that patients with localized disease may be successfully treated with very potent topical corticosteroids. Those with generalized disease in which topical therapy is not feasible can be treated with systemic steroids.

- Prednisone at an initial dose of 0.5 to 0.75 mg/kg/day (depending on disease severity and overall health of the patient) is started and continued till active inflammation, blistering and pruritus have stopped which mostly happens in about 6–8 weeks (Fig. 4.3). The steroids are then tapered gradually and are usually stopped completely in 3–6 months. Doses of prednisolone >0.75 mg/kg/day showed no added benefit over lower doses and had an increased incidence of adverse effects.

- Considering the risk of both short- and long-term systemic corticosteroid therapy in elderly population, every effort should be made to find the minimum dosage of systemic corticosteroids required to suppress disease.

- With only a few exceptions, all elderly patients started on systemic corticosteroids should also start calcium, vitamin D, and bisphosphonate therapy.

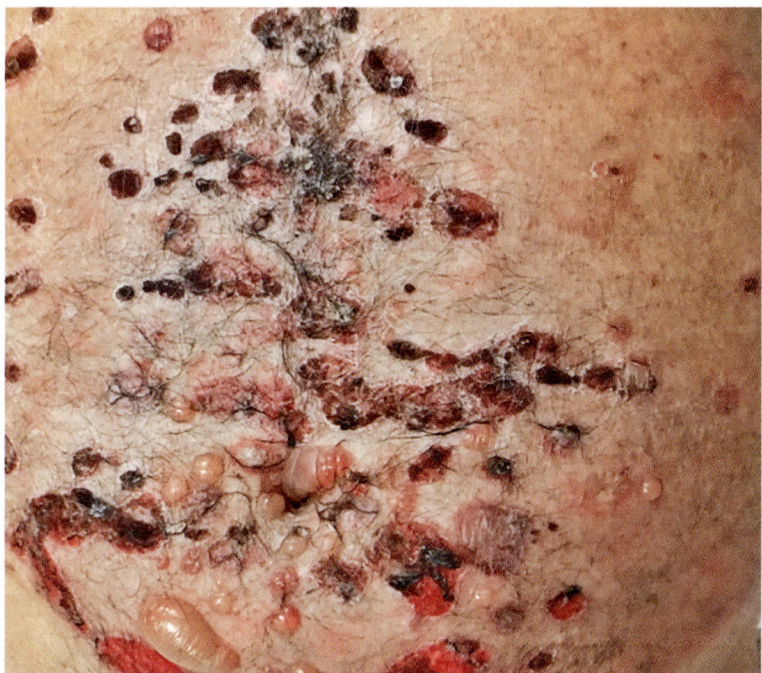

Fig. 4.3: Bullous pemphigoid: Hemorrhagic crusts and tense bullae with few urticarial wheals in a case of bullous pemphigoid.

---

[d]Kirtschig G, Middleton P, Bennett C, Murrell DF, Wojnarowska F, Khumalo NP. Interventions for bullous pemphigoid. Cochrane Database Syst Rev 2010;10:CD002292.

Lupus Erythematosus

- Systemic corticosteroids are not commonly used in the milder forms of lupus, however severe cutaneous disease or internal organ involvement necessitate their use (Fig. 4.4). Some common manifestations requiring systemic steroid therapy include:
  - Lupus nephritis
  - Neuropsychiatric disease
  - Severe refractory thrombocytopenia
  - Haemolytic anaemia
  - Severe vasculitis
  - Cardiopulmonary disease
- These agents may also be used to bridge the gap between the initiation and the achievement of peak levels of antimalarials which form the mainstay of management of cutaneous lupus.
- Low to moderate doses daily with a quick taper in 2–4 weeks is generally used.
- Initial dose is usually in the range of 0.4–0.6 mg/kg/day which can be increased to doses as high as 1.5 mg/kg/day. However, in cases requiring such high doses, pulse therapy with either dexamethasone or methylprednisolone has been found to be a good alternative.[40]
- Steroids have been found to prevent relapses in clinically silent but serologically active patients and thus, moderate dose systemic steroid therapy may be considered in these situations.[41]

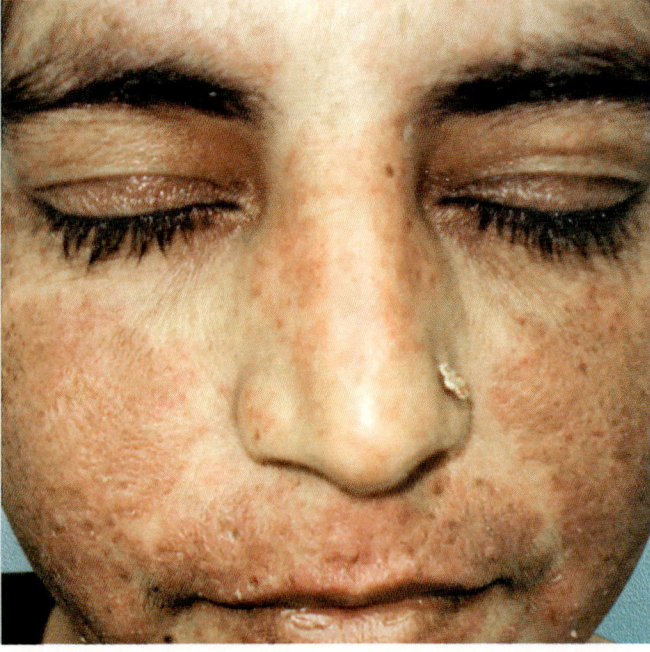

Fig. 4.4: Lupus erythematosus: Erythematous plaques involving bilateral cheeks, supraorbital areas, upper lips and dorsum of nose. Note the characteristic sparing of nasolabial folds.

Dermatomyositis

- Corticosteroids are the mainstay therapy for acute as well as long-term management of patients with dermatomyositis (Figs 4.5 to 4.8). High dose therapy (1 mg/kg) for the first 4–6 weeks to achieve control the disease and then gradual tapering till the lowest effective dose is reached by the next 6–9 months is the preferred therapy.[42]

- Pulse methylprednisolone therapy (1 g for three days) and dexamethasone pulse therapy can be used in extremely sick patients.[40,43]

- Muscle enzymes usually normalize in about 4–6 weeks and muscle strength recovers later in about 3 months. Resolution of skin manifestations varies from patient to patient and may be rapid in some and protracted in others.[44]

- Corticosteroid tapering generally begins after normalization of muscle enzyme, however, some clinicians may continue higher doses until complete recovery of muscle strength. A slower tapering over few months is recommended in dermatomyositis.[e]

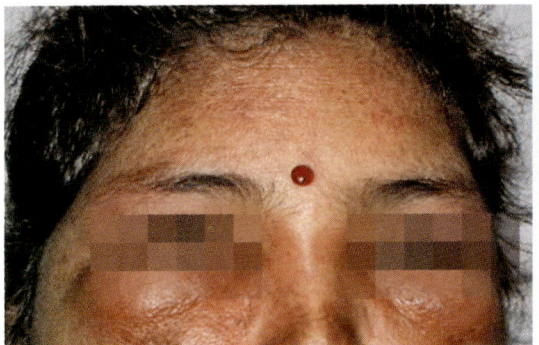

Fig. 4.5: Heliotrope rash in a patient of dermatomyositis.

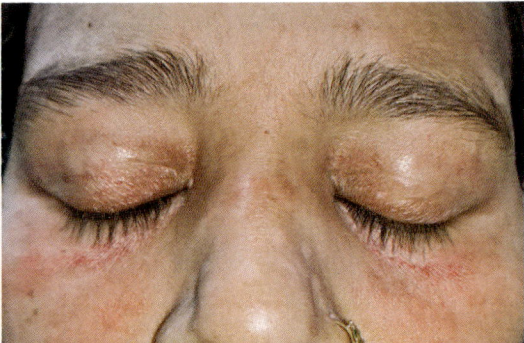

Fig. 4.6: Dermatomyositis: Macular violaceous erythema and edema in periorbital areas associated with proximal muscle weakness.

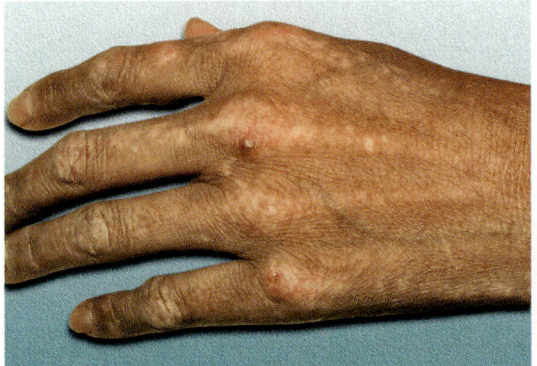

Fig. 4.7: Gottron papules and sign in a patient of dermatomyositis.

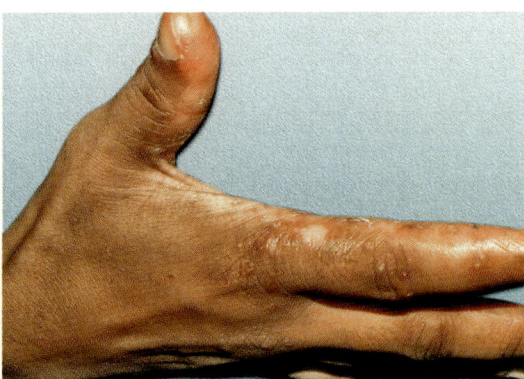

Fig. 4.8: Mechanic hands in a patient of dermatomyositis.

---

[e]**A suggested schedule is as follows:** 10 mg decrements every week till a dose of 40 mg/day, 5 mg decrements every week till a dose of 20 mg/day, 2.5 mg decrements every week till a dose of 10 mg/day and 1 mg decrements every week till a dose of 5 mg/day.

- Careful clinical monitoring for muscle weakness, extramuscular complications and steroid toxicity is warranted. Steroid myopathy and disease flare can cause a clinical conundrum for the treating dermatologists. Electromyography showing fibrillation potentials and sharp waves indicate active myositis and may be a useful investigation. Empirically lowering prednisone dose and seeing response has also been tried.

Neutrophilic Dermatosis

Sweet's Syndrome

- Sweet syndrome is often idiopathic, but may be associated with malignancy, inflammatory bowel disease, infection, medication, radiation, and pregnancy (Figs 4.9 to 4.11). Treatment of the underlying associated condition or discontinuation of the causative medication may lead to resolution of skin lesions.
- Systemic corticosteroids have been found extremely effective in Sweet's syndrome with response being so dramatic that it is included in the diagnostic criteria for the condition.[46]
- A review of the literature regarding treatment for Sweet syndrome showed that corticosteroid therapy (oral prednisone 0.5–1.5 mg/kg daily tapered over 4–6 weeks) results in rapid relief of systemic symptoms (within 1–2 days) and skin lesions within 3 to 9 days.[47–50]

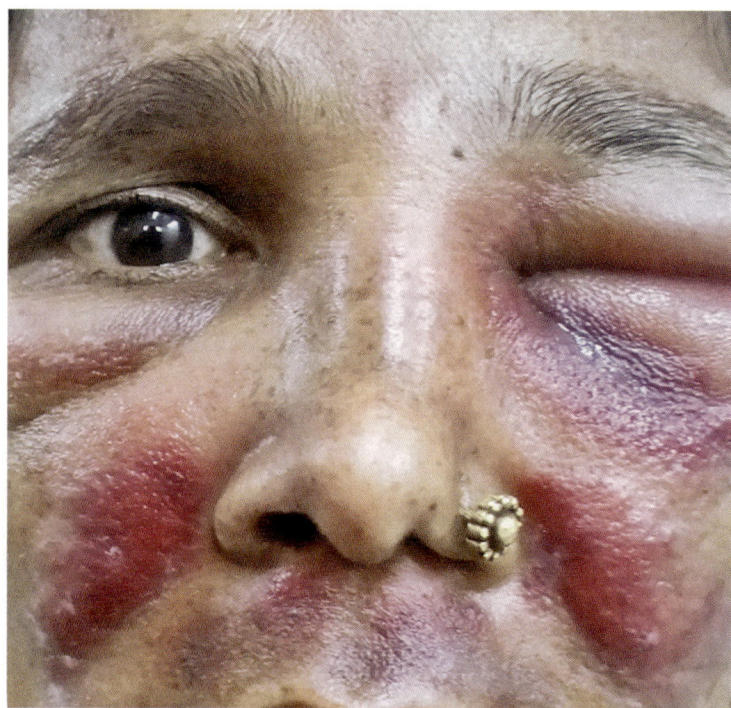

Fig. 4.9: Sweets syndrome: Erythematous tender nodules and plaques associated with fever and neutrophilia.

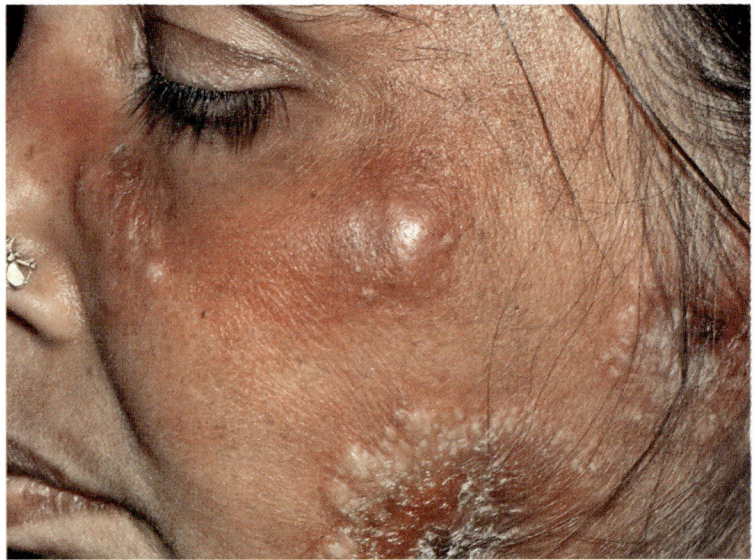

Fig. 4.10: Erythematous edematous plaques with blistering and ulceration in a patient of sweets syndrome.

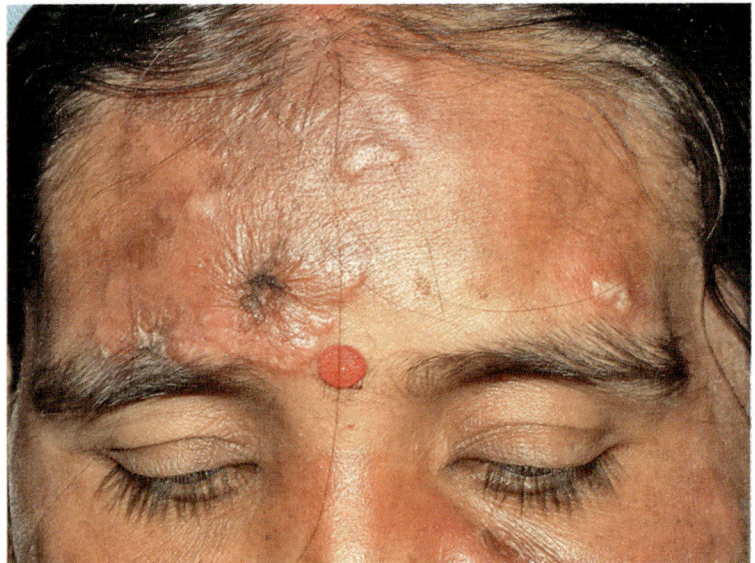

Fig. 4.11: Erythematous edematous plaques on forehead in a patient of sweets syndrome.

Pyoderma Gangrenosum (PG)

- PG results in painful rapidly progressive necrotic ulcers associated with disfiguring scarring (Fig. 4.12).
- Though, no treatment is always effective, the most consistent results are reported with systemic corticosteroids and ciclosporin.[51,52]
- The response to systemic corticosteroids is dramatic and is included in the diagnostic criteria of PG.

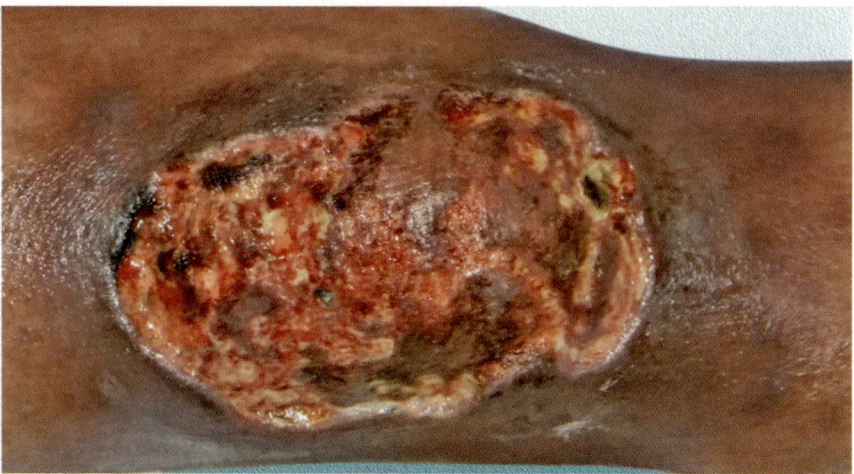

Fig. 4.12: Pyoderma gangrenosum: A large painful ulcer over the lower leg with necrotic floor, violaceous border and surrounding erythema.

- Prednisone (0.5–1 mg/kg/day) is used to achieve quick control which is evident in about one week of starting therapy. Ulcers stabilize and show signs of healing within 1–2 weeks with significant decrease in pain as well.[53] After this intensive phase, the steroid can be tapered down and the patient can be maintained on dapsone (100 mg/day). Intravenous dexamethasone methylprednisolone pulse therapies are useful in extensive disease.[54]

Vasculitis

Idiopathic Cutaneous Small Vessel Vasculitis (CSSV)

- Acute (<4 weeks) and uncomplicated CSSV are self-limited and require only supportive care. However, patients developing cutaneous necrosis, ulceration or hemorrhagic blisters require systemic corticosteroids (Fig. 4.13).[55]
- Use of prednisone (0.5 mg/kg/day) limits complications such as scarring, secondary infection and chronic wounds. Treatment is continued at this dose until new lesions (1–2 weeks) cease to form and then the steroids are tapered quickly over a period of 3–6 weeks.
- Patients having recurrence require steroid-sparing immunomodulatory agents as do patients not responding within 2 weeks.

Urticarial Vasculitis

- Urticarial lesions with vasculitis on histopathology with hypocomplementemia define this disease entity. Systemic corticosteroids are indicated in moderately severe disease and in combination with other immunomodulatory drugs for severe disabling disease.[56–58]
- Prednisone is started at a dose of 0.5–1 mg/kg/day and shows symptomatic improvement within a few days, however assessment of response should be

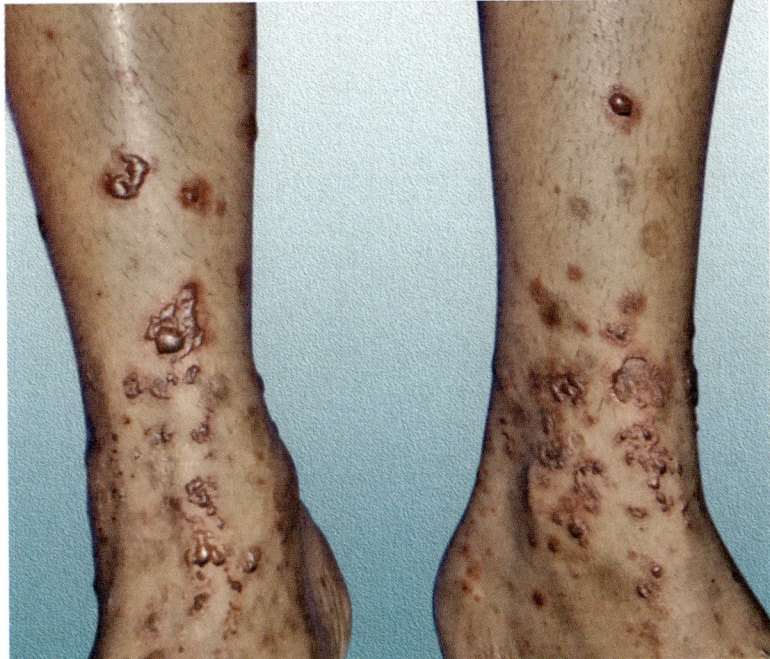

Fig. 4.13: Small vessel vasculitis: Purpuric macules over the bilateral lower legs associated with vesiculation.

made at two weeks of starting the treatment. Patients not having good control may need a higher dose up to 1.5 mg/kg/day.[59,60]

- Steroids are tapered slowly every 1–2 weeks to the lowest maintenance dose.

Leprosy[61–63]

Type 1 Reactions

- Increased cell mediated immunity against *Mycobacterium leprae* bacilli manifests as type 1 leprosy reaction. Neuritis commonly presenting as nerve tenderness, severe inflammation in skin lesions and nerve function impairment require treatment with systemic corticosteroids (Figs 4.14 and 4.15).
- Corticosteroids are vital in preventing permanent nerve damage. Prednisone (initial dose 1 mg/kg/day) along with rest and immobilization of the limb is the mainstay of therapy. Treatment has to be continued after resolution of acute attack for up to 4 weeks and then slowly tapered at the rate of 2.5 mg/week and then stopped.
- The duration of steroid therapy is an important determinant of success of therapy and should be long enough to cover the period during which the antigen load is high enough to mount an immune response. It generally ranges from 3 to 6 months in tuberculoid leprosy, 4 to 9 months in borderline tuberculoid leprosy, 6 to 12 months in borderline leprosy and 6 to 24 months in borderline lepromatous leprosy.
- Patients planned for nerve decompression are to be operated under steroid cover.

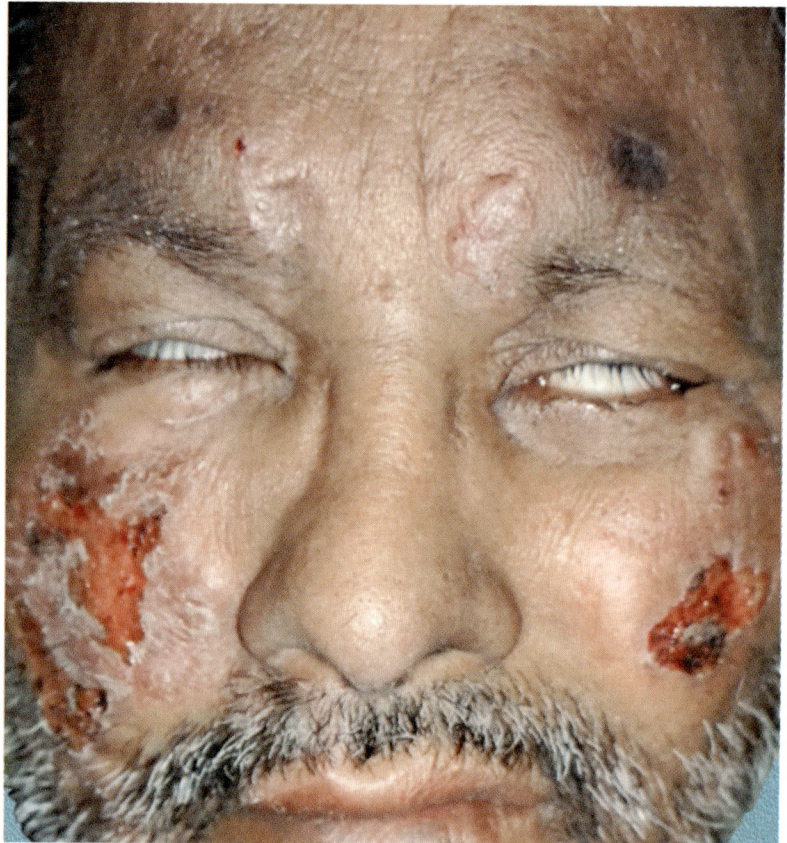

Fig. 4.14: Type 1 reaction—a case of borderline tuberculoid leprosy presenting with erythema, edema and ulceration of the existing plaques associated with fever and facial nerve palsy.

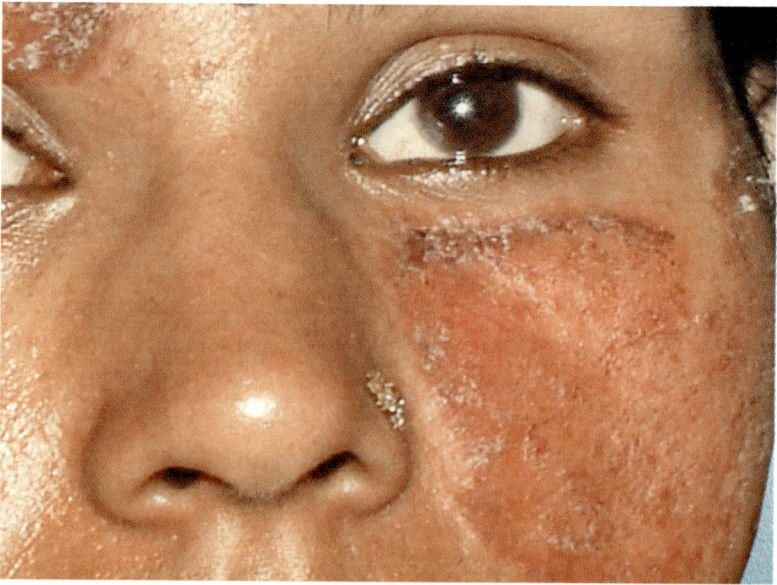

Fig. 4.15: Borderline tuberculoid Hansen's disease with type 1 reaction.

Type 2 Reactions

- Systemic corticosteroids are the first line therapy in severe type 2 reaction (Figs 4.16 and 4.17). Prednisolone should be started with 0.5 to 1 mg/kg/day till clinical improvement, and then tapered every week by 5 to 10 mg over 6 to 8 weeks. A maintenance dose of 5 to 10 mg may be needed for several weeks to prevent recurrence.[64]
- The duration of therapy in type 2 reaction is shorter as compared to type 1 reaction and corticosteroids can be tapered off within one month as the acute phase type 2 reaction is generally short lasting and the risk of steroid dependence is high.

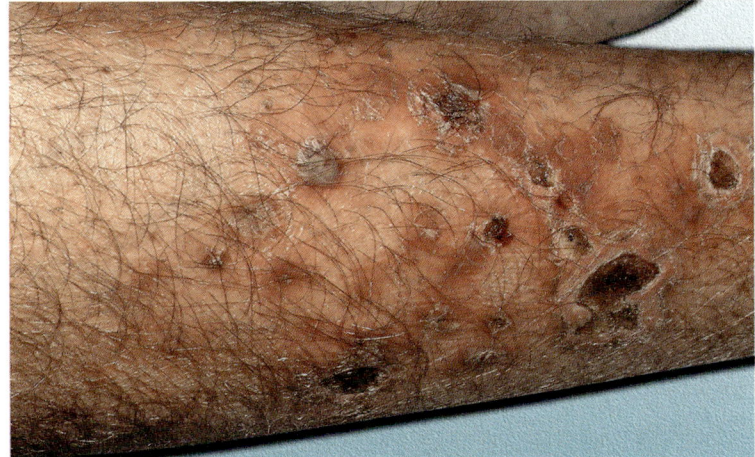

Fig. 4.16: Vesicular and necrotic lesions in type 2 reaction in Hansen's disease.

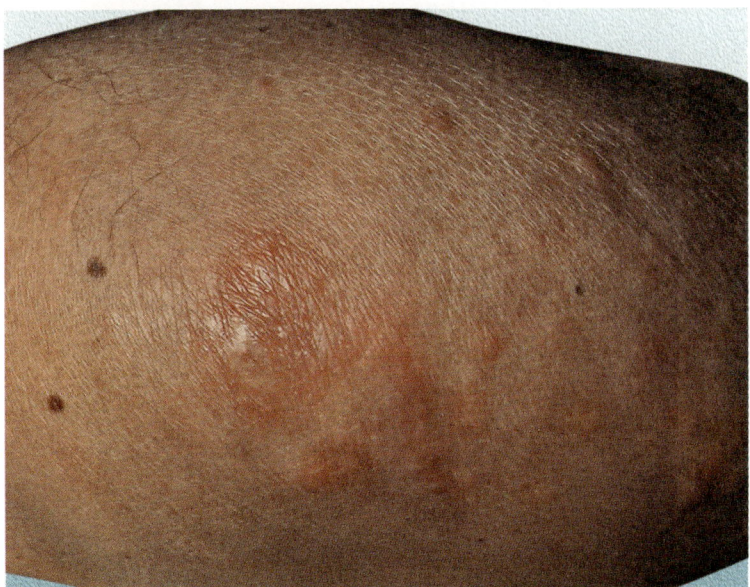

Fig. 4.17: Erythematous tender nodules in type 2 reaction in Hansen's disease.

Contact and Atopic Dermatitis

- Allergen avoidance and topical steroids are the mainstay of management however systemic steroids play an important role when the disease is severe (>10% body surface area) and/or involves the face and genitals (Figs 4.18 to 4.20).

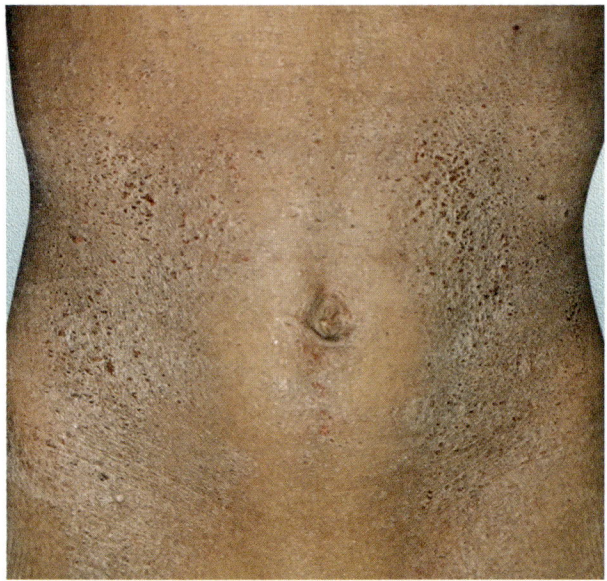

Fig. 4.18: Atopic dermatitis: Itchy hyperpigmented eczematous plaques over the trunk.

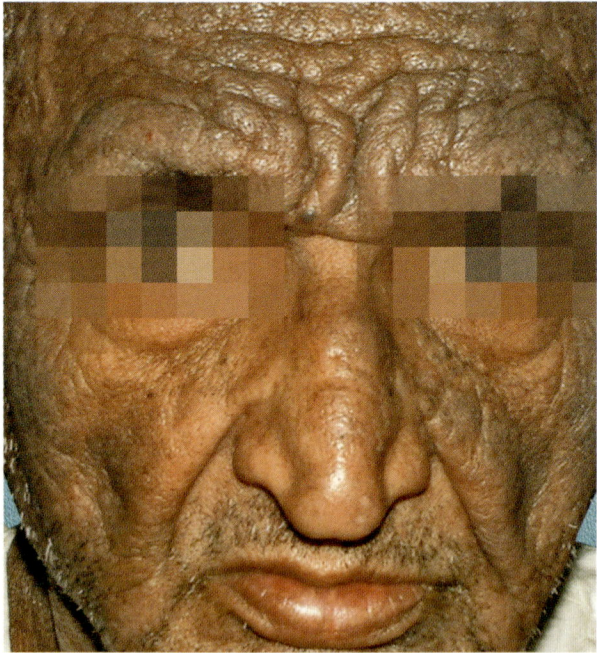

Fig. 4.19: Chronic actinic dermatitis to parthenium resulting in lichenified plaque over forehead and cheeks.

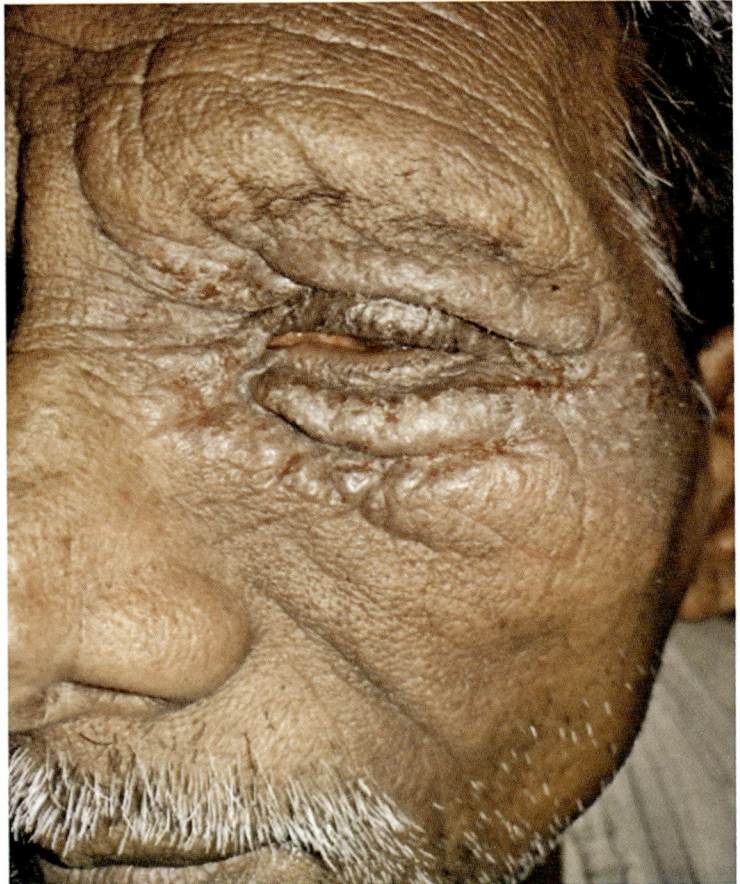

Fig. 4.20: Contact dermatitis to eyedrops resulting in erythematous oozy plaque in periorbital location associated with edema.

- Oral prednisolone started at a dose of 0.75–1 mg/kg/day tapered over next one month to lowest maintenance dose is the recommended regimen.[65,66] Short course of systemic steroids is also useful for rapid improvement in dyshidrotic eczema and nummular dermatitis.

REFERENCES

1. Sulek K. [Nobel prize for Edward Calvin Kendall, Thaddeus Reichsteinand Philip Showalter Hench in 1950 for their discoveries related toadrenal cortex hormones, their structure and biological activity]. Wiad Lek. 1968;21:1885–7.

2. Sulzberger MB, Witten VH. The effect of topically applied compound F in selected dermatoses. J Invest Dermatol. 1952;19:101–2.

3. Centennial Paper. November 1951 (Arch Dermatol Syphilol: Cortisone acetate administered orally in dermatologic therapy by Marion B. Sulzberger, Victor H. Witten and Stanley N. Yaffe. Arch Dermatol. 1983;119:858–64.

4. Freyberg RH, Traeger CH, Patterson M, Squires W, Adams CH. Problems of prolonged cortisone treatment for rheumatoid arthritis; further investigations. J Am Med Assoc. 1951;147:1538–43.

5. Herzog HL, Nobile A, Tolksdorf S, Charney W, Hershberg EB, Perlman PL. New antiarthritic steroids. Science. 1955;121:176.

6. Stafford RO, Barnes LE, Bowman BJ, Meinzinger MM. Glucocorticoid and mineralocorticoids activities of delta1-fluorohydrocortisone. Proc Soc Exp Biol Med. 1955;89:371–4.

7. Peterson RE. Metabolism of adrenocorticosteroids in man. Ann N Y Acad Sci. 1959;82:846–53.

8. Nugent CA, Eiknes K, Samuels LT, Tyler FH. Changes in plasma levels of 17-hydroxycorticosteroids during the intravenous administration of adrenocorticotropin (ACTH). IV. Response to prolonged infusions of small amounts of ACTH. J Clin Endocrinol Metab. 1959;19:334–43.

9. Sherlock JE, Letteri JM. Effect of hemodialysis on methylprednisolone plasma levels. Nephron. 1977;18:208–11.

10. Milsap RL, George DE, Szefler SJ, Murray KA, Lebenthal E, Jusko WJ. Effect of inflammatory bowel disease on absorption and disposition of prednisolone. Dig Dis Sci. 1983;28:161–8.

11. Frey FJ, Frey BM. Altered plasma protein-binding of prednisolone in patients with the nephrotic syndrome. Am J Kidney Dis. 1984;3:339–48.

12. Milsap RL, Plaisance KI, Jusko WJ. Prednisolone disposition in obese men. Clin Pharmacol Ther. 1984;36:824–31.

13. Renner E, Horber FF, Jost G, Frey BM, Frey FJ. Effect of liver function on the metabolism of prednisone and prednisolone in humans. Gastroenterology. 1986;90:819–28.

14. Pratt WB, Morishima Y, Murphy M, Harrell M. Chaperoning of glucocorticoid receptors. Handb Exp Pharmacol. 2006;172:111–38.

15. Zhang G, Zhang L, Duff GW. A negative regulatory region containing a glucocorticosteroid response element (nGRE) in the human interleukin-1beta gene. DNA Cell Biol. 1997;16:145–52.

16. Rhen T, Cidlowski JA. Anti-inflammatory action of glucocorticoids—new mechanisms for old drugs. N Engl J Med. 2005 Oct;353:1711–23.

17. Karin M, Liu Z g, Zandi E. AP-1 function and regulation. Curr Opin Cell Biol. 1997 Apr;9:240–6.

18. Auphan N, DiDonato JA, Rosette C, Helmberg A, Karin M. Immunosuppression by glucocorticoids: inhibition of NF-kappa B activity through induction of I kappa B synthesis. Science. 1995;270:286–90.

19. Göttlicher M, Heck S, Herrlich P. Transcriptional cross-talk, the second mode of steroid hormone receptor action. J Mol Med (Berl). 1998;76:480–9.

20. Scheinman RI, Cogswell PC, Lofquist AK, Baldwin AS. Role of transcriptional activation of I kappa B alpha in mediation of immunosuppression by glucocorticoids. Science. 1995;270:283–6.

21. Borson DB, Gruenert DC. Glucocorticoids induce neutral endopeptidase in transformed human tracheal epithelial cells. Am J Physiol. 1991;260:L83–9.

22. Tobler A, Meier R, Seitz M, Dewald B, Baggiolini M, Fey MF. Glucocorticoids downregulate gene expression of GM-CSF, NAP-1/IL-8, and IL-6, but not of M-CSF in human fibroblasts. Blood. 1992;79:45–51.

23. Liu D, Ahmet A, Ward L, Krishnamoorthy P, Mandelcorn ED, Leigh R, et al. A practical guide to the monitoring and management of the complications of systemic corticosteroid therapy. Allergy, Asthma Clin Immunol. 2013;9:30-xx.

24. Tanner AR, Caffin JA, Halliday JW, Powell LW. Concurrent administration of antacids and prednisone: Effect on serum levels of prednisolone. Br J Clin Pharmacol. 1979;7:397–400.

25. Uribe M, Casian C, Rojas S, Sierra JG, Go VL. Decreased bioavailability of prednisone due to antacids in patients with chronic active liver disease and in healthy volunteers. Gastroenterology. 1981;80:661–5.

26. Stjernholm MR, Katz FH. Effects of diphenylhydantoin, phenobarbital, and diazepam on the metabolism of methylprednisolone and its sodium succinate. J Clin Endocrinol Metab. 1975;41:887–93.

27. Czock D, Keller F, Rasche FM, Häussler U. Pharmacokinetics and pharmacodynamics of systemically administered glucocorticoids. Clin Pharmacokinet. 2005;44:61–98.

28. Frey BM, Frey FJ. Phenytoin modulates the pharmacokinetics of prednisolone and the pharmacodynamics of prednisolone as assessed by the inhibition of the mixed lymphocyte reaction in humans. Eur J Clin Invest. 1984;14:1–6.

29. Evans PJ, Walker RF, Peters JR, Dyas J, Riad-Fahmy D, Thomas JP, et al. Anticonvulsant therapy and cortisol elimination. Br J Clin Pharmacol. 1985;20:129–32.

30. Petereit LB, Meikle AW. Effectiveness of prednisolone during phenytoin therapy. Clin Pharmacol Ther. 1977;22:912–6.

31. Harman KE, Albert S, Black MM, British Association of Dermatologists. Guidelines for the management of pemphigus vulgaris. Br J Dermatol. 2003;149:926–37.

32. Chams-Davatchi C, Esmaili N, Daneshpazhooh M, Valikhani M, Balighi K, Hallaji Z, et al. Randomized controlled open-label trial of four treatment regimens for pemphigus vulgaris. J Am Acad Dermatol. 2007;57:622–8.

33. Chams-Davatchi C, Mortazavizadeh A, Daneshpazhooh M, Davatchi F, Balighi K, Esmaili N, et al. Randomized double blind trial of prednisolone and azathioprine, vs. prednisolone and placebo, in the treatment of pemphigus vulgaris. J Eur Acad Dermatol Venereol. 2013;27:1285–92.

34. Ioannides D, Apalla Z, Lazaridou E, Rigopoulos D. Evaluation of mycophenolate mofetil as a steroid-sparing agent in pemphigus: a randomized, prospective study. J Eur Acad Dermatol Venereol. 2012;26:855–60.

35. Beissert S, Mimouni D, Kanwar AJ, Solomons N, Kalia V, Anhalt GJ. Treating pemphigus vulgaris with prednisone and mycophenolate mofetil: a multicenter, randomized, placebo-controlled trial. J Invest Dermatol. 2010;130:2041–8.

36. Mimouni D, Nousari CH, Cummins DL, Kouba DJ, David M, Anhalt GJ. Differences and similarities among expert opinions on the diagnosis and treatment of pemphigus vulgaris. J Am Acad Dermatol. 2017;49:1059–62.

37. Ratnam K V, Phay KL, Tan CK. Pemphigus therapy with oral prednisolone regimens. A 5-year study. Int J Dermatol. 1990;29:363–7.

38. Femiano F, Gombos F, Scully C. Pemphigus vulgaris with oral involvement: evaluation of two different systemic corticosteroid therapeutic protocols. J Eur Acad Dermatol Venereol. 2002 Jul;16:353–6.

39. Mentink LF, Mackenzie MW, Tóth GG, Laseur M, Lambert FPG, Veeger NJGM, et al. Randomized controlled trial of adjuvant oral dexamethasone pulse therapy in pemphigus vulgaris: PEMPULS trial. Arch Dermatol. 2006;142:570–6.

40. Pasricha JS. Pulse therapy as a cure for autoimmune diseases. Indian J Dermatol Venereol Leprol. 2003;69:323–8.

41. Tseng C-E, Buyon JP, Kim M, Belmont HM, Mackay M, Diamond B, et al. The effect of moderate-dose corticosteroids in preventing severe flares in patients with serologically active, but clinically stable, systemic lupus erythematosus: findings of a prospective, randomized, double-blind, placebo-controlled trial. Arthritis Rheum. 2006;54:3623–32.

42. Troyanov Y, Targoff IN, Tremblay J-L, Goulet J-R, Raymond Y, Senécal J-L. Novel classification of idiopathic inflammatory myopathies based on overlap syndrome features and autoantibodies: analysis of 100 French Canadian patients. Medicine (Baltimore). 2005;84:231–49.

43. Drake LA, Dinehart SM, Farmer ER, Goltz RW, Graham GF, Hordinsky MK, et al. Guidelines of care for dermatomyositis. American Academy of Dermatology. J Am Acad Dermatol. 1996;34:824–9.

44. Joffe MM, Love LA, Leff RL, Fraser DD, Targoff IN, Hicks JE, et al. Drug therapy of the idiopathic inflammatory myopathies: predictors of response to prednisone, azathioprine, and methotrexate and a comparison of their efficacy. Am J Med. 1993;94:379–87.

45. Robinson LR. AAEM case report #22: polymyositis. Muscle Nerve. 1991;14:310–5.

46. Rochet NM, Chavan RN, Cappel MA, Wada DA, Gibson LE. Sweet syndrome: clinical presentation, associations, and response to treatment in 77 patients. J Am Acad Dermatol. 2013;69:557–64.

47. O'Connor Reina C, Garcia Iriarte MT, Rodriguez Diaz A, Gomez Angel D, Garcia Monge E, Sanchez Conejo-Mir J. Tonsil cancer and Sweet's syndrome. Otolaryngol Head Neck Surg. 1998;119:709–10.

48. Cohen PR, Kurzrock R. Sweet's syndrome: a review of current treatment options. Am J Clin Dermatol. 2002;3:117–31.

49. von den Driesch P. Sweet's syndrome (acute febrile neutrophilic dermatosis). J Am Acad Dermatol. 1994;31:535–56.

50. Mahajan VK, Sharma NL, Sharma RC. Sweet's syndrome from an Indian perspective: a report of four cases and review of the literature. Int J Dermatol. 2006;45:702–8.

51. Reichrath J, Bens G, Bonowitz A, Tilgen W. Treatment recommendations for pyoderma gangrenosum: an evidence-based review of the literature based on more than 350 patients. J Am Acad Dermatol. 2005;53:273–83.

52. Binus AM, Qureshi AA, Li VW, Winterfield LS. Pyoderma gangrenosum: a retrospective review of patient characteristics, comorbidities and therapy in 103 patients. Br J Dermatol. 2011;165:1244–50.

53. Chow RK, Ho VC. Treatment of pyoderma gangrenosum. J Am Acad Dermatol. 1996;34:1047–60.

54. Prystowsky JH, Kahn SN, Lazarus GS. Present status of pyoderma gangrenosum. Review of 21 cases. Arch Dermatol. 1989;125:57–64.

55. Russell JP, Gibson LE. Primary cutaneous small vessel vasculitis: approach to diagnosis and treatment. Int J Dermatol. 2006;45:3–13.

56. Sanchez NP, Winkelmann RK, Schroeter AL, Dicken CH. The clinical and histopathologic spectrums of urticarial vasculitis: study of forty cases. J Am Acad Dermatol. 1982;7:599–605.

57. Callen JP, af Ekenstam E. Cutaneous leukocytoclastic vasculitis: clinical experience in 44 patients. South Med J. 1987;80:848–51.

58. O'Loughlin S, Schroeter AL, Jordon RE. Chronic urticaria-like lesions in systemic lupus erythematosus. A review of 12 cases. Arch Dermatol. 1978;114:879–83.

59. Venzor J, Lee WL, Huston DP. Urticarial vasculitis. Clin Rev Allergy Immunol. 2002;23:201–16.

60. Mehregan DR, Hall MJ, Gibson LE. Urticarial vasculitis: a histopathologic and clinical review of 72 cases. J Am Acad Dermatol. 1992;26:441–8.

61. Pai V V, Tayshetye PU, Ganapati R. A study of standardized regimens of steroid treatment in reactions in leprosy at a referral centre. Indian J Lepr. 84:9–15.

62. Naafs B. Treatment duration of reversal reaction: a reappraisal. Back to the past. Lepr Rev. 2003;74:328–36.

63. Van Veen NHJ, Lockwood DNJ, Van Brakel WH, Ramirez J, Richardus JH. Interventions for erythema nodosum leprosum. A Cochrane review. Lepr Rev. 2009;80:355–72.

64. Ridley MJ, Ridley DS. The immunopathology of erythema nodosum leprosum: the role of extravascular complexes. Lepr Rev. 1983;54:95–107.

65. Goodall J. Oral corticosteroids for poison ivy dermatitis. CMAJ. 2002;166:300–1.

66. Moe JF. How much steroid for poison ivy? Postgrad Med. 1999;106:21, 24.

5

Pulse Therapy

Neetu Bhari, Savera Gupta

SUMMARY

- Pulse therapy means administering suprapharmacologic dose of drug over a short period of time followed by withdrawing the drug completely until it is needed/administered again.
- High dose of drug helps to achieve rapid therapeutic effects which may not be achievable with the conventional daily doses, while the intermittent administration of drug minimizes side effects.
- In India, corticosteroid pulse therapy was first used in 1981 to successfully treat a patient with severe and recalcitrant Reiter's disease. Subsequently it was tried successfully in pemphigus vulgaris. The introduction of pulse therapy has revolutionized the therapy for pemphigus.
- Over years, pulse therapy has been used in various dermatological indications including immunobullous disorders, collagen vascular disorders and several others.
- Though, initially methylprednisolone was the corticosteroid most commonly used for pulse therapy, recent studies have shown that dexamethasone, a less expensive alternative, is as effective when used in 'pulsed doses' in many dermatologic and non-dermatologic indications.
- There are several corticosteroid pulse therapy regimens including dexamethasone pulse, methylprednisolone pulse, oral betamethasone pulse, oral mini pulse (betamethasone/dexamethasone), dexamethasone cyclophosphamide pulse, dexamethasone azathioprine pulse.
- Dexamethasone cyclophosphamide pulse (DCP) is the most frequently used regime of pulse therapy, especially in patients with pemphigus. It is given as a routine infusion, often in a day care or OPD setting, with the patient going home a few hours after completion of the infusion.
- DCP therapy consists of giving 100 mg dexamethasone intravenous in 500 ml of 5% dextrose as slow infusion over 2 hours, on 3 consecutive days and 500 mg of cyclophosphamide in same infusion on any one of the three days but by

convention on 2nd day. This constitutes 1 cycle of DCP. These patients also receive 50 mg cyclophosphamide daily orally between the pulses. Such DCPs are to be repeated every 28 days, counted from the first day of each DCP.

- Based on the response in pemphigus, the DCP therapy is classified into 4 phases, with the patient having active lesions in phase I, and being in clinical remission in phases II–IV.
- Based on patients' requirements, modifications in the basic DCP have been proposed in the regimen for pulse therapy for pemphigus. These include additional requirement of corticosteroids, omission of phase II, individualizing duration of therapy, modification of phase III, administration of mesna, prevention of corticosteroid-induced osteoporosis by calcium and vitamin D supplementation and management of concomitant diseases such as diabetes, hypertension, and infections.
- Because high doses of cyclophosphamide can lead to azoospermia/amenorrhoea, it is best avoided in unmarried patients and in those who have not yet completed their family and substituted with other immunosuppressive agents like azathioprine (daily 50 to 100 mg orally) or methotrexate (weekly 7.5 mg orally). These are known as dexamethasone azathioprine pulse (DAP) and Dexamethasone methotrexate pulse (DMP), respectively.
- Absolute contraindications of DCP include pregnant or lactating women, hypersensitivity to cyclophosphamide/corticosteroid, unmarried patients or reproductive age group whose family is not complete and bladder malignancy.
- A detailed clinical history and examination to look for duration of disease, extent and severity of disease, history of treatment taken in past, presence of concomitant systemic diseases and side effects of previous treatments is required prior to initiation of therapy.
- The laboratory evaluation consists of a complete hemogram, blood sugar, blood pressure, renal and liver function tests, serum electrolytes, urinalysis, X-ray of the chest, and electrocardiogram.
- Blood sugar and serum electrolytes are to be checked before each pulse. Pulse, respiratory rate, and blood pressure are monitored during infusion.
- Seven days after last pulse therapy, routine blood, urine tests and chest X-ray should be repeated. Test for pemphigus antibody levels can be repeated at this stage to monitor the immunological response of therapy. These investigations should be repeated once again after 7 days of completing phase III of pulse therapy.
- The major advantage of pulse therapy is that the side effects such as weight gain, cushingoid obesity, diabetes, hypertension, gastric hyperacidity, osteoporosis, cataract, acne, striae, hirsutism, etc. are less common as compared to conventional daily oral corticosteroids.
- However, some side effects like hiccups, facial flushing, headache, diarrhea and weakness are peculiar to corticosteroid pulse therapy. The other common

side effects of pulse therapy include generalized swelling, myalgia, hyperglycemia, hypokalemia, infections, mood and behaviour alteration and sleep disturbances.

INTRODUCTION

- Pulse therapy means administering suprapharmacologic dose of drug over a short period of time (in an intermittent manner), and then withdrawing the drug completely until it is needed/administered again.[1]
- High dose of drug helps to achieve rapid therapeutic effects which may not be achievable with the conventional daily doses, while the intermittent administration of drug minimizes side effects.
- Pulse corticosteroid therapy has been proposed as a means of rapidly controlling life-threatening or serious dermatologic diseases with minimal toxicity and allowing for less aggressive long term maintenance therapy.

HISTORY OF CORTICOSTEROID PULSE THERAPY

- First report of use of pulse administration of corticosteroids was in 1969 by Kountz and Cohn who used methylprednisolone[a] successfully to prevent renal graft rejection.[2]
- First report of dermatologic use of 'coticosteroid pulse therapy' was in 1982 by Johnson and Lazarus who used pulse doses of intravenous methylprednisolone to successfully treat a patient with pyoderma gangrenosum (PG).[3] In a subsequent report, Prystowsky et al[4] treated 8 patients with PG with corticosteroid pulse therapy, with 6 responding favourably.
- In India, Pasricha et al[5] were the first to use corticosteroid pulse therapy[b] in 1981 to successfully treat a patient with severe and recalcitrant Reiter's disease.
- Subsequently, it was tried successfully in pemphigus vulgaris, initially by Pasricha et al, and then by several others.[6–28] The introduction of pulse therapy has revolutionized the therapy for pemphigus and has since been used to treat a large number of patients at several centers in India and abroad.

MECHANISM OF ACTION

Corticosteroids exert their anti-inflammatory and immunosuppressive properties by genomic and non-genomic pathways. Depending on the concentration of corticosteroids used the effect seen is as follows:

- *At low concentrations (genomic effect)*: Corticosteroids form complexes with cytosolic GC receptors (GCR) to form GCR complex which activates the MAPK signalling pathway. The activated GCR complex moves to the nucleus that

---

[a]Post-transplantation, 1000 ml of physiologic saline which contained 1–2 g of methylprednisolone, 10,000 units heparin and 0.5 mg actinomycin D was infused over next 1 to 3 days at a rate of 3–20 ml per hour.

[b]With dexamethasone 100 mg, given intravenous for 3 consecutive days every 28 days. Dexamethasone, was used because of non-availability of methylprednisolone in India at that time.

activates the GC-responsive element which results in anti-inflammatory and immunosuppressive effects.

- *At high concentrations* (*genomic and nongenomic effects*): Corticosteroid intercalates with the cell membrane GCR causing rapid immunosuppression via apoptosis and induction of lipomodulin (which inhibits prostaglandins and leukotrienes). At high doses corticosteroids inhibit nuclear factor kappa B via "transrepression" (direct interaction of GC with transcription factors).

Mechanism of Action of corticosteroids in Pulse Therapy

- Clinical immunosuppressive effects that are observed when high dose of corticosteroids is administered occur too rapidly to be explained by the classic (genomic) mechanism of action alone, indicating that both genomic and non-genomic pathways are probably responsible for the effects of corticosteroid pulse therapy.

Indications: Over years, pulse therapy has been used in several dermatological indications (Table 5.1).[6–29]

CHOICE OF CORTICOSTEROID

- Conventionally, methylprednisolone (1000 mg) was the most commonly used corticosteroid for pulse therapy. However, recent studies have shown that dexamethasone, a less expensive alternative, is as effective when used in 'pulsed

Table 5.1: Indications of pulse therapy in dermatology	
Immunobullous disorders:	**Other diseases:**
• Pemphigus:	• Generalized lichen planus
– *P. vulgaris* and vegetans	• Neutrophilic dermatoses
– *P. foliaceus* and erythematosus	• Reiter's disease
– Paraneoplastic pemphigus	• Alopecia areata
• Bullous pemphigoid	• Resistant alopecia universalis
• Cicatricial pemphigoid	• Fast spreading extensive vitiligo
• Pemphigoid gestationis	• Sarcoidosis
• Chronic bullous dermatosis of childhood	• Multicentric reticulo-histiocytosis
• Epidermolysis bullosa acquisita	• Peyronie's disease
Collagen vascular diseases:	• Necrobiotic xanthogranuloma
• Lupus erythematosus	• Prurigo nodularis
• Systemic sclerosis	• Cytophagic histiocytic panniculitis
• Morphea (extensive, generalized, active linear)	• Eosinophilic fasciitis
• Dermatomyositis/polymyositis	• Cutaneous T cell lymphoma
	• Kawasaki's disease
	• Erythema multiforme major
	• Disseminated porokeratosis
	• Stevens-Johnson syndrome
	• Scleredema, scleromyxedema

doses' in many dermatologic and non-dermatologic indications.[30] The choice of dexamethasone made the treatment considerably more affordable and accessible to patients. Subsequently, betamethasone was used in suprapharmacological doses, with the advantage that it could be used orally.

- There was concern among some workers about the equivalence of 1000 mg of methylprednisolone and 100 mg of dexamethasone and some groups have administered pulses of 136 mg of dexamethasone.[13] However, a dose of 1000 mg of methylprednisolone is as arbitrary as a dose of 100 mg of dexamethasone, and in the absence of evidence that 136 mg pulses of dexamethasone are more effective, nearly all centres continue to use 100 mg boluses.[29]

PULSE THERAPY REGIMENS

Schedules and doses of corticosteroid pulse therapy are neither standardized nor sacrosanct, but the commonly used regimens include:
- Corticosteroid pulse therapy regimens:
  - Dexamethasone pulse (DP)
  - Methylprednisolone pulse (MP)
  - Oral betamethasone pulse (OBP)
  - Oral mini pulse (betamethasone/dexamethasone) (OMP)
- Combined corticosteroid and immunosuppressive pulse therapy regimens:
  - Dexamethasone cyclophosphamide pulse (DCP)
  - Dexamethasone azathioprine pulse (DAP)
  - Dexamethasone methotrexate pulse (DMP)

Dexamethasone Cyclophosphamide Pulse (DCP)[1]

This is the most frequently used regimen of pulse therapy, especially in patients with pemphigus (Figs 5.1 and 5.2).

Standard DCP Protocol

- Treatment consists of giving 100 mg[c] dexamethasone[d] intravenous in 500 ml of 5% dextrose[e] as slow infusion over 2 hours, on 3 consecutive days and 500 mg of cyclophosphamide in same infusion on any one of the three days but by convention on 2nd day. This constitutes 1 cycle of DCP. These patients also receive 50 mg cyclophosphamide daily orally between the pulses.
- Such DCPs are to be repeated every 28 days (nothing sacrosanct about the interval), counted from the first day of each DCP.

---

[c]In children less than 12 years of age, the dose of dexamethasone in pulse should be reduced to 50 mg.

[d]Dexamethasone is available as dexamethasone sodium phosphate 4.37 mg/ml (equivalent to 4 mg of dexamethasone phosphate), as 2 ml vials. For preparation of 100 mg of dexamethasone solution in 500 ml of 5% dextrose, 12 such vials are used.

[e]The reason for administration of dexamethasone in dextrose instead of normal saline is because steroids cause hypernatremia and hypokalemia.

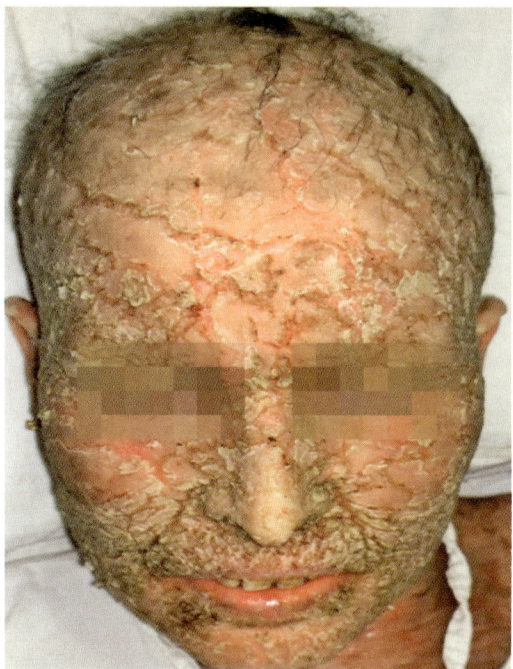
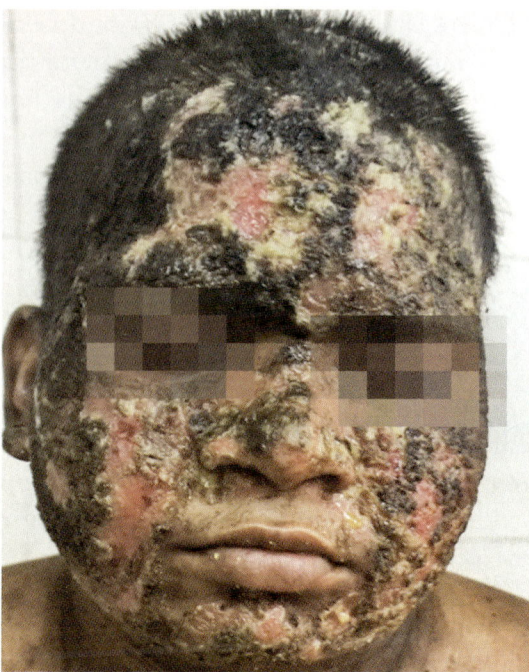

Fig. 5.1: Severe adherent purulent crusting and erosions requiring pulse therapy in a case of pemphigus foliaceus.

Fig. 5.2: Severe adherent purulent crusting and erosions requiring pulse therapy in a case of pemphigus foliaceus.

- There was initial alarm and anxiety about the large doses of corticosteroids and cyclophosphamide involved, and in the early days some centers would administer the therapy in the ICU under continuous cardiac monitoring. It is now given as a routine infusion, often in a day care or OPD setting, with the patient going home a few hours after completion of the infusion.

Phases of DCP Therapy[1,14]

- Based on the response in pemphigus, the DCP therapy is classified into 4 phases, with the patient having active lesions in phase I, and being in clinical remission in phases II–IV (Table 5.2).
  - *Phase I:* It is defined till the absence of new lesions, complete healing of the existing lesions, and the patient receives cyclophosphamide 50 mg orally per

Phase	Duration	Clinical lesions	DCP	Oral cyclophosphamide
I	Till clinical remission*	Yes	Yes	Yes
II	9 months	No	Yes	Yes
III	9 months	No	No	Yes
IV	Till relapse	No	No	No

Table 5.2: Phases of DCP therapy with respect to pemphigus

*The duration of phase I depends on several factors including the severity of disease especially mucosal lesions.

day in between the pulses with or without additional daily or interval corticosteroids.

- *Phase II*: It is defined as the period when the patient remains completely alright clinically but receives 9 more DCPs at exactly 28-day cycles along with 50 mg cyclophosphamide orally per day. Originally, the duration of phase II was 6 months.
- *Phase III*: It is defined as the period of complete withdrawal of DCP. During this phase patient receives only 50 mg cyclophosphamide orally per day for the next 9 months.
- *Phase IV*: It includes stoppage of all treatment for pemphigus and the patient is followed up once a year for at least 10 years to look for a relapse, if any.

Modified DCP Regimen

Based on patients' requirements, modifications in the basic DCP have been proposed in the regimen for pulse therapy for pemphigus.

- **Additional corticosteroid requirements:** In patients who continue to get new lesions in phase I in between the pulses (i.e. phase I is getting unduly prolonged), patients need to be given additional oral corticosteroids, but patient will be considered to be in phase I as long as he is receiving corticosteroids, even if there is clinical remission. Two strategies can be adopted:
  - *Interval dexamethasone pulse*: Patient can be given additional dexamethasone, 100 mg, administered on 1 or 2 (consecutive) day(s) in between 2 DCPs (usually 2 weeks after the previous DCP).
  - *Additional daily dose of oral corticosteroids*: If patient continues to develop lesions even earlier than 2 weeks after the DCP or if the skin and mucosal involvement is extensive, patient can be given a daily dose of oral corticosteroids in addition to the monthly DCPs with or without additional DPs.
- **Omitting phase II:** In a randomized controlled trial, 20 pemphigus patients who completed phase I of DCP were randomized to receive either standard phase II or were directly shifted to phase III. Since there were no statistically significant differences in clinical and biochemical parameters between 2 groups at 9 months of follow-up, it was proposed that phase II can actually be omitted.[31] However, further studies with larger sample size and longer follow up are required.
- **Individualizing duration of therapy:** Instead of a total of 18 months for phases 2 and 3; based on clinical severity, immunofluorescence, and response to therapy, the duration may be shortened or extended in quick/slow responders.[2]
- **Modification of phase III:** To reduce the cumulative dose, only a bolus dose of cyclophosphamide 500 mg IV can be administered every 4 weeks for 9 months instead of oral daily 50 mg.[32]

- **Administration of mesna:** Bladder toxicity is reduced by administration of IV mesna during IV doses of cyclophosphamide. The dose of mesna is equivalent to cyclophosphamide dose in 5 divided doses over 24 hours. Moreover, cyclophosphamide-induced hemorrhagic cystitis is prevented by infusion of 500 ml of 5% dextrose with IV cyclophosphamide. During the cyclophosphamide infusion, the patient is advised to empty the bladder half hourly during infusion until 2 hours after the infusion.
- **Prevention of corticosteroid-induced osteoporosis:** This can be done by administration of calcium supplementation (500 mg/day), vitamin D (400 IU/day), and bisphosphonate (e.g. alendronate).
- **For taking care of concomitant diseases**[14]
  - *Diabetes mellitus*: In addition to continuing the antidiabetic therapy, 8 units of insulin are added to each unit of 500 ml of 5% dextrose in which the dexamethasone has been mixed.
  - *Hypertension*: Anti-hypertensives need to be continued/started without interrupting the corticosteroid therapy and blood pressure should be monitored regularly.
  - *Secondary infection*: Pulse therapy can be given under cover of antibiotics/antifungals. If the skin lesions or mucosal ulcers are heavily infected and there is a risk of dissemination of the infection and toxemia or patient develops herpes simplex/zoster, the administration of the pulse therapy can be delayed till the infection has been controlled. Alternatively, first few pulses can be given with dexamethasone alone without cyclophosphamide to avoid severe immunosuppression. For concomitant tuberculosis infection, the patient may receive pulse therapy after having received 4 weeks of anti-tuberculous therapy first.

Dexamethasone Pulse (DP)

- Dexamethasone, 50–100 mg is given intravenous for 3 consecutive days every 28 days.
- It is given when patient cannot be given cyclophosphamide (e.g. patients in reproductive age whose family is not complete, or when patient[f] is intolerant to or has developed side effects to cyclophosphamide).
- DP can be combined with azathioprine and methotrexate.

Methylprednisolone Pulse

- Methylprednisolone, 500–1000 mg is given intravenous, for 3 consecutive days every 28 days.
- Biggest drawback of this therapy is the cost of methylprednisolone.

---

[f]Cumulative dose of cyclophosphamide: Dose of >12 g of cyclophosphamide is known to cause azoospermia and a dose more than 30 g increases the risk of ovarian failure.

Oral Betamethasone Pulse (OBP)

- Betamethasone, 100 mg given orally, for 3 consecutive days every 28 days.
- This therapy is advantageous as it circumvents the need for hospital admission.
- It is often combined with weekly methotrexate.

Oral Mini Pulse (OMP)

- Oral minipulse (betamethasone/dexamethasone): 5–10 mg given orally, once/twice (usually on consecutive days) every week.
- It is given in rapidly spreading vitiligo and extensive alopecia areata.

Dexamethasone Azathioprine Pulse (DAP)

- Because high doses of cyclophosphamide can lead to azoospermia/amenorrhea,* it is best avoided in unmarried patients and in those who have not yet completed their family and substituted with other immunosuppressive agents like azathioprine or methotrexate.
- In DAP, cyclophosphamide is replaced by daily oral azathioprine 50 to 100 mg in phases I to III.
- No bolus dose of azathioprine is given during the pulse.
- It is a viable option for unmarried patients and those who have not completed their family as azathioprine does not induce gonadal dysfunction.

Dexamethasone Methotrexate Pulse (DMP)

- Cyclophosphamide is replaced by 7.5 mg of oral weekly methotrexate[g] (three doses of 2.5 mg at 12 hours apart), during the three phases of pulse therapy.
- Apart from DAP, DMP can also be considered in patients who have not completed their family.
- DMP is recommended for patients not responding to DCP/DAP after 12 pulses in phase 1.

CONTRAINDICATIONS

Absolute Contraindications

DCP is contraindicated in the following patients:
- Pregnant or lactating women
- Hypersensitivity to cyclophosphamide/corticosteroids
- In reproductive age group, in those whose family is not complete
- Bladder malignancy

Relative Contraindications

DCP is relatively contraindicated in following patients:
- Uncontrolled hypertension

---

[g]Methotrexate: Always given with folic acid 5 mg weekly, usually on the day after the methotrexate is given.

- Uncontrolled diabetes mellitus
- Acid peptic disease
- Cardiovascular disease
- Psychiatric disturbance
- Severe active infections

EVALUATION OF PATIENTS ON CORTICOSTEROID PULSE THERAPY

Base Line Evaluation[14]

Clinical Assessment

- A detailed clinical history and examination to look for duration of disease, extent and severity of disease, history of treatment taken in past, presence of concomitant systemic diseases and side effects of previous treatments is required prior to initiation of therapy.
- In elderly patients, cardiac assessment should be done.

Laboratory Evaluation

- The laboratory evaluation consists of a complete hemogram (hemoglobin, total leukocyte and platelet counts and erythrocyte sedimentation rate), blood sugar, blood pressure, blood urea, serum creatinine, serum glutamate transaminases, serum sodium and potassium, urinalysis, X-ray of the chest, and electro-cardiogram.
- Other tests are indicated depending upon the concomitant disease and side effects of previous treatments.
- Histopathology and direct immunofluorescence (DIF) help in the diagnosis of pemphigus.
- Immunological tests (desmoglein 1 and 3 levels) can be done to determine the severity of disease.

Investigations to be Done during and after Therapy

- During phase I, clinical assessment should be repeated at each visit to look for response of the disease and any adverse effects associated with therapy.
- Check regular blood levels of sugar and electrolytes before each pulse.
- Monitor pulse, respiratory rate, and blood pressure during infusion.
- In case of an arrhythmia, the infusion is discontinued. Electrocardiography and electrolytes are measured, and abnormalities are corrected.
- Seven days after last pulse therapy, routine blood, urine tests and chest X-ray should be repeated. Test for pemphigus antibody levels can be repeated at this stage to monitor the immunological response of therapy.
- These investigations should be repeated once again after 7 days of completing phase III of pulse therapy.

ADVANTAGES OF PULSE THERAPY

- Pulse therapy has revolutionized the therapy of pemphigus and has shown to result in rapid control of the disease with faster healing of skin lesions in pemphigus (Table 5.3).
- The side effects such as weight gain, cushingoid obesity, diabetes, hypertension, gastric hyperacidity, osteoporosis, cataract, acne, striae, hirsutism, etc. are less common with dexamethasone pulse therapy as compared to conventional daily oral corticosteroids.
- Dexamethasone is more readily available and inexpensive as compared to methylprednisolone and the therapy can be administered in day care centres.

Table 5.3: Clinical trials and case series on DCP therapy in pemphigus			
Authors, years of publication	Adjuvant treatment	No. of patients	Results
Pasricha et al, 1992[8]	Cyclophosphamide, prednisolone	5	CR in all
Pasricha et al, 1995[10]	Cyclophosphamide	300	Of 227 patients who completed treatment, CR190 (84%), 10% remission on treatment, 5% active disease on treatment, 30% relapse, responded to further course of DCP
Rao et al, 2003[11]	Cyclophosphamide or azathioprine	41	CR 22/34 (51.8%) with DCP, 3/7 (42.8%), 6 relapses
Mahajan et al, 2005[12]	DCP group: Cyclophosphamide, prednisolone DP group: Azathioprine or dapsone Injectable triamcinolone acetonide group Azathioprine or dapsone Betamethasone oral mini pulse therapy (OMP) group: No adjuvant	DCP: 33 DP: 14 Injectable triamcinolone acetonide: 6 OMP: 2	DCP: CR 2, remission on treatment 11, 20 active disease on treatment DP: 3 patients remission on treatment, 11 active disease on treatment Injectable triamcinolone acetonide: only one patient completed treatment with CR, who relapsed in phase III OMP: Both patient CR followed by relapse
Pasricha et al, 2008[14]	Cyclophosphamide, betamethasone	143	123 patients completed treatment, all in CR
Appelhans et al, 1993[15]	Cyclophosphamide	20	CR 65%, PR 20%, no change 15%
Roy R et al, 1997[16]	Cyclophosphamide	37	Of 20 patients on treatment, CR 40%, 60% active disease
Toth et al, 2002[17]	Prednisolone	14	CR 7 (50%)

(Contd.)

Table 5.3: Clinical trials and case series on DCP therapy in pemphigus (*Contd.*)

Authors, years of publication	Adjuvant treatment	No. of patients	Results
Kanwar *et al*, 2002[18]	Cyclophosphamide, prednisolone	36	CR 88%, PR 22 %
Masood *et al*, 2003[19]	Cyclophosphamide, prednisolone	30	CR 45%, remission on treatment 33%
Pasricha *et al*, 2003[20]	Cyclophosphamide, prednisolone	500	384 patients completed treatment and all achieved CR
Sacchidan *et al*, 2003[21]	Cyclophosphamide, prednisolone	50	CR 12%, remission on treatment 50%, active disease 24%
Rose *et al*, 2005[22]	DCP: cyclophosphamide Methylprednisolone Azathioprine therapy (M/A): daily doses	DCP-11 M/A-11	DC pulse: 5/11 CR, 6/11 progression M/A: 9/11 CR, 1/11 progression, more relapses in M/A group
Momeni *et al*, 2007[23]	Cyclophosphamide	50	38 finished study, CR 55%, 26% healing stage, 13% partially healed, 5% died
Kandan *et al*, 2009[24]	Cyclophosphamide, prednisolone	65	CR 13 patients, 19 patients remission on treatment, 33 active disease
Sethy *et al*, 2009[25]	DCP plus oral cyclophosphamide (DCP+C) Cyclophosphamide plus oral prednisolone (CP+P)	DCP+C–15 CP+P–13	DCP+C:60% CR, CP+P:60% CR, comparable relapse rates
Zivanovic *et al*, 2010[26]	Cyclophosphamide	72	CR 43 patients, 13 no response, 9 lost follow up, 7 died
Hassan *et al*, 2014[27]	DCP, Dexamethasone Azathioprine Pulse (DAP), Dexamethasone Methotrexate Pulse (DMP)	DCP:30 DAP:12 DMP:5	DCP: CR in all, relapse in 3 DAP: High relapses, 5 in phase III, 4 in phase IV DMP: CR in 1 patient followed by relapse
Mentink *et al*, 2006[28]	Dexamethasone Pulse (DP) or Placebo Pulse (PP) with oral prednisolone and azathioprine	DP: 11, PP:9	DP: CR 8 of 11, PP:CR in all

DP: Dexamethasone pulse, DCP: Dexamethasone cyclophosphamide pulse, DAP: Dexamethasone azathioprine pulse, CP: Cyclophosphamide pulse, P: Prednisolone.
CR: Complete remission, PR: Partial remission.

OTHER INDICATIONS OF DCP

Autoimmune bullous diseases other than pemphigus: Other autoimmune bullous diseases as severe bullous pemphigoid, paraneoplastic pemphigus and cicatricial pemphigoid have shown good response to DCP therapy in small case series (Figs 5.3 to 5.6).[33–35]

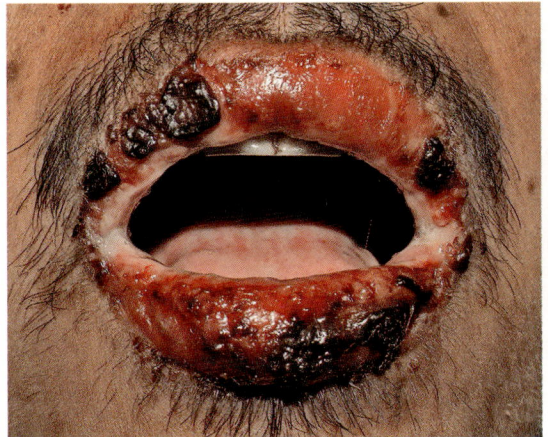

Fig. 5.3: Paraneoplastic pemphigus patient with severe recalcitrant mucosal erosions.

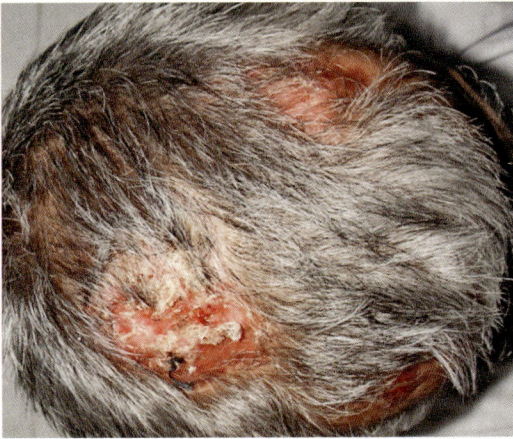

Fig. 5.4: Scarring lesion on scalp in a patient of cicatricial pemphigoid.

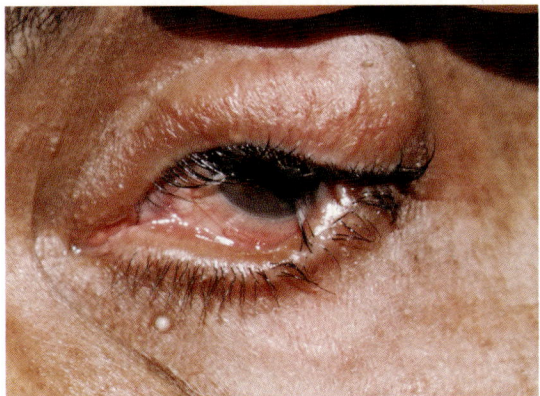

Fig. 5.5: Ocular scarring in a patient of cicatricial pemphigoid.

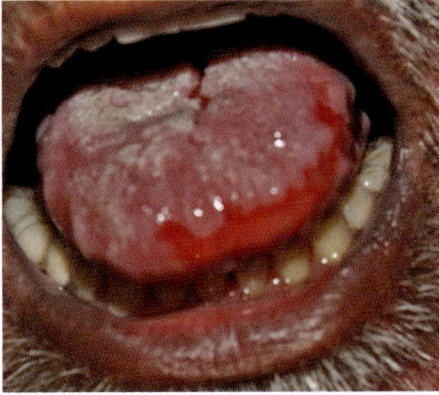

Fig. 5.6: Mucosa of cicatricial pemphigoid exhibiting sever scarring and erosions.

Collagen Vascular Disorders

- *Systemic Sclerosis (SSc):* Pasricha et al[36] (1990) reported the first case of SSc who was successfully treated with monthly dexamethasone pulses and subsequently published a series of 100 patients successfully treated initially with DP and later with DCP.[37] It has since been shown to improve various clinical parameters of SSc patients in many case series and trials.[38-43] It has been observed that rheumatological symptoms disappear within 3 months, skin starts softening within 3–6 months, dysphagia and dyspnoea improve substantially within 3–6 months, and though fingertip ulcers heal quickly, Raynaud's phenomenon is slow to respond (Figs 5.7 and 5.8).
- *Systemic lupus erythematosus (SLE):* Several studies have shown good response in various clinical (fever, malar rash, joint pain, oral ulceration, and occasionally in photosensitivity) and laboratory (renal function, proteinuria, ESR) parameters of LE when patients are treated with DCP/DP.[44] Response is early, observed in most patients after the 1st pulse in almost all the cases.

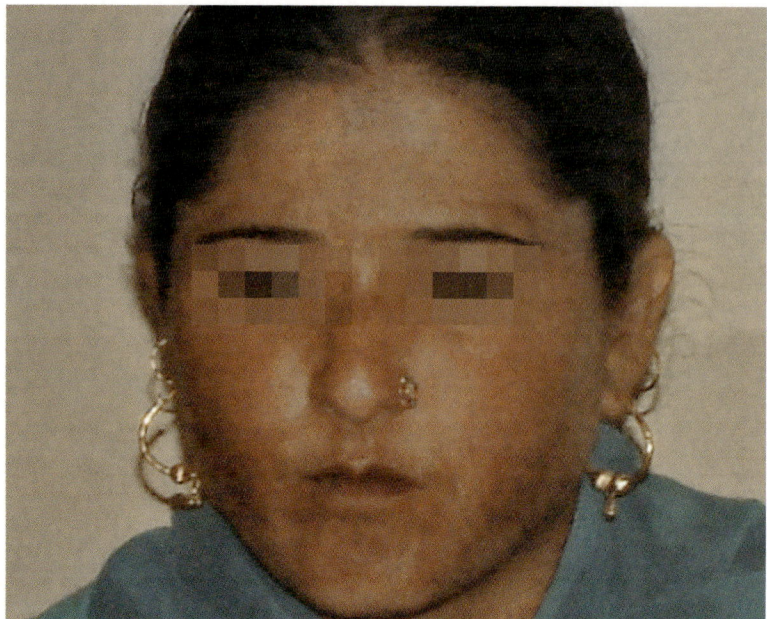

Fig. 5.7: Facial binding down of skin resulting in characteristic facies in a patient of systemic sclerosis.

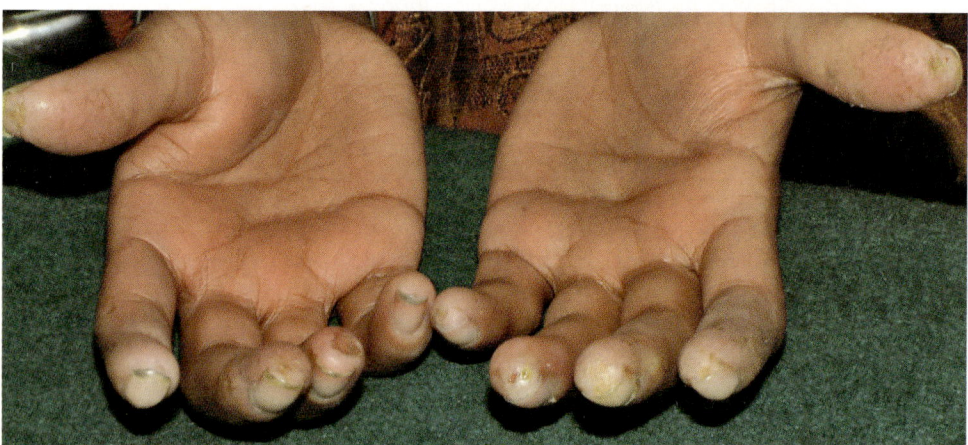

Fig. 5.8: Raynaud's phenomenon in a patient of systemic sclerosis.

Miscellaneous Conditions

- *Alopecia areata*: Pulsed doses of injectable and oral corticosteroids have shown to be beneficial in alopecia areata,[45] alopecia totalis and universalis.[46, 47] Short disease duration (<6 months), younger age at disease onset (<10 years) and multifocal disease are considered positive prognostic factors. However, studies with longer follow-up periods are required to evaluate the long-term remissions (Fig. 5.9).
- *Pyoderma gangrenosum*: Pasricha et al[48] had treated 3 patients with multiple, large necrotic ulcers on the extremities and trunk with 3 days DP given at 2-week intervals with an excellent response (Fig. 5.10).

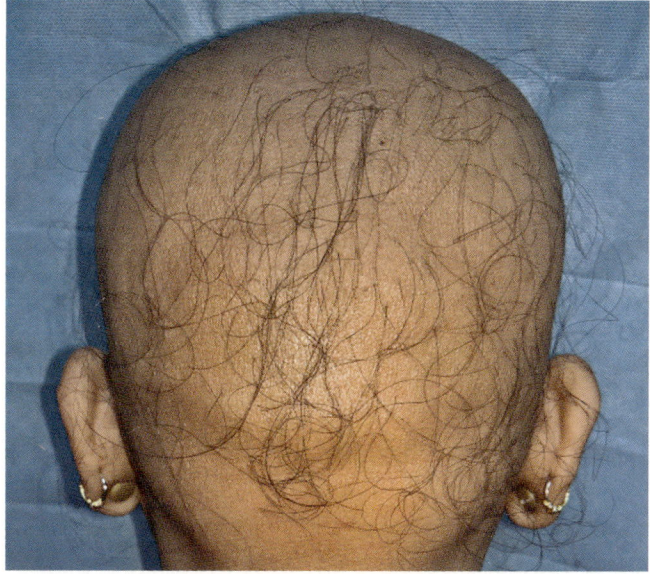

Fig. 5.9: Alopecia totalis resulting in loss of hairs over scalp and eyebrows.

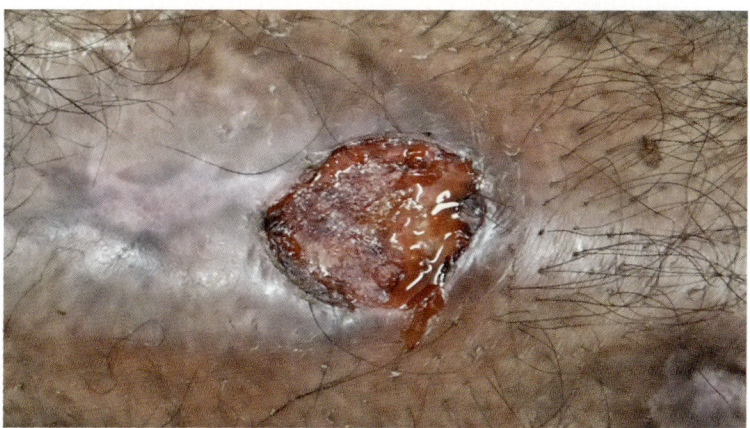

Fig. 5.10: Pyoderma gangrenosum ulcer with violaceous raised margin and granulating floor.

ADVERSE EFFECTS OF CORTICOSTEROID PULSE THERAPY

Though generally safe, some adverse effects are noted with administration of DP/DCP.[49] Many of these are infrequent compared to conventional daily oral corticosteroid therapy, but some like hiccups, facial flushing, headache, diarrhea and weakness are peculiar to corticosteroid pulse therapy. Fortunately, most patients are able to tolerate these symptoms, not warranting withdrawal of therapy.

- *Immediate adverse events*: Are noted during or within few hours of administration of DP/DCP and even other corticosteroid pulse therapies. Common (and specific to DCP/DP therapy) immediate complications include facial flushing, headache, diarrhea and weakness/numbness of feet. Patients also often complain of polyuria, tiredness, fever, chills and rigor, myalgia and arthralgia, headache, insomnia, dysguesia, nausea and vomiting. Irritability, anorexia, epigastric pain/dyspepsia, cough, dyspnea, chest pain, hypotension, sleep disturbances, mental confusion/psychosis, sweating, sore throat, facial puffiness and pedal edema, constipation, pruritus, urticaria, electrolyte abnormalities, cardiac arrhythmias[h] and seizures have also been reported, albeit rarely.

- *Delayed adverse events*: Are seen within few months to years of initiation of DP/DCP and other corticosteroid pulse therapies. The adverse events include:
  - Those which occur while patient is on corticosteroid pulse therapy include metabolic problems (weight gain, diabetes mellitus, hypertension, cushingoid habitus), infections (oral candidiasis, furuncles and cellulitis, dermatophytosis, Kaposi's varicelliform eruption, herpes zoster, molluscum contagiosum, HPV infections, reactivation of pulmonary tuberculosis and pneumonia), generalized hyperpigmentation, generalized pruritus, nail pigmentation, leukopenia, acneiform eruptions, haemorrhagic cystitis and deep vein thrombosis (Figs 5.11 to 5.14). Kumrah et al (2001) evaluated the pituitary adrenal function following DCP and found that 55% patients had suppressed hypothalamic-pituitary axis after 4 to 6 weeks of the last DCP of phase II. Though, the clinical significance of this finding is unclear, these patients may require corticosteroid supplementation during stress periods.[50]
  - Those which occur while patient is on therapy or may occur even on stopping therapy include cataract, menstrual disturbances/amenorrhea, azoospermia, diffuse scalp hair loss, avascular osteonecrosis of head of femur and osteopenia.

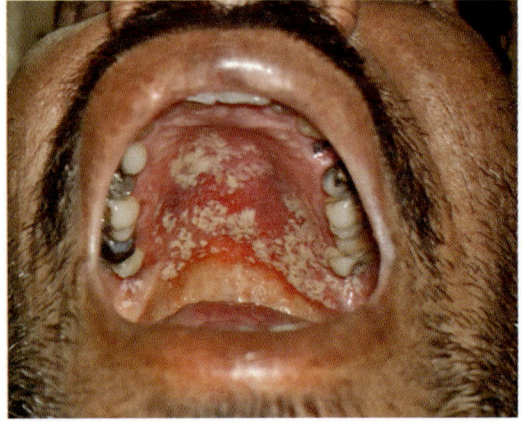 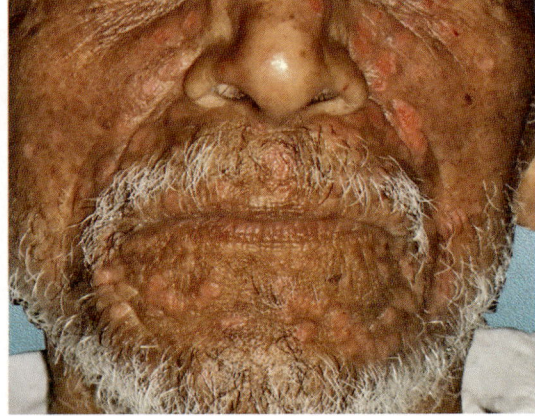

Fig. 5.11: Oral candidiasis following dexamethasone pulse therapy.

Fig. 5.12: Kaposi's varicelliform eruptions in a patient following dexamethason cyclophosphamide pulse therapy.

[h]Jain et al (2005) studied the cardiovascular side effects of DCP therapy in 30 patients and noticed that 2 patients developed asymptomatic ventricular arrhythmias and 10 patients developed sinus bradycardia. Acute cardiac complications are more commonly reported with methylprednisolone pulse therapy.

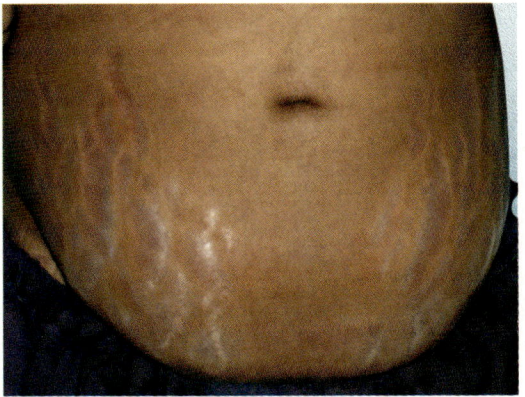

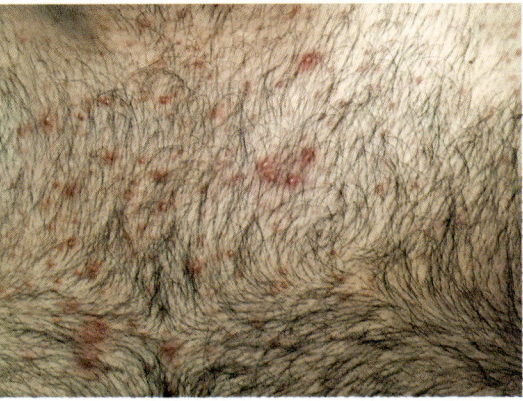

Fig. 5.13: Steroid pulse therapy induced cushingoid habitus and striae.

Fig. 5.14: Steroid pulse therapy induced acneiform eruptions.

REFERENCES

1. Pasricha JS. Pulse therapy in pemphigus and other diseases. 3rd ed. Pulse Therapy and Pemphigus Foundation. New Delhi; 2006.

2. Kountz SL, Cohn R. Initial treatment of renal allografts with large intrarenal doses of immuno-suppressive drugs. Lancet.1969;1:338–40.

3. Johnson RB, Lazarus GS. Pulse therapy: therapeutic efficacy in the treatment of pyoderma gangrenosum. Arch Dermatol. 1982;118:76–84.

4. Prystowsky JH, Kahn SN, Lazarus GS. Present status of pyoderma gangrenosum. Review of 21 cases. Arch Dermatol. 1989;125:57–74.

5. Pasricha JS, Gupta R. Pulse therapy with dexamethasone in Reiter's disease. Indian J Dermatol Venereol Leprol 1982;48:358–61.

6. Pasricha JS, Gupta R. Pulse therapy with dexamethasone-cyclophosphamide in pemphigus. Indian J Dermatol Venereol Leprol 1984;50:199–203.

7. Pasricha JS, Srivastava G. Cure in pemphigus-a possibility. Indian J Dermatol Venereol Leprol 1986;52:185–6.

8. Pasricha JS, Das SS. Curative effect of Dexamethason-Cyclophosphamide pulse therapy for the treatment of pemphigus vulgaris. Int J Dermatol 1992;31:875–877.

9. Pasricha JS, Khaitan BK, Raman RS, Chandra M. Dexamethasone-cyclophosphamide pulse therapy for pemphigus. Int J Dermatol 1995;34:875–882.

10. Pasricha JS, Khaitan BK. Curative treatment for pemphigus. Arch Dermatol 1996; 132:1518–1519.

11. Rao NP, Lakshmi TS. Pulse therapy and its modifications in pemphigus: A six year study. Indian J Dermatol Venereol Leprol 2003;69:329–33.

12. Mahajan VK, Sharma NL, Sharma RC, Garg G. Twelve year clinico-therapeutic experience in Pemphigus: A retrospective study of 54 cases. Int J Dermatol 2005; 44:821–7.

13. Kaur S, Kanwar AJ. Dexamethasone-cyclophosphamide pulse therapy in pemphigus. Int J Dermatol 1990; 29:37–4.

14. Pasricha JS, Poonam. Current regimen of pulse therapy for pemphigus: Minor modifications, improved results. Indian J Dermatol Venereol Leprol 2008:74:217–21.

15. Appelhans M, Bonsmann G, Orge C, Bröcker EB. Hautarzt. [Dexamethasone-cyclophosphamide pulse therapy in bullous autoimmune dermatoses]. 1993;44:143–7.

16. Roy R, Kalla G. Dexamethasone-Cyclophosphamide pulse (DCP) therapy in Pemphigus. Indian J Dermatol Venereol Leprol. 1997;63:354–6.

17. Toth GG, van de Meer JB, Jonkman MF. Dexamethasone pulse therapy in pemphigus. J Eur Acad Dermatol Venereol 2002;16:607–11.

18. Kanwar AJ, Kaur S, Thami GP. Long-term efficacy of dexamethasone-cyclophosphamide pulse therapy in pemphigus. Dermatology. 2002;204: 228–31.

19. Masood Q, Hassan I, Majid I, Khan D, Manzooi S, Qayoom S, et al. Dexamethasone cyclophosphamide pulse therapy in pemphigus: experience in Kashmir valley. Indian J Dermatol Venereol Leprol. 2003;69:97–9.

20. Pasricha J S. Pulse therapy as a cure for autoimmune diseases. Indian J Dermatol Venereol Leprol 2003;69:323–8.

21. Sacchidanand S, Hiremath NC, Natraj HV, Revathi TN, Rani S, Pradeep G, et al. Dexamethasone-cyclophosphamide pulse therapy for autoimmune-vesiculobullous disorders at Victoria hospital, Bangalore. Dermatol Online J. 2003;9:2.

22. Rose E, Wever S, Zilliken D, Linse R, Haustein UF, Bröcker EB Intravenous dexamethasone-cyclophosphamide pulse therapy in comparison with oral methylprednisolone-azathioprine therapy in patients with pemphigus: results of a multicenter prospectively randomized study.J Dtsch Dermatol Ges. 2005;3:200–6.

23. Momeni AZ, Iraji F, Aminjavaheri M, Emami MR, Momeni A. The use of oral cyclophosphamide with dexamethasone pulse therapy in the treatment of pemphigus vulgaris. J Dermatolog Treat. 2007;18:275–8.

24. Kandan S, Thappa DM. Outcome of dexamethasone-cyclophosphamide pulse therapy in pemphigus: A case series. Indian J Dermatol Venereol Leprol 2009;75:373–8.

25. Sethy PK, Khandpur S, Sharma VK. Randomized open comparative trial of dexamethasone-cyclophosphamide pulse and daily oral cyclophosphamide versus cyclophosphamide pulse and daily oral prednisolone in pemphigus vulgaris. Indian J Dermatol Venereol Leprol 2009;75:476–82.

26. Zivanovic D, Medenica L, Tanasilovic S, Vesic S, Skiljevic D, Tomovic M, et al. Dexamethasone-cyclophosphamide pulse therapy in pemphigus: a review of 72 cases. Am J Clin Dermatol. 2010;11: 123–9.

27. Hassan I, Sameem F, Masood QM, Majid I, Abdullah Z, Ahmad QM. Non comparative study on various pulse regimens (DCP, DAP and DMP) in pemphigus: Our experience. Indian J Dermatol 2014;59:30–4.

28. Mentink LF, Mackenzie MW, Tóth GG, Laseur M, Lambert FP, Veeger NJ, et al. Randomized controlled trial of adjuvant oral dexamethasone pulse therapy in pemphigus vulgaris: PEMPULS trial. Arch Dermatol. 2006;142:570–6.

29. Ramam M. Dexamethasone pulse therapy in dermatology. Indian J Dermatol Venereol Leprol 2003;69:319–22.

30. Menon V, Mehrotra A, Saxena R, Jaffery NF. Comparative evaluation of megadose methylprednisolone with dexamethasone for treatment of primary typical optic neuritis. Indian J Ophthalmol. 2007;55:355–9.

31. Parmar NV, Kanwar AJ, Minz RW, Parsad D, Vinay K, Tsuruta D, et al. Assessment of the therapeutic benefit of dexamethasone cyclophosphamide pulse *vs* only oral cyclophosphamide in phase II of dexamethasone cyclophosphamide pulse therapy: A preliminary prospective randomized controlled study. Indian J Dermatol Venereol Leprol 2013;79:70–6.

32. Ramam M. Prolonged antimicrobial and oral cyclophosphamide therapy in pemphigus: Need for caution. Indian J Dermatol Venereol Leprol. 2009;75:85.

33. Dawe RS, Naidoo DK, Ferguson J. Severe bullous pemphigoid responsive to pulsed intravenous dexamethasone and oral cyclophosphamide. Br J Dermatol. 1997;137:826–7.

34. Becker LR, Bastian BC, Wesselmann U, Karl S, Hamm H, Brocker EB. Paraneoplastic pemphigus treated with dexamethasone/cyclophosphamide pulse therapy. Eur J Dermatol 1998;8:551–3.

35. Axt M, Wever S, Baier G, Bogdan S, Hashimoto T, Bröcker EB, Zillikens D. [Cicatricial pemphigoid—a therapeutic problem]. Hautarzt. 1995;46:620–7.

36. Pasricha JS, Ramam M, Shah S. Reversal of systemic sclerosis with dexamethasone pulses. Indian J Dermatol Venereol Leprol 1990; 56: 40–2.

37. Pasricha J S. Systemic sclerosis and dexamethasone cyclophosphamide pulse therapy. Indian J Dermatol Venereol Leprol 2009;75:510–1.

38. Khaitan BK, Gupta S. Systemic sclerosis successfully treated with dexamethasone pulse therapy. Dermascan 1999;1:9–11.

39. Vatwani V, Palta SC, Verma N, Pathak PR, Singh RP. Pulse therapy in scleroderma, Indian Pediatr 1994;31:993–5.

40. Pai BS, Srinivas CR, Sabitha L, Shenoi SD, Balachandran CN, Acharya S. Efficacy of dexamethasone pulse therapy in progressive systemic sclerosis. Int J Dermatol 1995;34:726–8.

41. Sameem F, Hassan I, Ahmad QM, Khan D, Majeed I, Kamili MA, et al. Dexamethasone pulse therapy in patients of systemic sclerosis: is it a viable proposition? A study from Kashmir. Indian Journal of Dermatology. 2010;55:355–8.

42. Ahmad QM, Hassan I, Majid I. Evaluation of dexamethasone pulse therapy in systemic sclerosis. Indian J Dermatol Venereol Leprol. 2003;69:76–8.

43. Gupta R. Systemic sclerosis treated with dexamethasone pulse. Indian J Dermatol Venereol Leprol. 2003;69:191–2.

44. Dhabhai R, Kalla G, Singhi M K, Ghiya B C, Kachhawa D. Dexamethasone-cyclophosphamide pulse therapy in systemic lupus erythematosus. Indian J Dermatol Venereol Leprol 2005;71:9–13.

45. Friedland R, Tal R, Lapidoth M, Zvulunov A, Ben Amitai D. Pulse corticosteroid therapy for alopecia areata in children: a retrospective study. Dermatology. 2013;227:37–44.

46. Vañó-Galván S, Hermosa-Gelbard Á, Sánchez-Neila N, Miguel-Gómez L, Saceda-Corralo D, Rodrigues-Barata R, et al. Pulse corticosteroid therapy with oral dexamethasone for the treatment of adult alopecia totalis and universalis. J Am Acad Dermatol. 2016;74:1005–7.

47. Sharma VK, Gupta S. Twice weekly 5 mg dexamethasone oral pulse in the treatment of extensive alopecia areata. J Dermatol. 1999;26: 562–5.

48. Pasricha JS, Reddy R, Nandakishore Th, Khera V. Pyoderma gangrenosum treated with dexamethasone pulse therapy. Indian J Dermatol Venereol Leprol 1991;57:225–8.

49. Jain R, Kumar B. Immediate and delayed complications of dexamethasone cyclophosphamide pulse (DCP) therapy. J Dermatol. 2003;30:713–8.

50. Kumrah L, Ramam M, Shah P, Pandey RM, Pasricha JS. Pituitary-adrenal function following dexamethasone-cyclophosphamide pulse therapy for pemphigus. Br J Dermatol. 2001;145:944–8.

6

Complications of Systemic Steroids

Nikhil Mehta, Neetu Bhari

SUMMARY

- Glucocorticoids, by virtue of broad anti-inflammatory action through effect on multiple pathways, not only have multiple diverse indications for use, but also multiple diverse adverse effects.
- These adverse effects involve various systems.
- The adverse effects of glucocorticoid therapy depend upon the mode of administration, the dose and the duration for which the therapy is given.
- A high index of suspicion is required, particularly in patients on high dose or long-term treatment.
- More than 30–40% of patients receiving long-term glucocorticoid therapy have radiographic evidence of vertebral fractures while symptomatic fractures are seen in only one-third of these cases.
- High-dose glucocorticoid therapy decreases the effect of physiological growth hormone and impairs collagen synthesis. Use of systemic glucocorticoids in small doses for long term can cause significant growth suppression.
- Chronic glucocorticoid myopathy presents as a bilaterally symmetrical proximal muscle weakness starting in the lower extremities.
- Apart from development of new onset hyperglycemia or diabetes, glucocorticoid also worsen pre-existing diabetes resulting in difficulty in obtaining proper glycemic control.
- Long-term use of glucocorticoid and Cushing's disease exhibit similar type of lipid derangements in the form of increased total cholesterol and low-density lipoprotein cholesterol.
- Glucocorticoid-induced cushingoid syndrome is the commnest iatrogenic cause for this disease.
- With supraphysiological dose of glucocorticoids given for at least 4 weeks; hypothalamus, pituitary and adrenal secretion decreases via feedback mechanism.
- Long-term glucocorticoid therapy may also result in posteroid subcapsular cataract and gastrointestinal side effects.

- A pre-treatment baseline screening and regular screening for these adverse effects through history, examination and investigations as per guidelines is ideal.
- Each visit and renewal of prescription warrants an assessment for adverse effects, and treatment accordingly.

Dose

The European League Against Rheumatism (EULAR) defines the glucocorticoid dosing, on the basis of receptor saturation and side effects,[1] as:

Category	Dose (prednisolone equivalent per day)
Low	≤7.5 mg
Medium	7.5–30 mg
High	30–100 mg
Very high	>100 mg
Pulse dose	≥250 mg for one or a few days

A total cumulative dose is important as some studies indicate that long-term use of low doses of 5–7.5 mg/day can also cause significant adverse effects.[2]

Duration

The dosing can be classified as short-term, long-term or chronic based on the duration of use. Short-term dosing is considered when glucocorticoids have been used for less than 3 months.

Following is the list of potential adverse effects from the use of systemic corticosteroids.

1. Hypothalamic-pituitary-axis suppression	Steroid withdrawal syndrome Addisonian crisis
2. Metabolic	• Hyperglycemia • Dyslipidemia • Increased appetite • Weight gain • Cushingoid changes • Hypertension
3. Musculoskeletal	• Osteoporosis • Osteonecrosis • Myopathy (with muscle atrophy) • Hypocalcemia (indirectly)
4. Gastrointestinal	• Peptic ulcer disease • Bowel perforation • Fatty liver changes • Esophageal reflux • Nausea, vomiting

(Contd.)

5. Ocular	• Cataract • Glaucoma • Infections especially staphylococcal • Refraction changes (from corticosteroid induced hyperglycemia)
6. Psychiatric	• Psychosis • Agitation or personality change • Depression (prednisone phobia or dependency)
7. Neurologic	• Pseudotumor cerebri • Epidural lipomatosis • Peripheral neuropathy
8. Infectious	• Tuberculosis reactivation • Opportunistic-deep fungal, others • Prolonged herpes virus infections
9. Pediatric	• Growth impairment
10. Cutaneous	• Wound healing: Non-healing wounds, ulcers, striae, atrophy, telangiectasias • Pilosebaceous: Steroid acne, steroid rosacea • Vascular: Purpura, including actinic purpura • Infections: Staphylococcal, herpes virus infection • Hair effects: Telogen effluvium, hirsutism • Injectable: Fat atrophy, crystallization of injectable material • Other skin effects: Pustular psoriasis flare, acanthosis nigricans
11. Pulse therapy	• Flushing • Palpitations • Hiccups • Hyperglycemia • Hypertension • Electrolyte shifts • Cardiac dysrhythmias • Seizures • Generalized weakness • Psychosis, sleep disorder

OSTEOPOROSIS

Adverse effects on bone mass because of long-term use of glucocorticoid are classified as osteopenia and osteoporosis and are defined as below:

Category	T score on dual-energy X-ray absorptiometry (DEXA), S.D. below mean
Osteopenia	–1 to –2.5
Osteoporosis	<2.5

Osteoporosis can lead to fractures, which can present as acute back/or hip pain following trivial trauma. Osteoporosis due to long-term or chronic glucocorticoid therapy is the most prevalent form of secondary osteoporosis.

Mechanism of Action

Glucocorticoid induced osteoporosis has an early phase resulting from excessive bone resorption and a late phase secondary to decreased bone formation via its effect on osteoblasts.[3]

Glucorticoid use also results in a negative calcium balance as it inhibit calcium absorption from gastrointestinal tract and renal tubules resulting in excessive excretion. This leads to a subtle secondary hyperparathyroidism increasing the bone turnover.[4]

Features

More than 30–40% of patients receiving long-term glucocorticoid therapy have radiographic evidence of vertebral fractures while symptomatic fractures are seen in only one-third of these cases.[5,6]

There is predominance of vertebral and proximal femur fracture, due to marked trabecular bone loss because of its higher metabolic rate. Significant increase in the risk of fracture become apparent within 3 months of commencement of therapy and this risk further increases with increase in cumulative dose of glucocorticoid.

Though, long-term and high dose glucocorticoid therapy is implicated in causing osteoporosis and bone fractures, fractures can also be seen on doses as low as 2.5 mg of prednisone equivalent per day.[8] This fracture risk is reversible and decreases to baseline value after discontinuation of glucocorticoid therapy.[9]

Evaluation

A detailed history, clinical examination and evaluation is required (Table 6.1).

Table 6.1: Assessment of adverse effect of long-term glucocorticoid use on bone mass		
History	*Examination*	*Evaluation*
1. Dose and duration of use 2. Other significant risk factors such as • Malnutrition • Endocrine diseases as hypogonadism, secondary hyperpara-thyroidism and thyroid disease • Rheumatoid arthritis • Family history of hip fracture • History of alcohol abuse (significant if ≥3 units/ day) or smoking	1. Measurement of weight, height and muscle strength 2. Clinical evaluation for fracture as measurement of: • Bone tenderness • Joint deformity • Reduced space between lower ribs and upper pelvis	1. Bone mass density (BMD): within 6 months of starting glucocorti-coids in all patients >40 years of age or having any other risk factors for osteoporosis. FRAX (fracture risk assessment tool) is for all patients over 40 years of age within 6 months of starting glucocorticoids. A reassessment should be performed every year.

Management

a. *Risk Stratification*

Adults over the age of 40 years are stratified into low, moderate and high fracture risk using FRAX tool (Fig. 6.1).

A glucocorticoid adjusted FRAX 10 years hip fracture risk; ≤1%: low risk, 1–3%: moderate risk, and >3%: high risk.

Similarly, glucocorticoid adjusted FRAX 10 years risk for major osteoporotic fracture; <10%: low risk, 10–19%: moderate risk, and ≥20%: high risk.

Other points indicating to high fracture risk are prior history of osteoporotic fracture and DEXA T-score ≤–2.5 in men above 50 years of age and postmenopausal women.

b. *Treatment*

American College of Rheumatology (ACR) advises the following measures in patients receiving glucocorticoid therapy for prevention of osteoporosis (Fig. 6.2):

1. Daily calcium (1,000–1,200 mg/day) and vitamin D (600–800 IU/day; serum level ≥20 ng/ml) supplementation.
2. Lifestyle modifications (maintaining proper body weight, regular weight-bearing or resistance training exercise, smoking cessation, limiting alcohol intake).

For further treatment of osteoporosis:

Low fracture risk patients: no further treatment is recommended except yearly clinical reassessment and BMD every 2–3 years.

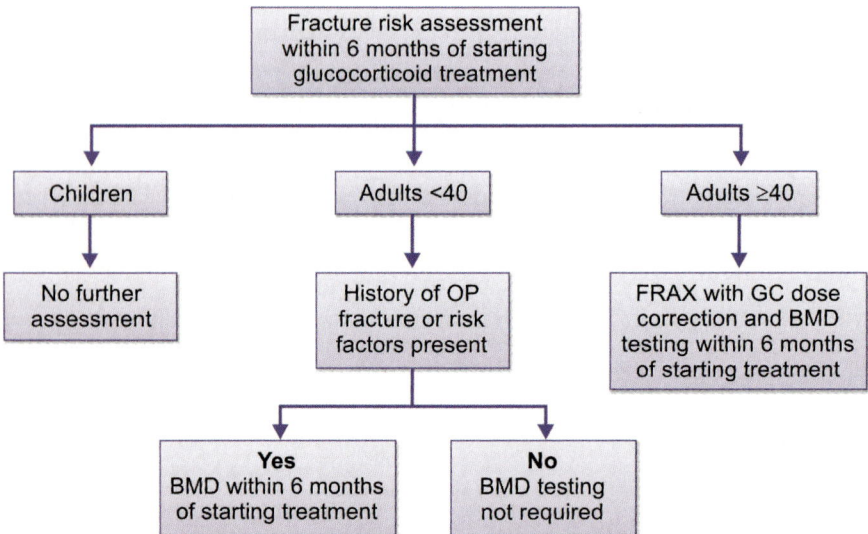

Fig. 6.1: Fracture risk evaluation in patients receiving long-term glucocorticoid therapy. (OP: Osteoporosis, BMD: Bone mass density, FRAX: Fracture risk assessment tool, GC: Glucocorticoids) *Adapted from*: American College of Rheumatology Guideline for the Prevention and Treatment of Glucocorticoid-induced Osteoporosis, 2017.

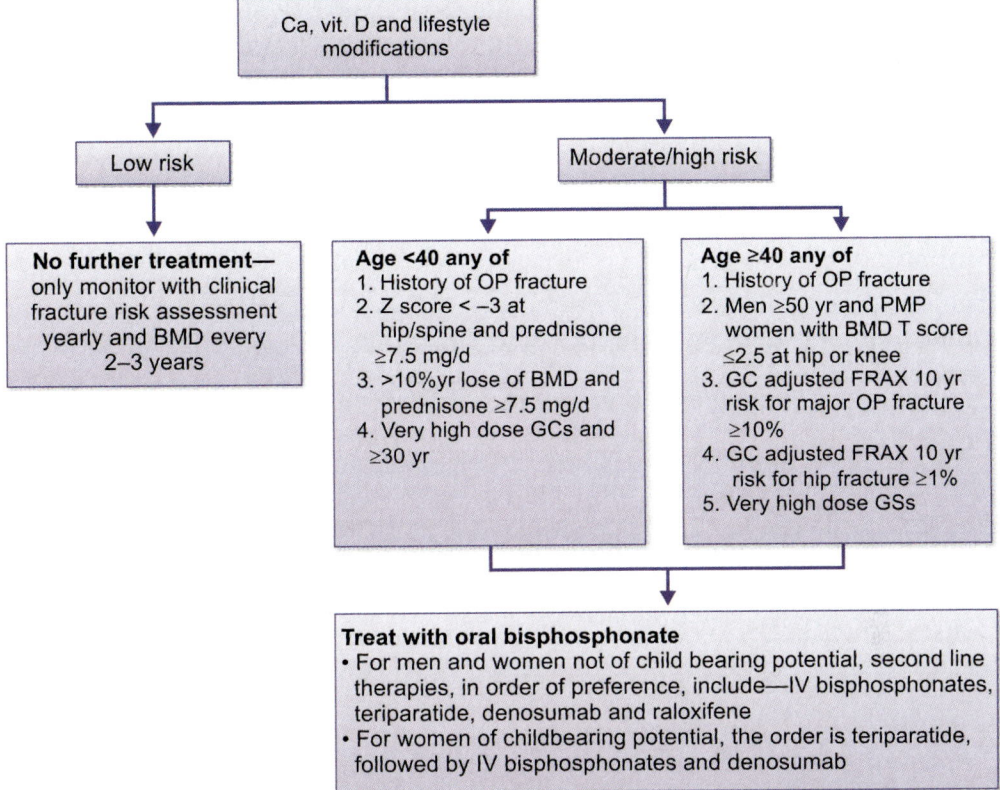

Fig. 6.2: Management of osteoporosis in patients receiving glucocorticoid therapy according to American College of Rheumatology.
Adapted from: American College of Rheumatology Guideline for the Prevention and Treatment of Glucocorticoid-induced Osteoporosis, 2017.

Moderate and high risk patients:

- Oral bisphosphonate is the first line of choice for treatment in men and women not of childbearing potential.
- Intravenous bisphosphonate is alternative first line treatment, preferred when there is low tolerance or compliance with oral dose.
- Teriparatide and denosumab are second line agents.
- Raloxifene can be used for postmenopausal women if no other therapy is available.
- For women of child-bearing potential, oral bisphosphonates and teriparatide are first and second line drugs respectively. Not enough evidence exists for safety of IV bisphosphonates and denosumab in pregnancy.

OSTEONECROSIS

Osteonecrosis is avascular necrosis of the bone marrow resulting in localised bone pain during activity. It most commonly occurs at the proximal femur. Distal femur and proximal tibia may also be involved. Chronic high-dose glucocorticoid therapy may result in osteonecrosis in 9–40% of patients and the risk increases with increase in dose.[10,11] A high dose for short term may also cause osteonecrosis.[12] Necrosis results from decreased blood supply to bone marrow, caused by increase bone marrow fat deposition due to glucocorticoids, which takes 6 to 12 months.[13] Other postulated mechanisms include fat embolism,[14] intravascular coagulation,[15] stress fractures, and osteocyte apoptosis due to glucocorticoids.

Evaluation

Evaluation for osteonecrosis is required in a patient on long term glucocorticoid therapy presenting with hip pain. An MRI (magnetic resonance imaging) is more sensitive to bone marrow changes than an X-ray.

Treatment

Treatment is conservative in early stages, including rest and reduced weight bearing. In late stages, it involves specialised orthopedic surgeries and may include a hip replacement.

GROWTH RETARDATION

High dose glucocorticoid therapy decreases the effect of physiological growth hormone and impair collagen synthesis.

Use of systemic glucocorticoids in small doses for long term can cause significant growth suppression.[16,17] Alternate day therapy can decrease this effect.

Compensatory growth spurt follows on discontinuing the glucocorticoid therapy and the final result is achievement of targeted height.

Evaluation and Treatment

Evaluation includes serial measurement of height to assess growth velocity.

Growth hormone therapy can be used in severe cases.[18,19]

MYOPATHY

Chronic glucocorticoid myopathy presents as a bilaterally symmetrical proximal muscle weakness starting in the lower extremities. The muscles are painless and nontender.[20] Glucocorticoids decreases the rate of protein synthesis and increases the protein breakdown which results to muscle atrophy.[21]

The acute form occurs frequently in ICU setting, presenting as rapidly progressive weakening of the proximal muscles, but can also involve distal muscles. Respiratory muscles may also be involved.[22] The chronic form of myopathy results in painless muscle weakness affecting the proximal muscles and it develop insidiously. It progresses very slowly and leads to muscle atrophy. This side effect is associated with long-term use of glucocorticoid in high doses, especially with fluorinated glucocorticoids.[21]

Evaluation and Treatment

Glucocorticoid induced myopathy is diagnosed clinically. It can be differentiated from inflammatory myopathy as in glucocorticoid induced myopathy muscle enzymes and electromyographic studies are generally normal[21] and muscle biopsy findings are non specific without any inflammation.

Patient may have increased urinary creatine excretion,[23] which is not found in inflammatory myopathy. No treatment to cure steroid induced myopathy exists, except tapering steroids. Patients take many months to recover and may not return to baseline.

HYPERGLYCEMIA AND DIABETES

Glucocorticoids cause steroid induced diabetes. The incidence of hyperglycermia induced by glucocorticoid therapy is 12% while glucocorticoid induced hypergly-cemia in hospital settings is almost 50%.[24–26] Up to 2% of incident cases of diabetes were associated with use of long-term glucocorticoid therapy in a primary care population.[27]

Proposed risk factors for glucocorticoid induced hyperglycemia and diabetes are:

- Higher cumulative dose and longer duration of glucocorticoid therapy,
- Previous history of diabetes or impaired glucose intolerance,
- A higher prevalence of comorbidities, and
- Older age[25]

Apart from development of new onset hyperglycemia or diabetes, glucocorticoid also worsen pre-existing diabetes resulting in difficulty in obtaining proper glycaemic control.

Postprandial hyperglycemia is a characteristic feature of intermediate acting glucocorticoid with once daily morning dose.[28–30] An alternate day regimen does not improve the risk of hyperglycemia and is difficult to implement in diabetic patients as a change in insulin will be required every alternate day.[31]

Mechanism of Action

1. Glucocorticoid increases gluconeogenesis in liver resulting in increased endogenous glucose synthesis.
2. Glucocorticoid decreases insulin secretion in pancreas by inhibiting beta cells.
3. Glucocorticoid reduces insulin sensitivity in skeletal muscle, decreasing peripheral glucose uptakes. Glucocorticoid also impair insulin sensitivity in adipose tissue further decreasing peripheral insulin uptake. They affect insulin sensitivity by modulating the activity of adipokines.[32]
4. Glucocorticoids induces insulin resistance via upregulation of nuclear peroxisome proliferator-activated receptor (PPARα).[33]

Patients return to their pretherapy glucose status within few months of stopping glucocorticoid therapy.

Due to insulin resistance, patients also develop hypertriglyceridemia so the diabetic diet should be further modified to decrease saturated and trans fat.

Evaluation

Blood sugar monitoring should be started with initiation of glucocorticoid therapy.[34]

Most of the patient develop hyperglycemia within initial 1–2 days of glucocorticoid therapy, thus early initiation of monitoring helps in timely detection of hyperglycemia with an effective management. If no derangement of blood sugar is noted in first 24–48 hours, the monitoring can be discontinued.[26]

Treatment

Management of glucocorticoid induced diabetes mellitus is different from nonsteroid induced diabetes. Insulin is used more frequently and at lower glucose levels than nonsteroid induced diabetes.

Preprandial glucose levels <200 mg/dL with no associated risk factors: Dietary changes and regular exercise with or without oral hypoglycemic agents. Metformin is usually less preferred for glucocorticoid induced diabetes mellitus because of associated comorbidities.

Preprandial glucose levels >200 mg/dL: Subcutaneous insulin with adjusted doses.[35] Larger doses may be required in the beginning due to insulin resistance.[36] The doses can be gradually reduced once glucose levels are controlled.[24,34] The further doses need to be adjusted with change in dose of glucocorticoids.

DYSLIPIDEMIA

Effect of glucocorticoid on lipid metabolism is multifactorial. Long-term use of glucocorticoid and Cushing's disease exhibit similar type of lipid derangements in the form of increased total cholesterol and low-density lipoprotein cholesterol.[37]

Evaluation and Treatment

A baseline lipid profile followed by regular monitoring should be done in patients receiving long-term glucocorticoid therapy. No specific guidelines exist about frequency of monitoring on long term for this purpose. Dyslipidemia can be prevented and managed as per the usual guidelines of general practise.

HPA AXIS SUPPRESSION

With any supra physiological dose given for at least 4 weeks; hypothalamus, pituitary and adrenal secretion decreases via feedback mechanism.

A systematic review has shown 37% prevalence of adrenal insufficiency in patient receiving glucocorticoid therapy. This insufficiency persisted in 15% of patients after 3 years of treatment cessation. The suppression was not related to dose and duration of therapy as it was seen at a dose as low as 5 mg of prednisolone equivalent and duration as less as 4 weeks.

Evaluation and Treatment

Less than 10 micrograms per decilitre of morning serum cortisol levels suggest HPA axis suppression.[38–40]

Generally, 10 mg/week tapering of glucocorticoid till reaching 40 mg/week, then 5 mg/week till reaching 10–20 mg/week, followed by 2.5 mg/week is helpful, but it can be modified according to individual needs. A rapid daily tapering can be done in patients experiencing severe adverse effects.[40]

Patients with adrenal suppression will require supplementation of stress dosing of glucocorticoid during major illnesses, surgeries or any other stressful conditions.

CUSHINGOID SYNDROME

Glucocorticoid induced cushingoid syndrome is the commnest iatrogenic cause for this disease. The clinical manifestation are identical to primary Cushing syndrome in the form of moon facies, central obesity, supraclavicular fat pads, muscle weakness involving proximal muscles, striae distensae and hypertension (Figs 6.3 to 6.6).[41]

Management includes reducing the dose and duration of glucocorticoid therapy.

CATARACT

A posterior subcapsular cataract is the most common type of cataract in patients of long term and/or high dose steroid use.

Cataract development is not decreased by alternate day therapy.

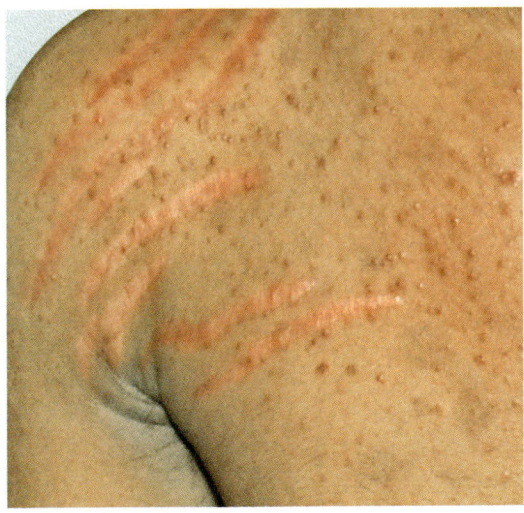

Fig. 6.3: Systemic steroid-induced striae and acneiform eruptions.

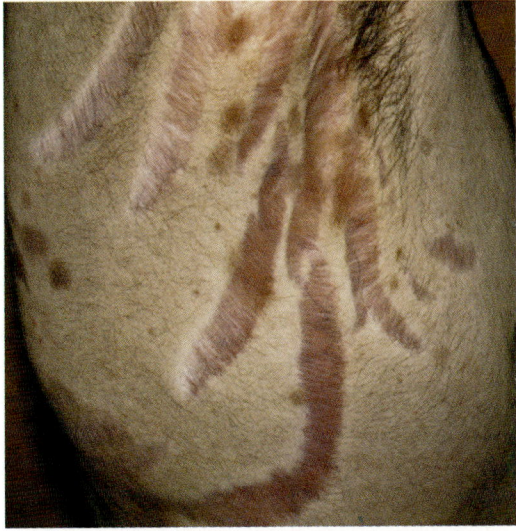

Fig. 6.4: Systemic steroid-induced striae.

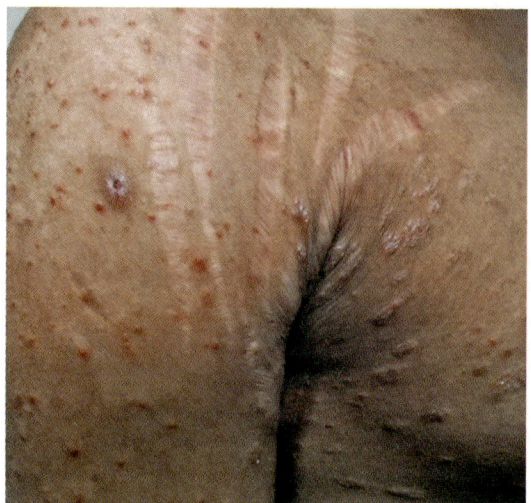
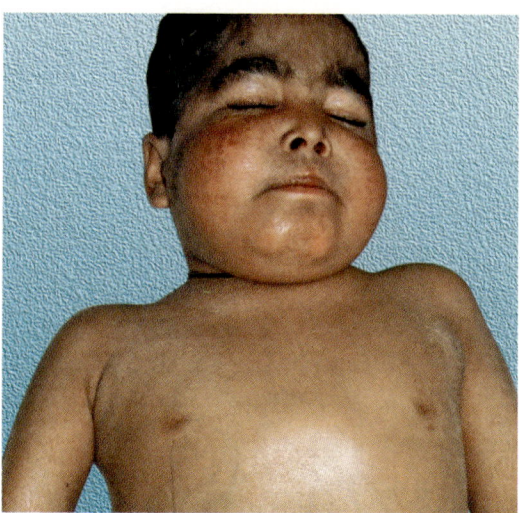

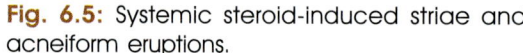

Fig. 6.5: Systemic steroid-induced striae and acneiform eruptions.

Fig. 6.6: Systemic steroid-induced cushingoid features.

Evaluation and Treatment

Patients on glucocorticoid therapy should be ophthalmologically evaluated every 6 to 12 months or even 3–4 times per year for patients on long term therapy.[42]

Cataract may progress despite discontinuing glucocorticoid therapy and require standard interventions.

GASTROINTESTINAL ADVERSE EFFECTS

Glucocorticoids conventionally have been associated with gastritis, GI bleeding, peptic ulcer disease, perforation and pancreatitis.

But the risk of these adverse effects with glucocorticoid monotherapy in absence of any other risk factor is minimal to low, with relative risk of gastrointestinal effects compared to control group ranging from 1.1 to 1.5.[43,44]

Various meta-analyses have found no significant increased risk (up to 40% more) in hospitalized patients of gastrointestinal bleeding and perforation as compared to placebo.[45,46] They indicate that peptic ulcer is a rare complication of systemic glucocorticoid therapy and occurs in 0.4–1.8% of patients.[47]

Despite the evidence from clinical studies, a majority of physicians believe that glucocorticoid monotherapy leads to significant increase in risk of ulcers,[48] in part due to evidence from experimental ulcers in animals.[49]

Glucocorticoids primarily decrease the regeneration and healing of gastrointestinal mucosa, which is compounded by simultaneous NSAID therapy. With simultaneous NSAIDS therapy the relative risk rises to 4.4.[1] Hence, a prophylactic therapy with proton pump inhibitors is advised for patients on glucocorticoid therapy with simultaneous NSAID therapy.[50]

Risk of acute pancreatitis is about 1.5 times more in patients using glucocorticoids as compared to control group. It is maximum from 4 to 14 days on starting glucocorticoids and gradually decreases after 14 days.[51] Patient on glucocorticoids is managed according to routine guidelines for acute pancreatitis.

REFERENCES

1. F. Buttgereit, J.A. Da Silva, M. Boers, et al. Standardised nomenclature for glucocorticoid dosages and glucocorticoid treatment regimens: current questions and tentative answers in rheumatology. 2002, Ann Rheum Dis,61:718–22.

2. Huscher D, Thiele K, Gromnica-Ihle E, et al. Dose-related patterns of glucocorticoid-induced side effects. Am Rheum Dis. 2009;68:1119–24.

3. Lukert BP, Raisz LG. Glucocorticoid-induced osteoporosis: pathogenesis and management. Ann Intern Med. 1990;112:352–64.

4. Canalis E. Mechanisms of glucocorticoid action in bone: implications to glucocorticoid-induced osteoporosis. J Clin Endocrinol Metab. 1996;81:3441–7.

5. Curtis J, Westfall AO, Allison J, et al. Population-based assessment of adverse events associated with long-term glucocorticoid use. Arthritis Rheum. 2006;55:420–6.

6. Angeli A, Guglielmi G, Dovio A, et al. High prevalence of asymptomatic vertebral fractures in post-menopausal women receiving chronic glucocorticoid therapy: a cross-sectional outpatient study. Bone. 2006;39:253–9.

7. Van Staa TP, Leufkens HG, Abenhaim L, Zhang B, Cooper C. Use of oral corticosteroids and risk of fractures. J Bone Miner Res. 2000;15:993.

8. Gluck OS, Murphy WA, Hahn TJ, Hahn B. Bone loss in adults receiving alternate day glucocorticoid therapy. A comparison with daily therapy. Arthritis Rheum. 1981;24:892.

9. Weinstein RS. Glucocorticoid-induced osteoporosis and osteonecrosis. Endocrinol Metab Clin North Am. 2012;41:595–611.

10. Davidson JK, Tsakiris D, Briggs JD, Junor BJ. Osteonecrosis and fractures following renal transplantation. Clin Radiol. 1985;36:27–35.

11. Taylor LJ. Multifocal avascular necrosis after short-term high-dose steroid therapy: a report of three cases. J Bone Joint Surg [Br]. 1984;66:431–3.

12. Hungerford DS, Lennox DW. The importance of increased intraosseous pressure in the development of osteonecrosis of the femoral head: implications for treatment. Orthop Clin North Am. 1985;16:635–54.

13. Jones JP. Fat embolism and osteonecrosis. Orthop Clin North Am. 1985;16:595–633.

14. Boettcher WG, Bonfiglio M, Hamilton HH, Sheets RF, Smith K. Nontraumatic necrosis of the femoral head. I. Relation of altered hemostasis to etiology. J Bone Joint Surg [Am]. 1970;52:312–21.

15. Simon D, Fernando C, Czernichow P, Prieur AM. Linear growth and final height in patients with systemic juvenile idiopathic arthritis treated with long-term glucocorticoids. J Rheumatol. 2002;29:1296–1300.

16. Allen DB, Mullen M, Mullen B. A meta-analysis of the effect of oral and inhaled corticosteroids on growth. J Allergy Clin Immunol. 1994;93:967–76.

17. Simon D, Lucidarme N, Prieur AM, Ruiz JC, Czernichow P. Effects on growth and body composition of growth hormone treatment in children with juvenile idiopathic arthritis requiring steroid therapy. J Rheumatol. 2003;30:2492–9.

18. Allen DB, Julius JR, Breen TJ, Attie KM. Treatment of glucocorticoid-induced growth suppression with growth hormone. National Cooperative Growth Study. J Clin Endocrinol Metab. 1998;83:2824–9.

19. Alshekhlee A, Kaminski HJ, Ruff RL. Neuromuscular manifestations of endocrine disorders. Neurol Clin. 2002;20:35–58.

20. Anagnos A, Ruffi RL, Kaminski H. Endocrine myopathies. Neurol Clin. 1997;15:673–96.

21. Van Balkom RH, van Der Heijden HF, van Herwaarden CL, Dekhuijzen PN. Corticosteroid induced myopathy of the respiratory muscles. Neth J Med. 1994;45:114–22.

22. Askari A, Vignos PJ Jr, Moskowitz RW. Steroid myopathy in connective tissue disease. Am J Med 1976; 61:485.

23. Gonzalez-Gonzalez JG, Mireles-Zavala LG, Rodriguez-Gutierrez R, Gomez-Almaguer D, Lavalle-Gonzalez FJ, Tamez-Perez HE, Gonzalez-Saldivar G, et al. Hyperglycemia related to high-dose glucocorticoid use in noncritically ill patients. Diabetol Metab Syndr 2013;5:18.

24. Donihi AC, Raval D, Saul M, Korytkowski MT, DeVita MA. Prevalence and predictors of corticosteroid-related hyperglycemia in hospitalized patients. Endocr Pract. 2006;12:358–62.

25. Fong AC, Cheung NW. The high incidence of steroid-induced hyperglycaemia in hospital. Diabetes Res Clin Pract. 2013;99:277–80.

26. Gulliford MC, Charlton J, Latinovic R. Risk of diabetes associated with prescribed glucocorticoids in a large population. Diabetes Care. 2006;29:2728–9.

27. Hirsch IB and Paauw DS. Diabetes management in special situations. Endocrinol Metab Clin North Am. 1997;26:631–45.

28. Gurwitz JH, Bohn RL, Glynn RJ, Monane M, Mogun H, Avorn J. Glucocorticoids and the risk for initiation of hypoglycemic therapy. Arch Intern Med. 1994;154:97–101.

29. Burt MG, Roberts GW, Aguilar-Loza NR, Frith P, Stranks SN. Continuous monitoring of circadian glycemic patterns in patients receiving prednisolone for COPD. J Clin Endocrinol Metab. 2011;96:1789–96.

30. Greenstone MA, Shaw AB. Alternate day corticosteroid causes alternate day hyperglycaemia. Postgrad Med J. 1987;63:761–4.

31. Clore JN, Thurby-Hay L. Glucocorticoid-induced hyperglycemia. Endocr Pract. 2009;15:469–74.

32. Perez A, Jansen-Chaparro S, Saigi I, Bernal-Lopez MR, Miñambres I, Gomez-Huelgas R. Glucocorticoid-induced hyperglycemia. J Diabetes. 2014;6:9–20.

33. Trence DL. Management of patients on chronic glucocorticoid therapy: an endocrine perspective. Prim Care. 2003;30:593–605.

34. Tamez-Pérez HE, Quintanilla-Flores DL, Rodriguez-Gutierrez R, Gonzales-Gonzales JG, Tamez-Peña AL.Steroid hyperglycemia: prevalence, early detection and therapeutic recommendations: a narrative review.World J Diabetes. 2015;6:1073–1081.

35. Umpierrez GE, Hellman R, Korytkowski MT, Kosiborod M, Maynard GA, Montori VM et al. Management of hyperglycemia in hospitalized patients in non-critical care setting: An endocrine society clinical practice guideline. Endocrine Society. J Clin Endocrinol Metab. 2012;97:16–38.

36. Hwang JL, Weiss RE. Steroid-induced diabetes: a clinical and molecular approach to understanding and treatment. Diabetes Metab Res Rev. 2014;30:96–102.

37. Arnaldi G, Scandali VM, Trementino L, Cardinaletti M, Appolloni G, Boscaro M. Pathophysiology of dyslipidemia in cushing's syndrome. Neuroendocrinology. 2010;92:86–90.

38. Joseph RM, Hunter AL, Ray DW, Dixon WG. Systemic glucocorticoid therapy and adrenal insufficiency in adults: A systematic review. Semin Arthritis Rheum. 2016;46(1):133–141.

39. Fauci AS. Alternate-day corticosteroid therapy. Am J Med. 1978;64:729–31.

40. Ackerman GL and Nolsn CM. Adrenocortical responsiveness after alternate-day corticosteroid therapy. N Engl J Med. 1968;278:405–9.

41. Hopkins RL, Leinung MC. Exogenous Cushing's syndrome and glucocorticoid withdrawal. Endocrinol Metab Clin North Am. 2005;34:371–84.

42. Renfro L, Snow JS. Ocular effects of topical and systemic steroids. Dermatol Clin. 1992;10:505–12.

43. Piper JM, Ray WA, Daugherty JR, Griffin MR. Corticosteroid use and peptic ulcer disease: role of nonsteroidal anti-inflammatory drugs. Ann Intern Med. 1991;114:735.

44. Messer J, Reitman D, Sacks HS, Smith H Jr, Chalmers TC. Association of adrenocorticosteroid therapy and peptic-ulcer disease. N Engl J Med. 1983;309:21.

45. Conn HO, Poynard T. Corticosteroids and peptic ulcer: meta-analysis of adverse events during steroid therapy. J Intern Med. 1994;236:619–32.

46. Narum S, Westergren T, Klemp M. Corticosteroids and risk of gastrointestinal bleeding: a systematic review and meta-analysis. BMJ Open, 2014;4:e004587.

47. Dorlo TP, Jager NG, Beijnen JH, Schellens JH. [Concomitant use of proton pump inhibitors and systemic corticosteroids]. Ned Tijdschr Geneeskd. 2013; 157:A5540.

48. Martínek J, Hlavova K, Zavada F, Seifert B, Rejchrt S, Urban O et al. "A surviving myth"— corticosteroids are still considered ulcerogenic by a majority of physicians. Scand J Gastroenterol. 2010;45:1156–61.

49. Carpani de Kaski M, Rentsch R, Levi S, Hodgson HJ. Corticosteroids reduce regenerative repair of epithelium in experimental gastric ulcers. Gut. 1995;37:613–6.

50. Scarpignato C, Gatta L, Zullo A, Blandizzi C. Effective and safe proton pump inhibitor therapy in acid-related diseases - A position paper addressing benefits and potential harms of acid suppression. BMC Medicine. 2016;14:179.

51. Sadr-Azodi O, Mattsson F, Bexlius TS, Lindblad M, Lagergren J, Ljung R. Association of oral glucocorticoid use with an increased risk of acute pancreatitis: a population-based nested case-control study. JAMA Intern Med. 2013;173:444.

7

Topical Steroid Abuse: Indian Perspective

Neha Taneja, Vishal Gupta

SUMMARY

- Topical steroid abuse is becoming rampant in India. Easy availability as over-the-counter drugs makes topical steroids vulnerable to their misuse. Other factors leading their abuse include wrong prescription, fraudulent marketing by pharmaceutical companies, use as 'fairness creams' and 'all-purpose' creams.
- There are several irrational combinations of topical steroids with antifungals and antibiotics available freely in the market.
- Common reasons for topical steroid abuse include their use as 'fairness creams', treatment for acne, fungal infections, pruritus, and as a cosmetic or skin cream for any type of rash.
- Betamethasone valerate is one of the most commonly abused steroid.
- Topical steroid damaged facies, a newly described entity associated with TSs abuse, is now being increasingly recognized.
- IADVL has formed a task force, IADVL Task force Against Topical Steroid Abuse (ITATSA) with main aims of raising public awareness, running media campaigns, forming study groups for doctors, highlighting the problem in journals, and meeting with central and state authorities.
- By including topical steroids under schedule H, their sale can be regulated. A coordinated approach among drug regulator, physicians, pharmacists and patients is vital to prevent misuse of TCs in India. Proper education, sensitization, regularization of prescriptions and strict legal rules and actions are essential to curb the topical steroid abuse menace.

INTRODUCTION

- Abuse is defined as inappropriate or excessive use of a drug. In recent years, there has been a dramatic increasein topical steroid abuse.
- Topical steroids (TSs), which came into existence more than 50 years ago have been used for decades to treat various dermatological disorders and are among the most commonly prescribed medications in dermatology.

- Various properties of TSs such as vasoconstrictive, immunosuppressive, anti-proliferative, anti-pruritic, atrophogenic, melanopenic and sex-hormone like effects lead to rapid response in many dermatoses including infections. Unfortunately these effects have now become responsible for the myriad deleterious effects of TSs.
- In India, their free availability over the counter (OTC) without prescription has made them prone for abuse, increasing the risk of local and systemic side effects. Betamethasone valerate is the most favored preparation, being popular due to the misconception of it being fairness and anti-acne cream.

HISTORICAL ASPECTS OF TOPICAL STEROIDS AND THEIR ABUSE

- Sulzberger in 1951, introduced the first TS, topical hydrocortisone, then known as "Compound F". An year later, in 1952, an article on the utility of topically applied compound F in dermatology was published by Sulzberger and Witten.
- A large number of modifications of the original Compound F (Hydrocortisone) were discovered in rapid succession. Based on their vasoconstrictive properties, they have been variously classified, viz. Fluorohydrocortisone (1955); Triamcinolone acetonide (1958); Fluocinolone acetonide (1961); Betamethasone (1963); Clobetasone propionate (1974); Clobetasone butyrate (1978); Fluticasone (1990); Halobetasone (1990); Mometasone (1991) and a host of other molecules.
- Approved dermatological indications of TSs as per the information available on the Central Drugs Standard Control Organization (CDSCO) website are listed in Table 7.1. Considering the list of approved TSs, it seems that their off-label use is a common clinical practice in India. More serious concern is their inappropriate use in symptomatic treatment for various dermatological disorders like acne, primary bacterial and fungal infections, undiagnosed skin rash and as fairness cream by non-registered practitioners or on the advice of pharmacist at chemist shops.

How does Misuse of Steroids Occur?

The reasons for rampant TSs abuse vary from wrong prescription, dubious marketing by pharmaceutical companies, free availability as OTC drugs, use of cosmetic and ayurvedic products that contain unlabeled depigmenting agents and steroids, availability of TSs in various irrational combinations and lack of regulations regarding the manufacturing of irrational combinations.[2,5]

VARIOUS STAGES OF STEROID MISUSE[6]

The misuse of TSs occurs at various levels such as manufacturing, marketing, prescription, sales and end-use by patients and laymen.[6]

- *Manufacturing misuse:* Many pharmaceutical companies often market products which they think would be innovative and attractive to the prescriber, to increase their sales. But in the long run such products do more harm than good. Examples

Table 7.1: TSs approved in India and their indications[7]

Approved TSs	Indications as single agent	Indications as fixed-dose combination
Beclomethasone	Not specified	Topical treatment of bacterial and fungal infections
Betamethasone	Psoriasis, contact dermatitis, atopic dermatitis, neurodermatitis, senile pruritus	Keratosis, ichthyosis, lichen planus, dry scaly condition of skin, psoriasis vulgaris, superficial bacterial and fungal infections associated with steroid-responsive dermatoses
Clobetasol	Not specified	Dry hyperkeratotic steroid-responsive dermatoses, superficial bacterial infections including contact dermatitis, seborrheic dermatitis and infective eczema
Clobetasone	Mild eczema, dermatitis, steroid-responsive dermatoses	Not approved
Dexamethasone	Not specified	Dermatological disorder complicated by bacterial and/or fungal infection
Fluocinolone	Not approved	Melasma of face in adults
Fluticasone	Inflammatory and pruritic manifestation of corticosteroid-responsive eczema, dermatitis	Not approved
Halcinonide	Indicated in the treatment of various common dermatoses	Not specified
Halobetasol	Corticosteroid-responsive dermatoses	Plaque psoriasis, superficial bacterial and fungal infections associated with steroid-responsive dermatoses
Hydrocortisone	Not specified	For treatment of patients with skin hyperpigmentation
Mometasone	Steroid-responsive dermatoses, atopic dermatitis, eczema	Treatment of moderate to severe melasma of face, plaque psoriasis, dermatoses with mixed infection

include modified Kligman's formula containing Mometasone for melasma, superpotent steroids with enhanced penetration and super potent steroids for use on scalp.

- *Marketing misuse:* TSs are often introduced to non-dermatologists without revealing the true aspects of its appropriate usage and information regarding side effects. Unfortunately such marketing practices may not be strictly illegal, leading to abuse of TSs. Though it is illegal for a practitioner of alternative medicine to prescribe allopathic drugs, there is no legal restriction on promotion and sale of TSs by pharmaceutical companies to such practitioners. Hence TSs prescriptions coming from alternative medicine is common in India.

- *Prescription misuse*: Prescriptions of TSs by dermatologists may be incomplete with respect to quantity to be used, frequency, strength of TS, site and duration. Prescriptions of TSs by non-dermatologists ignore the important aspects like potency, site, duration and indication of these TSs. Also patients with TSs prescriptions tend to repeatedly buy the same drug from chemists without seeking medical advice.

- *Sales misuse*: Most TSs in India are available at very cheap prices since they come under drugs prices control order (DPCO), being sold as over-the-counter (OTC) products unlike the international market. Anyone can buy any TS from chemists for any ailment, without needing a medical prescription. Sales persons at chemist counters are considered equivalent to doctors by many lay persons who encourage buying of TSs to increase their sales. This results in TSs to be sold and misused freely without a dermatologist's prescription. In a questionnaire based study amongst 103 pharmacy students in Kerala, it was found that although several students were aware of the potential adverse effects of topical corticosteroids, there were gaps in the awareness about specific classes and adverse effects.

- *Misuse by lay persons*: Lay persons suffering from any dermatological disorder, tend to apply TSs recommended by their friends, neighbours or relatives. Even if their diseases aggravate on application of steroids, they do not consult dermatologists and continue to use steroids for long time increasing the risk of side effects. Another situation where steroids are commonly misused is their use as fairness cream. Mometasone, hydroquinone, and tretinoin containing skin lightening agent's usage has become very popular especially in India resulting in their aggressive marketing and prescription not just by dermatologists but all physicians resulting in their widespread abuse.[2]

COMMONLY ABUSED STEROIDS AND INDICATIONS FOR THEIR MISUSE

- Betamethasone valerate (0.1%), fluocinolone acetonide (0.1%) and betamethasone dipropionate (0.05%) are the major steroids being abused. In few recent studies, clobetasol propionate (0.05%) is found to be the most commonly abused TS.

- In May 2015, the greatest increase in sales was that of a combination containing clobetasol, ornidazole, ofloxacin, and terbinafine (Panderm Plus Cream).

- A modified version of the original triple combination of Kligman's formula containing a potent topical corticosteroid such as mometasone in addition to hydroquinone and tretinoin (Skinlite), intended for patients with melasma topped the sales in 2015, with total sales of ₹ 2.74 billion. Despite the fact that mometasone can cause severe cutaneous adverse effects if used inappropriately, these combinations are easily available over-the-counter.

- Some combination products are marketed and used as whitening creams, while others in combination with antifungal and antibiotics are promoted as 'all-purpose' creams.
- Indications for which TSs are misused include acne, pigmentation, fungal infection, pruritus, and as a cosmetic or skin cream for any type of rash.[5]
- Earlier their use as fairness creams was the most common reason for abuse, but now superficial fungal infections are emerging as the leading cause of steroid abuse. A questionnaire-based cross-sectional observational study in Rajasthan found the main reasons for using TS was fungal infection (52.43%). Tinea incognito (49.5%) and acne (30.3%) were the most common adverse effects of TSs abuse.

POPULATION COMMONLY ABUSING TOPICAL STEROIDS

- TSs abuse is more common in the younger generation who in the pursuit of looking good and fair, try to procure TSs OTC and use it indiscriminately.[2]
- Another vulnerable population is dark colored races, in whom TSs have acquired the reputation of being cheap fairness, anti-acne and anti-blemish agents.
- People staying in rural areas, where there is lack of qualified dermatologists and chemists are their point of first contact for any dermatoses.

SALE OF TOPICAL STEROIDS IN INDIAN MARKET

- In the Indian market, more than 1000 brands of TSs are being sold. The sale of TSs at the end of December 2013 was ₹ 14 billion, showing an annual growth of 16%. This accounted for 82% of the topical dermatology market, reflecting clearly their popularity. In 2014–15, the market in India was worth ₹ 15.55 billion, 11% higher than 2013.[10]
- Data suggests that 85% of the market (₹ 13.22 billion in 2014–15) comprises "steroid cocktails," which are FDCs of topical corticosteroids and one or two antibiotics and antifungals. Sales of such irrational combinations grew 26% in 2014–15, compared with the previous year, when the market was worth ₹ 10.5 billion.
- The top selling combination in 2013 was that containing beclomethasone, neomycin and clotrimazole, which was surpassed by combination product containing clobetasol, ofloxacin, ornidazole and terbinafine in 2014–15. Another high selling combination is that of modified Klingman formula, containing mometasone with hydroquinone and tretinoin.
- According to IMS health data, most prescriptions for TSs and combinations come from dermatologists followed by general practitioners, obstetrician and gynecologists, pediatricians and physicians.

MAGNITUDE OF STEROID ABUSE PROBLEM IN INDIA

- In India all drug combinations are considered new drugs for the first four years and, therefore, need approval from the Drug Controller General of India after safety and efficacy data have been presented. After approval, the state licensing authorities allow manufacture and sale throughout the country.[10]

- According to Indian laws, topical corticosteroids like clobetasol, clobetasone, fluticasone, and mometasone, can be sold in India only after prescription from a registered medical practitioner. Though all steroids are included in schedule H of the Drugs and Cosmetics Rules, 1945, a footnote confusingly excludes topical preparations and eye ointments from the list. Thus, the status of these drugs is interpreted as "over-the-counter". This needs to be revised urgently so as to prevent their rampant misuse. Moreover, existing laws are poorly implemented. Many of India's 800,000 pharmacists sell steroid creams without a prescription, ignoring the box warnings.[10]

- A study done at rural tertiary care teaching hospital in Maharashtra concluded that 28% of 500 prescriptions had TSs, out of which 98% were very potent corticosteroids; and in 85% of cases, the basis of prescribing TSs could not be established.

- In a study conducted in Bengaluru, to know the awareness among people about various commonly available TSs and their combinations, they found that 81% of the patients had heard about at least one of the topical steroids or its combinations and 61% had used these creams for various reasons. 52% of the patients complained of some form of side effect after using these creams. These medicines were recommended by general practitioners in 49.5% patients and pharmacists in 11.6% patients.[5]

- More than 100 fixed-dose combinations (FDCs) of TSs with other agents (antibacterial, antifungal, keratolytic, etc.) are available in our country. Though not scientific and rational, FDCs are widely abused due to their easy availability and propensity to provide quick symptomatic relief in many dermatoses. Surprisingly, out of these hundreds of available formulations, only 27 feature among the CDSCO's approved list of FDCs from 1961 to July 2014 in India. Also, none of the three best-selling dermatology FDCs in India in 2013 is in the updated list of approved FDCs by the CDSCO.[7] Non-inclusion of these in the list of approved FDCs on Indian regulator's website means that their manufacturing and marketing has not been permitted in the country. Furthermore, the pharmaceutical companies are marketing non-approved FDCs and the regulator needs to take stern steps to regulate dermatological drug market in the country.

- The situation in India is complicated by certain factors such as:
  - The number of dermatologists in India is currently approximately 8500, of which more than 80% practice in urban areas. The population of India is 1.3 billion, out of which about two-thirds live in villages. This clearly indicates

that not enough dermatologists are available to meet the needs of Indian population living in rural area. Because of this, untrained non-physicians, ayurvedic and homeopathic practitioners and unqualified charlatans treat dermatological diseases by prescribing TSs.[13] The top prescribers of topical steroids in India, after dermatologists, are general practitioners, gynaecologists, paediatricians, and consulting physicians.[10]

– Lack of awareness about medication among the general public, particularly in a developing country like ours, is another major concern which results in consumption of prescription drugs as non-prescription drugs.[6]

– The higher authorities have failed to regulate unscrupulous pharmacists who act as quasi dermatologists and are guilty of dispensing superpotent topical steroids either alone or in combination to the unsuspecting public.

– TSs are Schedule H drugs according to Drugs and Cosmetics (D and C) Act 1940, which means that they have to be sold strictly only after prescription of a registered medical practitioner. However, only few TSs such as clobetasol propionate, clobetasone 17- butyrate, fluticasone propionate and mometasone furoate are included in this list. Further, TS combinations are also not included in the list. From the analysis of the affidavit filed in the Supreme Court in November 2013 in a drug pricing case by All India Drug Action Network and others vs Union of India and others, 99.8% of topical steroids have not been included in Drug Price Control Order.[10,13]

– In India, there is obsessiveness amongst people for fair skin color. But none of the TSs or their FDCs in the CDSCO list has been approved for fairness of the skin. TSs such as hydrocortisone 1%, mometasone 0.1% and fluocinolone 0.01% in FDCs with hydroquinone and tretinoin are approved for management of melasma. This is being exploited by pharmaceutical marketing companies and beauticians, who use these FDCs for promoting fairness amongst people.

– The easy OTC availability of TCs at chemist shops across the country without any valid prescription is further compounding this problem of abuse.

– In India, patients with prescriptions often repurchase drugs and share them with friends and relatives with similar symptoms to save the cost and inconvenience of a dermatological consultation.

SIDE EFFECTS OF TSs

General Side Effects

• Prolonged and unsupervised TSs use is associated with several cutaneous side effects such as telangiectasia, cutaneous atrophy, striae, hyper-/hypopigmentation, steroid modified tinea which can be extensive or pustular (Fig. 7.1), tinea incognito or tinea pseudoimbricata (Fig. 7.2), impetigo incognito, perioral dermatitis (Fig. 7.3), infantile gluteal granuloma and pyodermas.

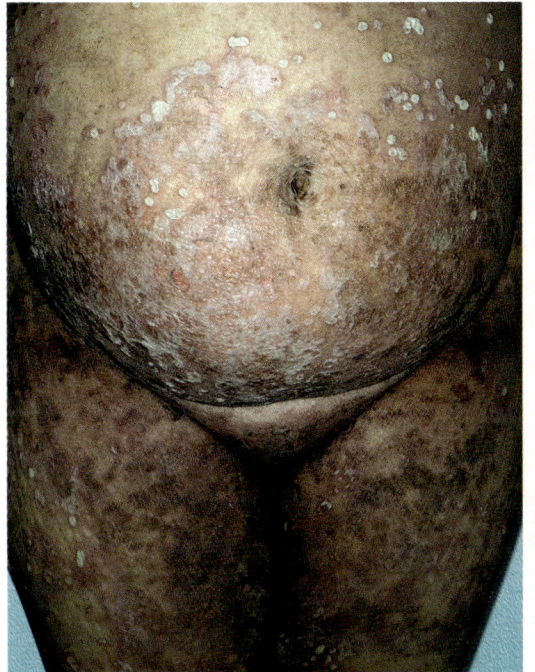

Fig. 7.1: Extensive pustular tinea corporis and cruris.

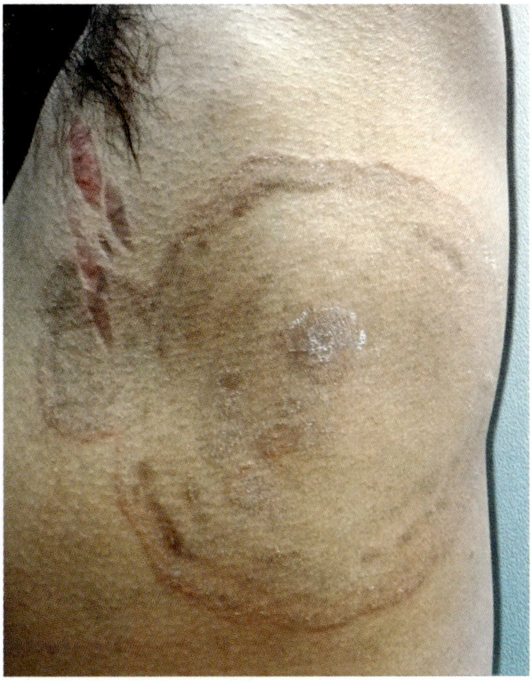

Fig. 7.2: Tinea pseudoimbricata: Multiple concentric rings. Also note the striae.

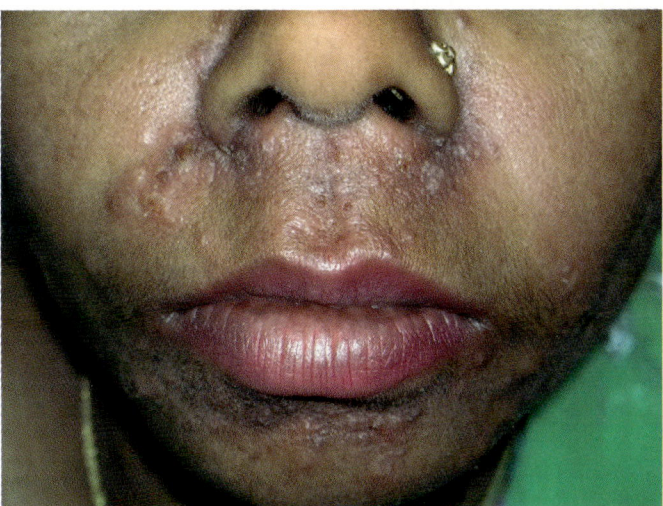

Fig. 7.3: Perioral dermatitis: Inflammatory papules and papulo-pustules around the nose and lips.

- These side effects are more likely to occur when superpotent TSs are applied on face, flexural skin and on areas with a thin skin (e.g. genitalia). Children are especially liable to these side effects due to their relatively thin skin.
- Hypopigmentation due to TSs use results from impaired melanocyte function. This side effect is particularly seen with triamcinolone because of its tendency to aggregate owing to its large molecular size.

- Both epidermis and dermis can show atrophic changes after TSs use. Microscopically, atrophy begins to occur within 3–14 days of steroid application. Initially there is thinning of epidermis due to reduction in epidermal cell size, which reflects a decreased metabolic activity. With continuous use, there occurs reduction in cell layers: Stratum granulosum is almost lost and stratum corneum becomes thin. Synthesis of stratum corneum lipids and keratohyalin granules and formation of corneodesmosomes are also reduced.
- Dermal atrophy occurs due to decreased fibroblast growth and reduced synthesis of collagen. Intertriginous areas are particularly susceptible to these side effects because the skin at these sites is thinner, has increased moisture and elevated temperature due to occlusion. The atrophy may be reversible on stoppage of TS, but may take several months.

Side Effects on Face

- Another major aspect of TSs abuse is its use as cosmetic by dark skinned people, particularly in combination with bleaching creams, to make the skin fair. TS damaged facies is a newly described entity associated with TSs abuse.
- Common side effects of steroid abuse on face are:[1,9,16,17]
  - Steroid dependence
  - Red burning skin syndrome
  - Status cosmeticus
  - Acneiform eruption
  - Hypertrichosis
  - Demodicidosis
  - Facial plethora
  - Perioral dermatitis
  - Telangiectasias (Fig. 7.4)

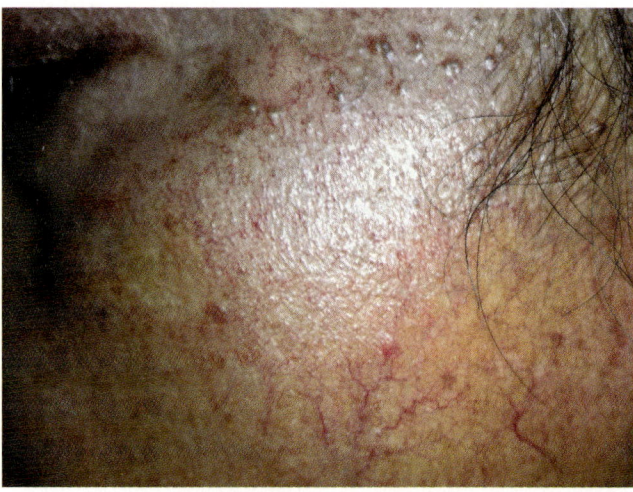

Fig. 7.4: Telangiectasias on the cheek. There is background blotchy hypopigmentation as well.

- Steroid rosacea (synonyms—light-sensitive seborrheid, rosacea-like dermatitis, steroid dermatitis resembling rosacea, steroid-induced rosacea): This entity refers to development of dermatitis following repeated or chronic unsupervised application of TSs which resembles rosacea. This results not only with abuse of TSs, but also with excessive regular use of fluorinated steroids on face. It initially presents as development of erythematous papules which dry up and evolve into diffuse erythema, pustules and nodules (Fig. 7. 5). It requires many months for it to develop, but also depends on the steroid potency.
- Topical steroid damaged/dependent face (TSDF): This is a recently described entity, which often results from an unsupervised continuous application of TSs on the face long after resolution of the primary dermatosis for which the TS was first prescribed. It is characterised by occurrence of severe rebound erythema, burning and scaling (Fig. 7.6) on the face whenever TS application is attempted to be stopped. Another feature of TSDF is development of flares of photosensitivity, papules, and pustules. Therefore, patients get caught up in a vicious cycle of more and more potent TSs to avoid these rebound effects associated with withdrawal, becoming addicted to topical steroids in the process.

- Less known cutaneous side effects of TSs include:[16]
  - Hypertrichosis
  - Cutaneous dyschromias
  - Delay in wound healing
  - Flare of skin infections

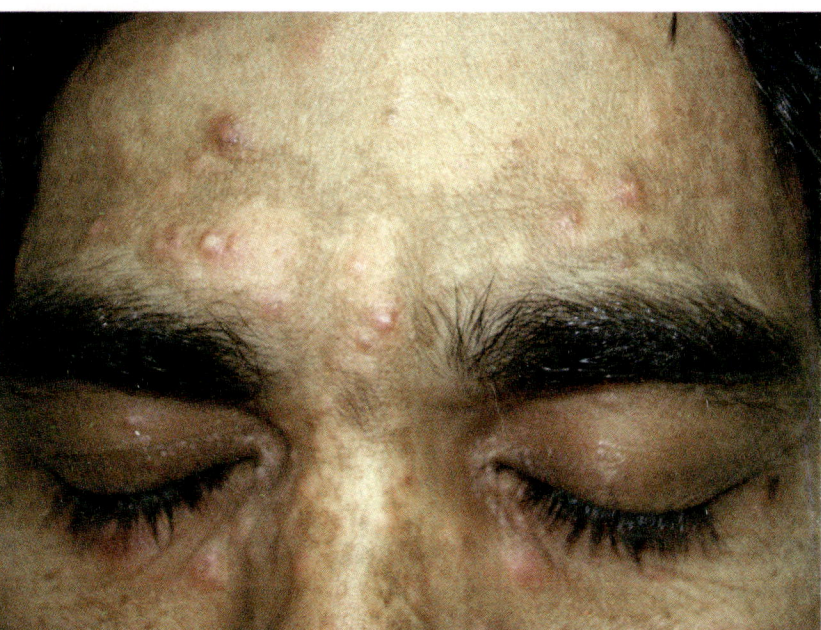

Fig. 7.5: Steroid rosacea: Inflammatory papules and pustules on the face. Patient had been applying potent topical steroids for melasma.

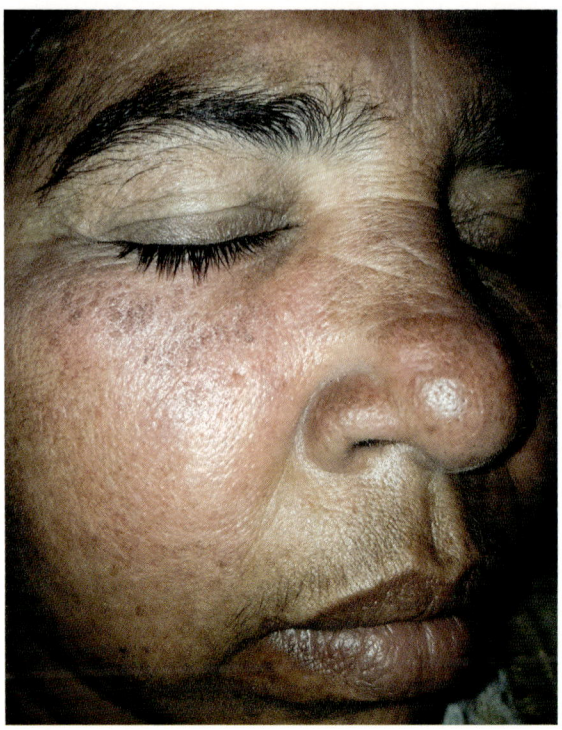

Fig. 7.6: Topical steroid dependant face: Ill-defined facial erythema and mild scaling.

Ocular Complications

Ocular complications of TSs abuse include steroid induced open angle glaucoma with reversible increased intraocular tension, irreversible glaucomatous cupping of the optic disc and visual field defects.

Systemic Side Effects

Systemic side effects of TSs are known to occur when superpotent or potent TSs are used for a long time on areas with thin skin, e.g. face and on raw/inflamed surfaces.[16]

The systemic side effects of TSs include:
- Ocular—cataract (posterior cortical), open angle glaucoma
- Endocrine—Cushing disease, mineralocorticoid effects especially with hydrocortisone and 9-α-fluoroprednisolone
- Impaired glucose tolerance
- Reduced bone mineral density
- Decreased growth rate
- Electrolyte imbalance
- Edema
- Hypocalcemia
- Hypertension
- Suppression of the HPA axis

Factors causing HPA suppression are as mentioned below:[16]

- Applying TSs over large areas
- Using higher concentrations of TSs
- Using TSs under occlusion
- Increased application of moderately potent TSs
- Increased steroid penetration (especially in atopics)
- Modest use of more potent derivatives

This can cause iatrogenic Cushing disease, corticosteroid-related Addison crises, growth retardation and death. The HPA axis recover spontaneously in a fortnight.

AWARENESS CAMPAIGN IN INDIA AGAINST STEROID ABUSE

- The *Indian Journal of Dermatology* in 2006, published the first major article about TSs abuse from India.
- In the same year, a thread was initiated in the ACAD IADVL group of IADVL, named "Topical steroid misuse menace" to highlight the problem. A delegation of IADVL which was led by Dr Suresh Joshipura, the then President of IADVL and Dr Koushik Lahiri, the then Hon. General Secretary of IADVL submitted a memorandum on this issue of steroid abuse to the Union Minister of Health and to the Ministry of Chemicals and Fertilizers.
- Since the first report on topical steroid abuse, an increasing number of articles have been published from India, highlighting the issue of steroid misuse and abuse. Patients presenting with steroid abuse are being actively discussed in ACAD IADVL. Facebook group named "No steroid cream on face without a doctor's prescription" has been created where dermatologists post photographs and discuss this issue. The issue is also discussed in lay print, electronic and social media.[6]

IADVL Task Force Against Topical Steroid Abuse (ITATSA)

- The Indian Association of Dermatologists, Venereologists, and Leprologists (IADVL) has formed a task force, IADVL Taskforce Against Topical Steroid Abuse (ITATSA), against TSs abuse, with main aims of raising public awareness, running media campaigns, forming study groups for doctors, highlighting the problem in journals, and meeting with central and state authorities.
- The task force has started to collect relevant data and has asked the drug controller to bring TSs under schedule H, disallowing their unrestricted sale, and has demanded explanation as to why the authorities authorise irrational combinations.[10]
- Another effort by ITATSA is the online petition, which is being given to the Ministry of Health and Family Welfare, Government of India and CDSCO, which stresses upon issues related to the indiscriminate sale of TCs without prescription in India due to unregulated market and also makes an effort to sensitize common people about the risks associated with their use.

Important Steps by IADVL Against TS Abuse

- **Pre-ITATSA**
  - 2006: Dr. Koushik Lahiri started a mail thread on IADVL ACAD group on the issue of TS abuse which was the first time this issue was discussed on a National platform.
  - 2007: Dr. Koushik Lahiri and Dr. Coondoo moved a proposal to stop OTC sale of TSs without prescription, in General body meeting at Chennai, which got passed.
  - 2008 (March): The term "Topical Steroid Damaged/Dependent Face (TSDF)" was coined by Dr. Koushik Lahiri on IADVL ACAD group.
  - 2008 (June): For the first time in the history of IADVL, Dr. Koushik Lahiri as the principal investigator initiated a countrywide multicentric study to analyze and assess the scenario of TSs abuse. The group of erudite and committed investigators from all areas of India, namely, Dr. Koushik Lahiri, Dr. Shyam Verma, Dr. Arijit Coondoo, Dr. CR Srinivas, Dr. Asit Mittal, Dr. Rajeev Sharma, Dr. Saumya Panda, Dr. Anil Abraham, Dr. Shyamanta Baruah, Dr. Manas Chatterjee, Dr. Muralidhar Rajgopalan and Dr. Abir Saraswat, formed the initial nidus for ITATSA.
  - 2011: The highly rated and quoted historic article on TS abuse based on the above mentioned mulicentric study was published in IJDVL.
  - 2012: Dr. Koushik Lahiri started the Facebook page "No steroid on Face without Dermatologists Prescription" which created history by many hits from all over the world.
  - 2014 (May 23rd): The petition at change. org was started.
  - 2014 (May 30th and 31st): IADVL Varanasi supported the movement and news were published in Dainik Jagaran. Also 250–500 signatures happened in 2 days.
  - 2014 (June 1st–5th): Writer Taslima Nasreen joined the crusade and tweeted supporting the cause. Also support came from IADVL Karnataka, NE, and WB branch. The signature mark crossed 1000.

- **IADVL Task Force Against Topical Steroid Abuse (ITATSA)**
  - 2014 (Juneto July): IADVL officially endorsed the movement and formed a dedicated taskforce ITATSA on 29th June 2014 (Dr. Abir Sarswat as Convenor and Dr. Koushik Lahiri as the Chair). Also Yahoo groups were formed and INSTEAD joined hands.
  - 2014 (August): ITATSA was endorsed by IADVL CC.
  - 2014 (September): ITATSA approached DCGI.
  - 2014 (October): IADVL appealed the industry partners to support the crusade against TSs misuse.
  - 2015 (February): ITATSA was endorsed by GB and Abbott Celebrity activity "Treat your skin right" program was unveiled. Also OPPI came forward in support.

- 2015 (March): ITATSA WhatsApp group was created.
- 2015 (April): Meeting was conducted with Dr. VK Subburaj (Secretary, Department of Pharmaceuticals), Dr. S Eswara Reddy (Joint Drug Controller General of India), Dr. Jagdish Prasad (Director General of Health Services), and Dr. GN Singh (DCGI).
- 2015 (May): DCGI issued circulars.
- 2015 (November and December): Follow up meetings were held with Dr. G N Singh (DCGI) and DCGI issued another circular.
- 2016 (February): New team was formed with Dr. Kiran Nabar initially and, later Dr. Rajeev Sharma as the Chairperson and Dr. Rajetha Damisetty as Convenor.
- 2016 (April to August): Follow-up meetings were held with DCGI.
- 2016 (August 12th): Gazette published including all the topical steroids under schedule H and deleting the footnote excluding topicals from the list.
- 2017 (January 14th): Dr. Shyam Verma took over as the Chairperson of ITATSA, Dr. Rajetha Damisetty continued as the Convener.

Studies on Topical Steroid Abuse

- Early reports of TS dependence or addiction were published in 1973 by Burry and in 1976 by Kligman and Frosch.[6]
- A landmark study in India by Saraswat *et al*, which screened 2926 patients with facial dermatosis, showed that steroid FDCs were used by 59.6% of patients and 14.8% of patients were using TSs over a long period in an unsupervised manner. This study revealed that most TSs abusers belonged to the 20–30 year age group, and Betamethasone valerate alone or in combination was most commonly abused. TSs use as a fairness/general purpose/after shave was in 29% and for acne was in 24% of the patients. The rural/suburban population and younger people used potent and superpotent TSs. Non-prescription TS use was in 59.3% and out of these, 90.3% were for potent/super-potent steroids. Among 40.7% physician prescriptions, 44.3% were from non-dermatologists. Adverse effects were seen in 90.5% TS users. Acne or acne exacerbation, and topical steroid dependent face were common side effects. In 93%, TS use was unnecessary, in excess, was of the wrong potency or was instituted without a diagnosis.[1]
- A study conducted in Bastar, Chattisgarh by Dey amongst 6723 new patients, revealed that lightening of skin colour was the main reason for using TSs followed by melasma and suntan. The commonest side effects were acne (38%), plethoric face with telangiectasia (19%), puffy face, and acneform eruptions with papulopustular lesions.[15]
- Another study by Jha *et al*, revealed that the majority (42.9%) of 410 patients studied self-prescribed TSs, 20% by their friends, family members, or neighbours, 18.2% by a non-dermatologist practitioner, 10.2% by a dermatologist, 8.5% were

recommended by beauty parlors. Steroid induced acne was the commonest adverse effect of topical steroids (42.9%) followed by hypopigmentation in 14.1%. The commonest abused TS was betamethasone valerate which was dispensed in 92 patients (22.4%) as fairness cream/anti-acne cream, Klingman formula in 43 patients (10.4%) for melasma/other hyperpigmented lesion, and TS containing antifungal/antibiotic cream in 41 patients (10%) for tinea faciei/other facial dermatoses.[3]

MANAGEMENT OF THE PROBLEM OF STEROID ABUSE IN INDIA

Measures need to be taken at different levels to prevent steroid abuse which include:

- *Senstization and education of general practitioners and pharmacists*: General practitioners and pharmacists are often the first point of contact for most of the patients. Training and sensitizing them regarding possible complications of these drugs and the extent of problem in the society would help in reduce the incidence of TSs related side effects.[5] Continuing medical education for residents in the dermatology department is also greatly needed. Also dissemination of information in this regard to the masses by means of mass media is of paramount importance.

- *Legal action*: Legislation/stronger implementation of existing laws is required to limit public access and advertising of potent TCs. A law should be enacted enforcing immediate ban on the non-prescription sale of TCs. The authorities should also be requested to ensure that such laws are strictly enforced both in "letter and spirit".[6]

- *Audit of prescriptions*: To reduce TSs related side effects especially with prolonged use, the rational use of TSs should include careful consideration of the patient's age, total area of application, quantity to be applied, efficacy of the selected steroid, and frequency of application. Hence, one step to achieve rational prescribing is periodic auditing of prescriptions.[14]

- *Proper prescriptions*: There should be more emphasis on rational and complete prescription of TSs. Principal factors to be taken into account while prescribing TSs are: (a) The site of application, (b) the potency of the drug, (c) age of the patient, (d) duration of application, and (d) indication for usage. The prescription pattern may be influenced by availability in the hospital pharmacy and choice of dermatologist. The medical community should prescribe with a social perspective in mind and should not follow practices which would be detrimental to the society. Regular continuing medical education and workshops to create awareness among dermatologists regarding this important issue will go a long way to ensure rational use of TSs. Topical calcineurin inhibitors (such as tacrolimus) greatly add to the armamentarium for treatment of inflammatory skin disorders and they should be considered, whenever feasible, especially on face, as these drugs are free of cutaneous and systemic side effects associated with TSs.

- *Education about dispensing TSs*: To achieve maximum effectiveness, patients must be encouraged to apply TSs appropriately. Dermatologists must inform the patients about the adverse effects of TS abuse on face. They should also explain the full details about proper use of TS. The use of fingertip unit method (FTU), which provides guidelines regarding the amount of ointment needed based on specific anatomic areas, should be practiced widely to reduce variations in the use of TSs and to encourage adherence to therapy.[14]

- *Revision of hospital formulary*: There is a need to revise hospital formulary where low-potency TSs should be included along with potent ones so that the latter can be avoided in conditions where they are unnecessary. The hospital authorities should make low-potency steroids available in the hospital pharmacy keeping in mind the adverse effects of potent steroids.

- *Evaluation of drug utilization pattern*: There is a need to do periodic evaluation of drug utilization pattern to enable suitable modification in the prescription of drugs to reduce the side effects and improve benefit.[14]

- *Sensitization of policy makers*: The potential hazards of TSs abuse need to be explained and discussed with policy makers in order to sensitize them to the grave problem of steroid abuse.[13]

- *Inclusion of TSs under schedule H*: The Indian government should bring TSs, except for those with low potency; under schedule H to ensure their production and sale are regulated.[8] Perhaps stringent regulations, similar to the recently issued new Schedule H1 to curb the growing menace of antibiotic resistance in India, are required to regulate TC drug market in India.

- *Tackling the issue of skin fairness*: The "fairness of the skin" has been specified under Schedule J of Drugs and Cosmetics Act, 1940. According to this "no drug may purport or claim to prevent or cure or may convey to the intending user thereof any idea that it may prevent or cure one or more of the diseases or ailments specified in this schedule."[19] Hence, there should be proper check on the advertisement of the drugs which claim to promote fairness of the skin. Furthermore, according to the Drugs and Magic Remedies (Objectionable Advertisements) act, 1954, section 4 (Prohibition of Misleading Advertisements Relating to Drugs), no one can advertise a drug which (a) directly or indirectly gives a false impression regarding the true character of the drug or (b) makes a false claim for the drug.

REFERENCES

1. Saraswat A, Lahiri K, Chatterjee M, Barua S, Coondoo A, Mittal A, et al. Topical corticosteroid abuse on the face: A prospective, multicenter study of dermatology outpatients. Indian J Dermatol Venereol Leprol 2011;77:160–6.

2. Sinha A, Kar S, Yadav N, Madke B. Prevalence of Topical Steroid Misuse Among Rural Masses. Indian J Dermatol 2016 Jan-Feb?61(1):119.

3. Jha AK, Sinha R, Prasad S. Misuse of topical corticosteroids on the face: A cross-sectional study among dermatology outpatients. Indian Dermatol Online J 2016;7:259–63.

4. Hengge UR, Ruzicka T, Schwartz RA, Cork MJ. Adverse effects of topical glucocorticosteroids. J Am Acad Dermatol 2006;54:1–18.

5. Nagesh TS, Akhilesh A. Topical Steroid Awareness and Abuse: A Prospective Study among Dermatology Outpatients. Indian J Dermatol 2016 Nov-Dec?61(6):618–621.

6. Coondoo A. Topical Corticosteroid Misuse: The Indian Scenario. Indian J Dermatol 2014 Sep-Oct;59(5):451–455.

7. Kumar S, Goyal A, Gupta YK. Abuse of topical corticosteroids in India: Concerns and the way forward. J Pharmacol Pharmacother 2016;7:1–5.

8. Ashique KT, Kaliyadan F, Mohan S. Knowledge, Attitudes and Behavior Regarding Topical Corticosteroids in a Sample of Pharmacy Students: A Cross Sectional Survey. Indian Dermatol Online J 2018 Nov-Dec;9(6):432–4.

9. Rathi S. Abuse of topical steroid as cosmetic cream: A social background of steroid dermatitis. Indian J Dermatol 2006;51:154–5.

10. Verma SB. Topical corticosteroid misuse in India is harmful and out of control. BMJ 2015;351:h6079.

11. Meena S, Gupta LK, Khare AK, Balai M, Mittal A, Mehta S, Bhatri G. Topical corticosteroids abuse: A clinical study of cutaneous adverse effects. Indian J Dermatol 2017;62:675.

12. Mahe A, Ly F, Aymard G, Dangou JM. Skin diseases associated with the cosmetic use of bleaching products in women from Dakar, Senegal. Br J Dermatol 2003;148:493–500.

13. Verma SB. Sales, status, prescriptions and regulatory problems with topical steroids in India. Indian J Dermatol Venereol Leprol 2014;80:201–3.

14. Rathod SS, Motghare VM, Deshmukh VS, Deshpande RP, Bhamare CG, Patil JR. Prescribing practices of topical corticosteroids in the outpatient dermatology department of a rural tertiary care teaching hospital. Indian J Dermatol 2013;58:342–5.

15. Dey VK. Misuse of topical corticosteroids: A clinical study of adverse effects. Indian Dermatol Online J 2014;5:436–40.

16. Coondoo A, Phiske M, Verma S, Lahiri K. Side-effects of topical steroids: A long overdue revisit. Indian Dermatol Online J 2014;5:416–25.

17. Chohan SN, Suhail M, Salman S, Bajwa UM, Saeed M, Kausar S, et al. Facial abuse of topical steroids and fairness creams: a clinical study of 200 patients. Journal of Pakistan Association of Dermatologists 2014;24(3):204–211.

18. Mehta AB, Nadkarni NJ, Patil SP, Godse KV, Gautam M, Agarwal S. Topical corticosteroids in dermatology. Indian J Dermatol Venereol Leprol 2016 Jul-Aug;82(4):371–8.

19. Ljubojeviae S, Basta-JuzbaSiae A, Lipozeneiae J. Steroid dermatitis resembling rosacea: Aetiopathogenesis and treatment. J Eur Acad Dermatol Venereol 2002;16:121–6.

20. Sneddon I. Adverse effect of topical fluorinated corticosteroids in rosacea. Br Med J 1969;1:671–3.

21. Mandapati JS, Metta AK. Intraocular pressure variation in patients on long-term corticosteroids. Indian Dermatol Online J 2011;2:67–9.

22. Ministry of Health and Family Welfare. GSR 588(E). Central Drugs Standard Control Organization, India. [Last accessed on 2019 May 18]. Available from: http://cdsco.nic.in/writereaddata/588E30th Aug 2013.pdf.

8

Steroid Use in Emergency Dermatoses

Eswari L, Deepika Yadav

SUMMARY

- Steroids are considered the first-line treatment for various dermatological emergencies such as severe cutaneous adverse drug reactions, extensive pemphigus, severe angioedema, acute erythroderma and generalized pustular psoriasis of pregnancy.
- Role of steroids is unclear in SJS/TEN, few studies point towards their early use in appropriately high doses and for short duration.
- Systemic steroids should be started early in DRESS and require a gradual taper over months to prevent flare-up.
- Systemic steroids remain the cornerstone of treatment for severe flares or extensive pemphigus vulgaris. If response is unsatisfactory with daily oral steroids, pulsed steroids may be tried.
- A short course of systemic steroids may be given in acute urticaria not responding to antihistamines. Long-term steroids should not be given in urticaria.
- Patients with angioedema affecting the eyelids, lips or tongue may be given a short course of oral steroids for rapid relief. Laryngeal edema or anaphylaxis requires IV hydrocortisone, in addition to epinephrine and airway management.
- Corticosteroids can also be used in erythroderma, especially dermatitis, for quick disease control. Systemic steroids are avoided in psoriatic erythroderma.
- Systemic steroids are regarded as the first-line treatment for generalized pustular psoriasis of pregnancy. Steroids are also indicated in retinoic acid syndrome, a rare life-threatening complication of retinoid treatment in psoriasis.
- Acne fulminans should be initially treated with systemic steroids. Oral isotretinoin should be given in a low-dose and only after disease control with steroids, as there is a risk of worsening the disease.

INTRODUCTION

Contrary to popular perception, dermatologists do deal with medical emergencies. Dermatological emergencies exist, and can even be fatal. Some examples include severe cutaneous drug reactions, acute urticaria and/or angioedema/anaphylaxis and extensive pemphigus. Corticosteroids are an important drug in the armamentarium of agents available to deal with these situations. Though corticosteroids have often been used in these situations, there is no consensus regarding the timing, dose and duration of corticosteroids. Further, though the role of corticosteroids is not in doubt in some conditions such as extensive pemphigus or severe angioedema, its use is controversial in others such as Stevens-Johnson syndrome or toxic epidermal necrolysis. In this chapter, we shall discuss the therapeutic status of corticosteroids in some of the commonly encountered dermatological emergencies.

A. ROLE OF STEROIDS IN STEVENS-JOHNSON SYNDROME/TOXIC EPIDERMAL NECROLYSIS

- Stevens-Johnson syndrome (SJS)/toxic epidermal necrolysis (TEN) is a potentially fatal idiosyncratic reaction, caused most commonly by drugs and occasionally by other triggers like infections. There is <10% of total body surface area (TBSA) involvement in SJS, >30% TBSA involvement in TEN, whereas it is 10–30% TBSA in SJS/TEN overlap.[1]

- Pathophysiology of SJS/TEN is not completely understood, but extensive apoptosis leading to keratinocyte death has been proposed as the main mechanism. CD8-positive T cells,[2] macrophages, inflammatory cytokines (including TNF-α) and enzymes (perforin and granzyme B)[3] play an important role both in the epithelial necrosis and epithelial detachment. Some suggest that apoptosis is mediated principally through activation of the Fas receptor by increased Fas ligand expression.[4] Interferon-γ upregulation of keratinocytes also plays a role.[5] Granulysin, a component of cytotoxic T-cell and NK/T-cell, is considered to be the major cytotoxic molecule resulting in epidermal necrosis.[6]

- Diagnosis of SJS/TEN is primarily clinical, and is based on temporal correlation of mucocutaneous eruption with drug exposure (usually after 1–3 weeks). Skin lesions in SJS/TEN can be purpuric macules, flat atypical targets, raised atypical targets, or typical targets (Fig. 8.1). Usually, at least 2 mucosae are affected (Fig. 8.2).

- Prognosis differs greatly depending primarily on when the culprit drug is stopped and how much body surface area is affected. The mortality in SJS ranges from 1 to 3%, and can be as high as 25–35% in TEN.[7] A prognostics scoring system, SCORTEN, was developed based on 7 clinical and laboratory variables to assess the patient's severity of illness (Table 8.1). SCORTEN score at 72 hours is considered to be of greater prognostic importance than that at 24 hours.

Management of SJS/TEN

Management of SJS/TEN involves early identification and removal of the trigger(s) along with supportive skin and eye care, pain control, maintaining fluid and electrolyte balance, and prevention/treatment of infections.

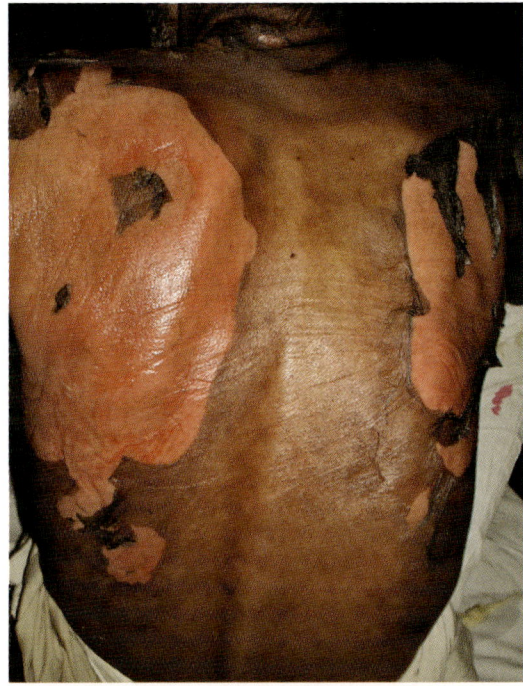

Fig. 8.1: Extensive peeling of skin in a patient of toxic epidermal necrolysis.

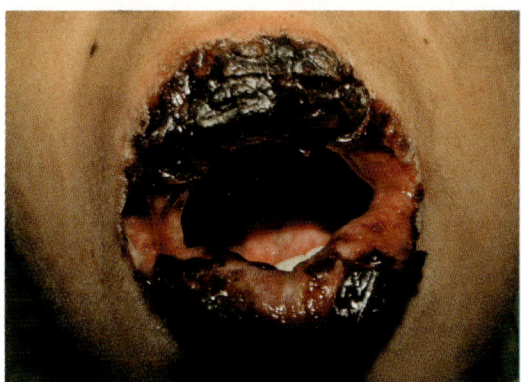

Fig. 8.2: Severe mucosal crusting in a patient of Stevens-Johnson syndrome.

Table 8.1: Score of toxic epidermal necrosis: SCORTEN			
Risk factors		No. of risk factors	Mortality rate (%)
Age	>40 years	0–1	3.2
Associated malignancy	Yes	2	12.1
Heart rate (beats/min)	>120	3	35.3
Serum urea (mmol/L)	>10	4	58.3
Detached or compromised body surface	>10%	5 or more	>90
Serum bicarbonate (mEq/L)	<20		
Serum glucose (mmol/L)	>14		

As the barrier function of skin is lost in SJS/TEN, it is frequently complicated by infections, and fluid and electrolyte imbalance. Patients are at a risk of hypovolemic shock, local and systemic infections, including sepsis and multiorgan failure. Urgent restoration of barrier function of skin and mucosae is paramount.[8]

Rationale of Using Steroids

- SJS/TEN is an immunologically mediated drug reaction, therefore, immunomodulatory drugs have an important role to switch off the initial cascade of events and preventing further skin damage. Examples of these agents include steroids, IVIg, cyclosporine and TNF-alpha inhibitors (like infliximab), with steroids perhaps being the most commonly used worldwide.
- For maximum benefit, steroids should be started as early as possible, preferably within 3–5 days of onset of disease and given in adequate doses.[9]

Controversial Status of Steroids in SJS/TEN

Though there is no consensus on the use of steroids in management of SJS/TEN owing to the lack of randomized clinical trials (RCTs), steroids have traditionally been the mainstay of treatment of SJS/TEN. However, there are several aspects of steroid use that are unclear, mainly the timing (whether in early or late disease), dose, and duration of therapy. Steroids are often given too late, in too low a dose, and for too long. There are several studies supporting the use of systemic steroids in the treatment of SJS/TEN.[1,10]

Positive Effects of Steroids

Use of steroids early in the disease has the following benefits:
- Halting the immunological cascade;
- Decreasing the extent of skin necrosis;
- Reduce the local factors like pain, itching, discomfort and fever;
- Minimise the extent of internal organ damage and
- Reduce the overall mortality and morbidity.

Negative Effects of Steroids

Prolonged or delayed use of steroids can have adverse effects like:
- Increased risk of secondary infection or sepsis;
- Altered wound healing;
- Gastrointestinal bleed;
- Uncontrolled blood sugar levels;
- Elevated blood pressure.

Quality of Studies on Systemic Steroids in SJS/TEN

- Corticosteroids have been used in the treatment of SJS/TEN for a long time all around the world. In fact prior to 1970, they were the mainstay of treatment apart from supportive care. During 1970, a few case series emerged which pointed towards the adverse effects of steroid use in SJS/TEN and their association with increased mortality. However, it is to be noted that these studies had several discrepancies regarding the steroid dose, duration of treatment and timing of steroid initiation. Since then, many studies have shown benefit of steroids over supportive care alone (Table 8.2). SJS/TEN being a rare condition, all these studies suffer from several deficiencies: retrospective, uncontrolled, small sample size and heterogeneous inclusion criteria. Lack of good-quality studies is a major limitation, and the same was expressed by Law et al, in their review of 6 retrospective studies. They concluded that out of these 6 studies, only one showed marginal benefit of steroids in decreasing the mortality in SJS/TEN.[1] Notably, none of the studies reported any adverse effect secondary to steroid use. In another recent review including 11 studies, there was a trend towards the beneficial role of steroids in SJS/TEN, however it was not statistically significant (OR: 0.54, 95% CI: 0.29–1.01).[10]

- Regarding the dose, route of administration and duration of steroid use, there again exists a lot of heterogeneity. Methylprednisolone, prednisolone and dexamethasone have all been used in various studies in doses of 1–2 mg/kg/day for former two, and 16–24 mg/day for the latter. Most of these were given parenterally (intravenous or intramuscular) initially followed by oral administration as maintenance. Duration of steroid treatment has also varied from few days to up to 3–4 weeks.
- Some authors have used steroids in pulse form (methylprednisolone 1000 mg or dexamethasone 100 mg for 2–3 days) with encouraging results. The rationale behind pulsed steroids being that early use of extremely high dose steroids will terminate the initial immune mechanisms, thereby halting the further chain of events leading to keratinocyte apoptosis.
- There are a few studies reporting additional benefit of combination treatment (with agents such as IVIg and cyclosporine) as compared to steroids alone.
- Apart from preventing skin necrosis, steroids have also been found to reduce ocular morbidity.

Limitations of Studies[1,9,10]

- *Study design:* Most of the studies available are retrospective in nature. Few of these which are prospective, are non-randomised uncontrolled studies. The results are also different based upon whether the study was conducted in a burn unit managed by surgeons or dermatology units with latter favouring steroids use and former were against. This introduces a bias and, therefore, the results of these studies should be interpreted in the context of these limitations.

Table 8.2: Various studies using steroids for the treatment of SJS-TEN

Study	Nature of study	Number of cases	Dose and duration of corticosteroid	Time since initiation of therapy	TBSA involved (%)	Mortality	Comments
Murphy et al, 1997[11]	Retrospective case series	44	Variable	>7 days	52.4	36%	Delayed presentation and severe disease associated with increased mortality
Schulz et al, 2000[12]	Retrospective case series	34	Variable	NA	>20%	38% (13/34)	Steroid use was not significantly associated with increased mortality
Tripathi et al, 2000[13]	Retrospective case series	67	Methylprednisolone 160–240 mg, tapering and total duration variable	NA	NA	1.4% (1/67)	One death was not due to SJS/TEN. No increased mortality with steroids
Ducic et al, 2002[14]	Retrospective case series	29	Variable	NA	>20%	44.8% (13/29)	No increase in mortality with steroids
Kim et al, 2005[15]	Retrospective case series	21	Intravenous methylprednisolone 250–1000 mg then tapered to oral prednisolone, duration NA	NA	48.7%	28.5% (6/21)	No significant difference in actual (6) vs predicted mortality based on SCORTEN (5.97), so no added advantage of use of steroids

(Contd.)

Table 8.2: Various studies using steroids for the treatment of SJS-TEN (*Contd.*)

Study	Nature of study	Number of cases	Dose and duration of corticosteroid	Time since initiation of therapy	TBSA involved (%)	Mortality	Comments
Kardaun et al, 2007[16]	Retrospective case series	12	Intravenous Dexamethasone (100 mg)-cyclophospha-mide (500 mg) pulse in 3 patients; Dexamethasone 1.5 mg/kg for 3 days	2.8 days	26.7	8.3% (1/12)	Actual mortality (1/12) was less than predicted mortality based on SCORTEN (4/12). Pulsed steroids were found to be useful in reducing mortality.
Schneck et al, 2008[17]	Retrospective Multicentre case series	159	Prednisolone [maximum dose: 250 mg (100–500 mg)] for a median period of 4 days (2–12)	4 days (2–5)	NA	18% (28/159)	Overall odd ratio with steroid use was 0.4 (0.2–0.9). No added advantage with steroid over supportive care alone.
Yang et al, 2009[18]	Retrospective case series	45	Intravenous Methylpredni-solone 1–1.5 mg/kg, duration not mentioned	5.8 days	41	22% (10/45)	Actual death (10) > predicted death (8.63) based on SCORTEN. IVIG plus corticosteroid arm was better than corticosteroid alone.

(Contd.)

Table 8.2: Various studies using steroids for the treatment of SJS-TEN (Contd.)

Study	Nature of study	Number of cases	Dose and duration of corticosteroid	Time since initiation of therapy	TBSA involved (%)	Mortality	Comments
Chen et al, 2010[19]	Retrospective case series	58	Intravenous Hydrocortisone (100–700 mg) or methylpredni-solone (40–80 mg) for 7–14 days	NA	NA	3.4% (2/58)	Actual mortality (2) < predicted mortality (4.2) based on SCORTEN. Combination of IVIg and steroids better than steroids alone.
Hirahara et al, 2013[20]	Retrospective case series	8	Intravenous methylpredni-solone 1000 mg/day for 3 days followed by oral prednisolone 0.8–1 mg/kg/day with gradual tapering	3–10 days	5–80%	0 (0/8)	Observed mortality (0) <predicted mortality (1.6) based on SCORTEN.
Pasricha et al, 1996[21]	Retrospective case series	5	Intravenous dexamethasone 16–24 mg/day for 7–10 days	NA	NA	0 (0/15)	Beneficial role of steroids in early phase.
Das et al, 2013[22]	Propspective case series	14	Intravenous Dexamethasone 1 mg/kg till decreased and stopped 5 days after resolution of erythema	NA	>30	0 (0/14)	Steroids effective in early phase

(Contd.)

Table 8.2: Various studies using steroids for the treatment of SJS-TEN (Contd.)

Study	Nature of study	Number of cases	Dose and duration of corticosteroid	Time since initiation of therapy	TBSA involved (%)	Mortality	Comments
Rai et al, 2008[23]	Retrospective case series	3	Intravenous dexamethasone 100 mg for 2–4 days followed by cyclosporine 2 mg/kg/day for 2 weeks	NA	>30%	0 (0/3)	
Singh et al, 2013[24]	Retrospective case series using cyclosporine; Compared with historical controls treated with steroids	11-cyclosporine; 6-steroid	Cyclosporine 3 mg/kg/day × 7 days, tapered over next 7 days; Controls treated with injectable dexamethasone followed by oral prednisolone ≥ 1 mg/kg/day	2.63 days in cyclosporine group; 2.16 days in steroid group	23.36% in cyclosporine group; 22.2% in steroid group	0/11 in cyclosporine; 33% (2/6) in steroid group	Actual mortality (2) > predicted mortality using SCORTEN (0.51) in steroid group. No actual mortality in cyclosporine group as against predicted mortality of 1.1.

NA: Not available
TBSA: Total body surface area

- *Inclusion criteria and outcome assessment parameters*: There is a lot of heterogeneity in the inclusion criteria, such as the day of onset of treatment, body surface area involvement and SCORTEN at baseline. Similarly, the outcome parameters are also variable: some studies have reported only the actual mortality while others have compared it with predicted mortality using SCORTEN (Table 8.2). Several clinically meaningful end-points such the time to re-epithelialization, reduction in erythema, healing of mucosal erosions and duration of hospital stay are also mentioned only in some studies. Further, there are a lot of inconsistencies in the nature of supportive treatment, making it difficult to compare the results of one study with another, and translating these into clinical practice.
- *Adverse events*: Data on adverse effects of steroids, especially the short term side effects have not been reported in many studies.

Scope for Research

There is a need for multicentre studies with large sample size conducted in randomised controlled manner to address the following issues.
- Are steroids beneficial in SJS/TEN?
- Optimal dose, duration and type of steroid?
- Ideal time since onset of disease for starting steroids?
- Role of combining steroids with other agents like cyclosporine or IVIG?

SIG-CADR Recommendations

For the management of SJS/TEN IADVL's special interest group on cutaneous adverse drug reactions (SIG-CADR) recommends steroids (with a level of evidence II and grade of recommendation B):[9]
- Use of steroid should be individualised based on the patient characteristic. Ideally if there is no contraindication like sepsis, secondary infection, immunosuppression like HIV, uncontrolled blood sugar levels; steroids can be used in treatment of SJS/TEN.
- Start steroids as early as possible, preferably within 3 days of onset of symptoms and up to 7 days.
- Initial high doses such as 1–2 mg/kg/day of methylprednisolone or prednisolone or 16–24 mg of dexamethasone. Consider pulsed steroid if there is continued progression of disease (methylprednisolone 1000 mg or dexamethasone 100 mg for 2–3 days).
- Parenteral route of administration to be preferred initially, shift to oral once patient's condition improves.
- Monitor response to treatment by examining number of new lesions, perilesional erythema and pain in lesions. Taper and stop steroids according to response within 10–14 days.

B. ROLE OF STEROIDS IN MANAGING SEVERE CUTANEOUS DRUG REACTIONS (OTHER THAN SJS/TEN)

Adverse drug reactions can be uncomplicated like urticaria or exanthema and complicated reactions like SJS/TEN and drug reaction with eosinophilia and systemic symptoms (DRESS). They can be seen with a variety of drugs including antibiotics, aromatic anticonvulsants, NSAIDs, anti-tubercular drugs and sulfa drugs. These reactions are seen more commonly in immunocompromised individuals, especially in people with human immunodeficiency virus (HIV) as they are on multiple therapies like, drugs for opportunistic infections, anti-tubercular drugs, prophylactic drugs to prevent infection like sulphonamides and dapsone, as well as anti-retroviral drugs.

Complicated/Severe Cutaneous Adverse Drug Reactions[25]

- Stevens-Johnson syndrome/toxic epidermal necrolysis
- Drug reaction with eosinophilia and systemic symptoms (DRESS)/drug induced hypersensitivity syndrome (DIHS)
- Acute generalised exanthematous pustulosis (AGEP)
- Drug induced anaphylaxis
- Extensive fixed drug eruption (FDE)

Markers of Severe Cutaneous Adverse Drug Reactions

- Facial edema
- Lymph node enlargement
- Bullous or pustular lesions
- Skin tenderness
- Peeling of skin and/or a positive Nikolsky sign
- Mucosal erosions
- Systemic features like fever, malaise
- Deranged laboratory parameters like increased total leucocyte count, peripheral blood eosinophilia, atypical lymphocytes, increased liver function tests, elevated creatinine.

Severe cutaneous adverse drug reactions have been found to cause a lot of morbidity and even mortality, if not managed appropriately and in time. Mainstay of treatment is early withdrawal of suspected drug and if necessary, initiation of oral steroids.

Role of Steroids in DRESS

DRESS presents with generalised maculopapular rash along with yellowish discoloration of the sclera due to deranged liver functions (Fig. 8.3). Steroids remain the cornerstone of treatment for DRESS apart from stopping the suspected drug. They not only improve the cutaneous lesions but also ameliorate the systemic manifestations as evidenced by improvement of laboratory parameters.

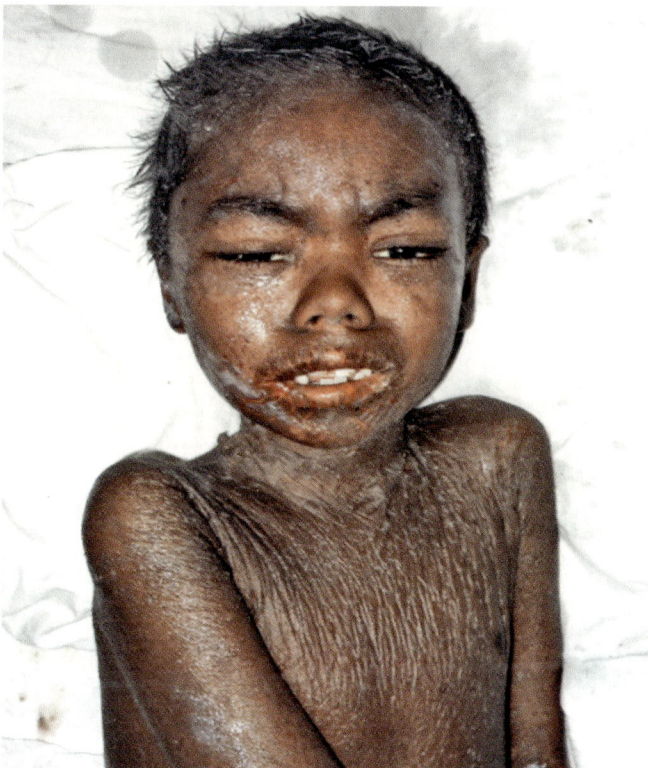

Fig. 8.3: DRESS requiring systemic steroids.

Usually, oral prednisolone in the dose of 1 mg/kg/day is initiated and the response can be expected within a few days of initiation.[26] Unlike SJS/TEN, steroid tapering is very slow in DRESS, decreased by 10 mg every 6–8 weeks, in order to prevent relapse.

Response to treatment should be monitored using clinical features like disappearance of rash, absence of fever, malaise, lymphadenopathy, reduction in laboratory abnormalities like peripheral eosinophilia, atypical lymphocytes, and liver or renal function tests.

In case the patient fail to respond to high dose corticosteroid, pulsed steroids in the form of IV methylprednisolone 1 gm for 3 consecutive days can be resorted to, or another agent like cyclosporine A can be added.

Role of Steroids in AGEP

The usually implicated drugs in AGEP include aminopenicillins, macrolides, quinolones, sulphonamides and calcium channel blockers. It manifests as generalised erythema and multiple pustules, with a flexural predilection (Fig. 8.4).

It can be easily managed by withdrawing the causative drug and no systemic treatment is generally required as it is benign and self-limiting.[27]

However, in severe cases, a short course of oral steroids may be tried.

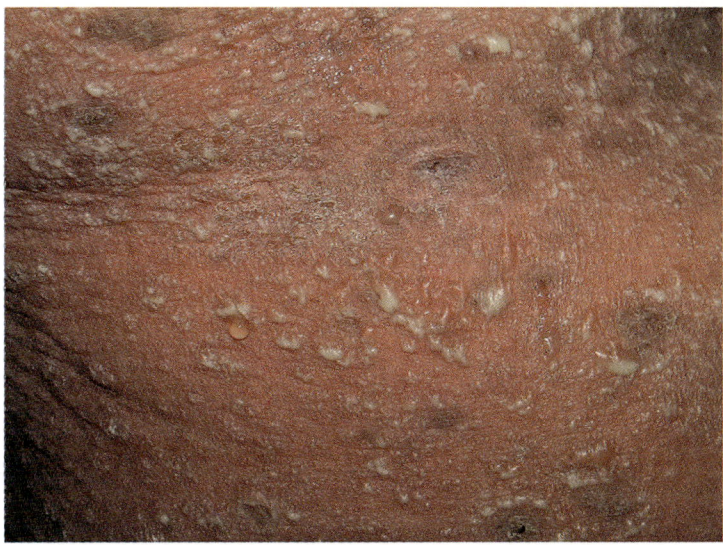

Fig. 8.4: Acute generalized exanthematous pustulosis.

Role of Steroids in Drug Induced Angioedema or Anaphylaxis

Drug induced angioedema can be caused by any drug, however the commonly implicated ones include NSAIDs and ACE inhibitors. Management includes withdrawing the culprit drug, and oral antihistamines generally suffice for the management of angioedema. However, if the angioedema affects important sites such periorbital area, lips or tongue, a short course of oral steroids should be given.

Laryngeal edema can present as choking sensation, wheezing or difficulty in breathing and should be treated as anaphylaxis.

Anaphylaxis should be considered if the patient develops urticaria or angioedema, along with features of laryngeal edema/bronchospasm, hypotension or gastrointestinal symptoms. Management of anaphylaxis includes removing the offending trigger/drug, securing the airway, IV hydrocortisone and IM epinephrine. Once stable, patient should be discharged on a short course of oral steroids to protect against the late phase of anaphylactic reaction.

It is important to remember that steroids have no role in the management of hereditary angioedema (C1 esterase inhibitor deficiency).

Role of Steroids in Extensive Fixed Drug Eruption

Fixed drug eruptions are usually not severe, presenting as solitary to few dusky erythematous round-to-oval skin lesions.

However, sometimes patients can develop bullous fixed drug eruption with multiple lesions, usually after a continuous re-exposure to the offending drug. It can even mimic SJS/TEN clinically. However, it can be differentiated on the basis of prior history of classical FDE, well-defined rounded border of lesion and relative sparing of mucosae.

Since the skin involvement is extensive, a short course of oral steroid like prednisolone 0.5–1 mg/kg/day for 7–10 days can be given to provide quick relief.

Steroids for Drug Reactions in HIV

Cutaneous adverse drug reactions are more common in HIV rather than general population. Sulfonamide drugs are the most implicated in HIV-infected patients,[28] followed by nevirapine (NVP). In a study from South Africa, cutaneous adverse reactions were seen in 10.7% cases (266/2489) in HIV infected individuals on anti-retroviral therapy (ART).[29] However, only 0.5% (12 cases) had SJS/TEN. Nevirapine was the most commonly implicated drug in the study found in 63.4% of all cases and 4.6% of SJS/TEN cases. Management of cutaneous adverse drug reactions in HIV positive individuals remains largely the same as immunocompetent people.

The offending drug likely ART is not stopped if the drug reaction seems to be mild in severity (for example, a maculopapular exanthem), as it is likely to self-resolve in few days despite continuing ART. However, if there is evidence of severe cutaneous involvement in the form of blistering, erythroderma, extreme itching, mucosal involvement and/or systemic features like high grade fever, pain abdomen, jaundice, elevated transaminases (>5 times), the suspected drugs should be immediately stopped and the patient should receive systemic corticosteroids depending on the nature and severity of drug reaction.[30] The CD4 count should preferably be on the higher side, however despite being on lower sides, short steroids do not impair the immune functions adversely.

Treatment of patients with corticosteroids within the first 24 h of TMP-SMX hypersensitivity has been shown to be of benefit.[31] Prophylactic use of corticosteroids or antihistamines to prevent hypersensitivity reactions to nevirapine has not been recommended as it can increase the risk of developing the rash.[32,33]

Early short course steroids can be given in patients with SJS/TEN with no adverse effect on the progression of HIV disease when the CD4 count is good enough (as per authors experience), although no original studies have been done in this regard.

C. ROLE OF STEROIDS IN EXTENSIVE PEMPHIGUS

Pemphigus is a group of autoimmune blistering disorders which presents with flaccid bullae and cutaneous erosions. Pemphigus foliaceus has only skin involvement, while pemphigus vulgaris usually has mucosal involvement as well. In extensive pemphigus, there can be large denuded areas of skin, placing the patient at risk of infection, sepsis, thermoregulatory disturbance and fluid and electrolyte imbalance. Pemphigus vulgaris has a higher risk of mortality, because of the deeper intraepidermal split presenting as frank moist erosions (Fig. 8.5).

Systemic steroids are the first-line drugs to achieve rapid disease control in pemphigus vulgaris. It is recommended to start with 0.5–1.5 mg/kg/day of oral prednisolone depending on severity. However, in extensive involvement, one may

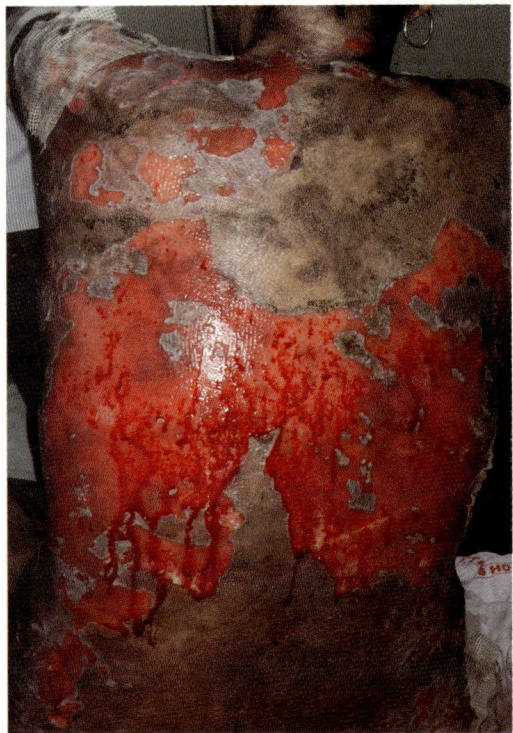

Fig. 8.5: Extensive pemphigus vulgaris: Large coalescing bleeding erosions on the back.

start with a higher dose and go up to 2 mg/kg in case of unsatisfactory response with the earlier doses.

If the total required dose of prednisolone is >100 mg/day or disease activity is not controlled with up to 2 mg/kg prednisolone, then pulsed steroids should be considered. Steroid pulse can be either IV methylprednisolone (1000 mg/day) or dexamethasone (100 mg/day) given for 3 consecutive days every month.[34] Oral prednisolone in dose of 0.5–1 mg/kg should continue along with the monthly pulses.

High-dose oral steroids or steroid pulses are sufficient to induce remission in pemphigus. Addition of cyclophosphamide to the dexamethasone pulse may be avoided early on in the disease when the skin barrier is impaired, as the additional immunosuppression puts the patients at risk of infections and hematological derangements. Cyclophosphamide can be added to steroid pulses later on when the patient comes out of the 'crisis' situation, as the purpose of adding cyclophosphamide is primarily to prolong the remission.

Sometimes, despite adequate treatment, the disease remains progressive or does not respond satisfactorily. Pemphigus can sometimes flare-up after receiving the first dose of rituximab. In such a situation, a one-day steroid interval pulse can be tried for quick disease control. These one-day steroid interval pulses can be given at weekly intervals, till satisfactory disease control (no new blisters, healing of established skin erosions) is achieved.

Patients with extensive pemphigus are at risk of secondary skin infection (which may be complicated by sepsis) because of skin detachment and therapeutic immunosuppression. Daily dressing under aseptic conditions and skin swab for pus culture sensitivity should be undertaken. Any skin infection should be appropriately treated with antibiotics, and a strict watch should be kept for warning signs of systemic infection. Patients should also be monitored for steroid associated side-effects like deranged blood sugar and raised blood pressure.

D. STEROIDS IN URTICARIA AND ANGIOEDEMA

Urticaria and angioedema are yet another emergency dermatoses with prevalence of former alone in about 50% of cases and latter alone in 10% respectively. Urticaria along with angioedema is seen in around 40% cases.[35] Both these conditions are mast cell mediated with histamine as the major mediator. Anti-histamines forms the major treatment modality. However, steroids may be indicated in severe cases to provide rapid control.

Steroids are Indicated in the Following Conditions

- When urticaria is refractory to treatment with escalated doses of antihistamines
- To gain control of the disease until other therapies can achieve control
- Pressure urticaria
- Angioedema

Role of Steroids in Managing Urticaria

- Sometimes for severe acute urticaria and angioedema, a short course of oral prednisolone 20–40 mg (0.5–1 mg/kg) per day might be necessary for disease control followed by tapering and termination within 2 weeks (Fig. 8.6).

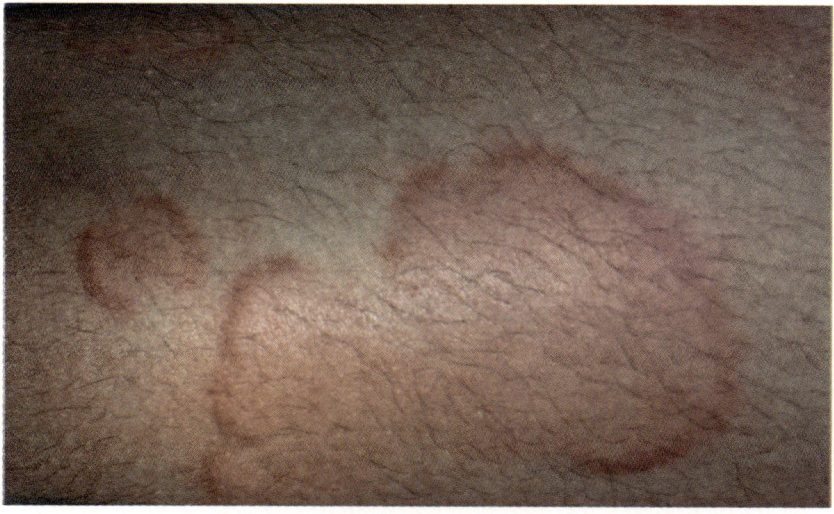

Fig. 8.6: Erythematous edematous wheals unresponsive to antihistamines.

- It is important to note that oral steroids should be used judiciously in urticaria; only when urticaria is severe, not controlled with antihistamines and only for a short duration (7–14 days).
- AAAAI/ACAAI Joint Task Force 2014[36] and EAACI/GA2LEN/EDF/WAO Guidelines 2017[37] do not promote use of long term steroids for the management of chronic spontaneous urticaria. However, for acute exacerbation of chronic spontaneous urticaria and acute urticaria, a short course of oral steroids for not more than 10 days may be tried till the time other agents takes control.

Role of Steroids in Managing Angioedema

- Most cases of angioedema can be managed with oral antihistamines.
- A short course of oral steroids (oral prednisolone 20–40 mg/day) can be tried for patients for a rapid response, or if it is causing any functional/cosmetic disability to the patient (for example, eyelid, lip or tongue swelling) (Fig. 8.7).
- Presence of laryngeal edema, is an indication for IV hydrocortisone. If the laryngeal edema is severe, then IM epinephrine and airway management are the mainstay of treatment along with supportive role of hydrocortisone (refer to management of anaphylaxis earlier).
- Topical steroids have no role in the management of urticaria or angioedema.

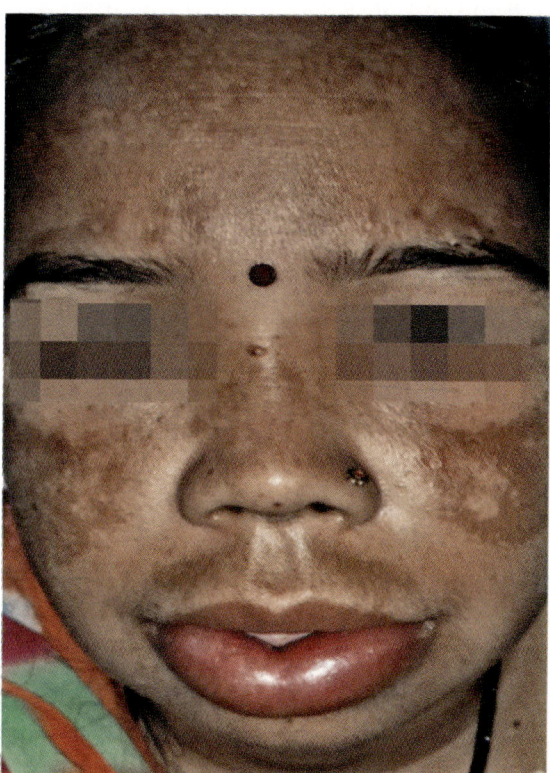

Fig. 8.7: Angioedema of periorbital area and lips requiring systemic steroids.

E. ROLE OF STEROIDS IN ERYTHRODERMA

Erythroderma refers to the extensive (usually >90%) skin involvement in the form of erythema and scaling. There are several causes of erythroderma in adults, common ones include endogenous/atopic dermatitis, psoriasis, cutaneous T-cell lymphoma, drug induced and idiopathic.

Management of erythroderma involves general skin care measures like liberal use of emollients, antihistamines, temperature regulation, maintaining fluid and electrolyte balance, and high-protein diet.

Most cases of erythroderma would require oral steroids to gain a rapid disease control. However, oral steroids are contraindicated in erythroderma secondary to psoriasis, so it must be ruled out prior to initiation of steroids.

Topical steroids can be an option for chronic stable erythroderma. However, high-potency steroids are generally avoided owing to the risk of systemic absorption through large areas of epidermal barrier defect.[38]

The usual dose is 0.5 mg/kg/day of prednisolone which can be increased or decreased depending on the response. Oral steroids are tapered gradually, by about 10 mg every 4 weeks. Another agent such as methotrexate, azathioprine or cyclosporine may be added to provide steroid-sparing effect.

Patients should be monitored for steroid side effects like raised blood pressure, blood sugar charting, bone mineral density and weight gain.[39]

F. ROLE OF STEROIDS IN SEVERE PSORIASIS

Systemic steroids are generally contraindicated in psoriasis, owing to the risk of flare-up when steroids are tapered or stopped abruptly.

However, systemic steroids are often considered to be the first-line drugs for generalized pustular psoriasis of pregnancy, at par with cyclosporine. Systemic steroids are pregnancy category C drugs.

Generalized pustular psoriasis of pregnancy, also known as impetigo herpetiformis, is a severe disease and can be associated with poor pregnancy outcomes. It manifests as multiple pustules, with lakes of pus and generalized erythema. Constitutional features such as fever, malaise are usually present.

In mild to moderate disease, oral prednisolone is started at the dose of 0.5–1 mg/kg.[40] In case of further progression, high dose of up to 2 mg/kg can be given, along with fetal monitoring as high dose steroids can affect fetus adversely. Steroids are continued till early postpartum period and then gradually tapered and stopped. Early tapering of steroids can be associated with relapse.

In addition to generalized pustular psoriasis of pregnancy, systemic steroids have also been tried for severe psoriasis/psoriatic erythroderma with metabolic complications (such as cardiovascular instability). Steroids are also indicated in retinoic acid syndrome, a rare life-threatening complication of retinoid treatment like acitretin in patients with psoriasis. It manifests as systemic complications like hypotension, pulmonary infiltrates, pleural and pericardial effusions, and renal failure.[41] It requires immediate withdrawal of the retinoid, and high-dose corticosteroids.

Indications of Systemic Steroids in Psoriasis[40,41]

1. Generalized pustular psoriasis of pregnancy.
2. Severe psoriasis/psoriatic erythroderma with metabolic complications, retinoic acid syndrome.

G. ROLE OF STEROIDS IN ACNE FULMINANS

Acne fulminans (AF) is a severe inflammatory variant of acne presenting as ulcerated, painful and crusted (hemorrhagic) lesions, usually accompanied with systemic features like fever and joint pains (Fig. 8.8).

Steroids are indicated in the initial management of AF, started alone at the dose of 0.5–1 mg/kg/day of oral prednisolone. It is continued for 2–4 weeks, followed by initiation of low dose isotretinoin (0.1 mg/kg/day). This dual therapy is continued for another 2–4 weeks, following which steroids are gradually tapered and stopped and isotretinoin to be hiked up to highest possible dose tolerated up to 1 mg/kg.

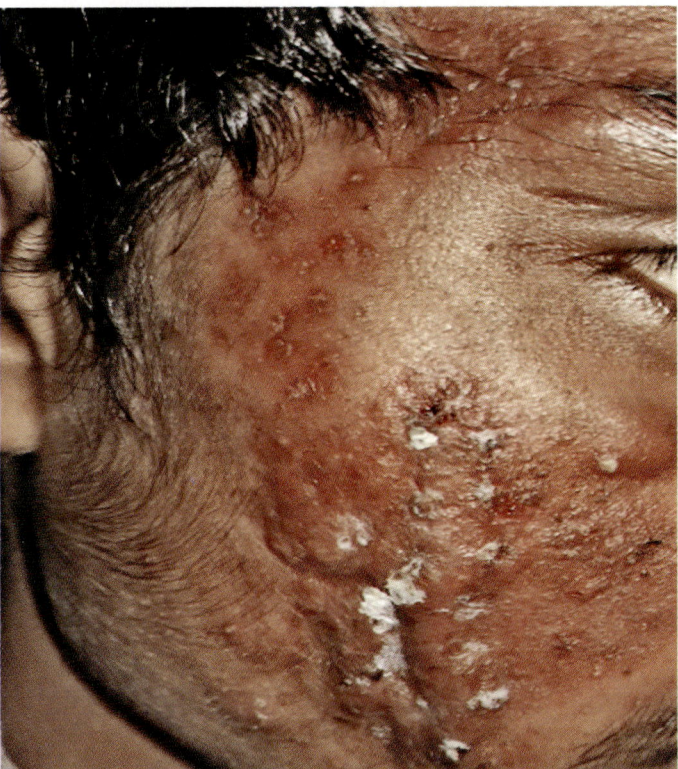

Fig. 8.8: Acne fulminans requiring systemic steroids.

There are no large-scale randomized controlled trials evaluating treatment for AF. Role of steroids lies in quickly controlling the severe inflammation during the initial phase.[42]

Oral isotretinoin alone should not be given in the treatment of acne fulminans, as it can further worsen the disease. It should only be initiated once the disease has been controlled with oral steroids.

REFERENCES

1. Law EH, Leung M. Corticosteroids in Stevens-Johnson Syndrome/toxic epidermal necrolysis: current evidence and implications for future research. Ann Pharmacother 2015;49:335–42.

2. Correia O, Delgado L, Ramos JP, Resende C, Torrinha JA. Cutaneous T-cell recruitment in toxic epidermal necrolysis. Further evidence of CD8+ lymphocyte involvement. Arch Dermatol 1993;129:466–8.

3. Posadas SJ, Padial A, Torres MJ, Mayorga C, Leyva L, Sanchez E, et al. Delayed reactions to drugs show levels of perforin, granzyme B, and Fas-L to be related to disease severity. J Allergy Clin Immunol 2002 ;109:155–61.

4. Abe R, Shimizu T, Shibaki A, Nakamura H, Watanabe H, Shimizu H. Toxic epidermal necrolysis and Stevens-Johnson syndrome are induced by soluble Fas ligand. Am J Pathol 2003;162:1515–20.

5. Viard I, Wehrli P, Bullani R, Schneider P, Holler N, Salomon D, et al. Inhibition of toxic epidermal necrolysis by blockade of CD95 with human intravenous immunoglobulin. Science 1998;282:490–3.

6. Schwartz RA, McDonough PH, Lee BW. Toxic epidermal necrolysis: Part I. Introduction, history, classification, clinical features, systemic manifestations, etiology, and immunopathogenesis. J Am Acad Dermatol 2013;69:173.e1-13; quiz 185–6.

7. Letko E, Papaliodis DN, Papaliodis GN, Daoud YJ, Ahmed AR, Foster CS. Stevens-Johnson syndrome and toxic epidermal necrolysis: a review of the literature. Ann Allergy Asthma Immunol Off Publ Am Coll Allergy Asthma Immunol 2005;94:419-36; quiz 436–8, 456.

8. Schwartz RA, McDonough PH, Lee BW. Toxic epidermal necrolysis: Part II. Prognosis, sequelae, diagnosis, differential diagnosis, prevention, and treatment. J Am Acad Dermatol 2013;69:187.e1-16; quiz 203–4.

9. Gupta LK, Martin AM, Agarwal N, D'Souza P, Das S, Kumar R, et al. Guidelines for the management of Stevens-Johnson syndrome/toxic epidermal necrolysis: An Indian perspective. Indian J Dermatol Venereol Leprol 2016;82:603–25.

10. Zimmermann S, Sekula P, Venhoff M, Motschall E, Knaus J, Schumacher M, et al. Systemic Immunomodulating Therapies for Stevens-Johnson Syndrome and Toxic Epidermal Necrolysis: A Systematic Review and Meta-analysis. JAMA Dermatol 2017;153:514–22.

11. Murphy JT, Purdue GF, Hunt JL. Toxic epidermal necrolysis. J Burn Care Rehabil 1997;18:417–20.

12. Schulz JT, Sheridan RL, Ryan CM, MacKool B, Tompkins RG. A 10-year experience with toxic epidermal necrolysis. J Burn Care Rehabil 2000;21:199–204.

13. Tripathi A, Ditto AM, Grammer LC, Greenberger PA, McGrath KG, Zeiss CR, et al. Corticosteroid therapy in an additional 13 cases of Stevens-Johnson syndrome: a total series of 67 cases. Allergy Asthma Proc 2000 ;21:101–5.

14. Ducic I, Shalom A, Rising W, Nagamoto K, Munster AM. Outcome of patients with toxic epidermal necrolysis syndrome revisited. Plast Reconstr Surg 2002;110:768–73.

15. Kim KJ, Lee DP, Suh HS, Lee MW, Choi JH, Moon KC, et al. Toxic epidermal necrolysis: analysis of clinical course and SCORTEN-based comparison of mortality rate and treatment modalities in Korean patients. Acta Derm Venereol 2005;85:497–502.

16. Kardaun SH, Jonkman MF. Dexamethasone pulse therapy for Stevens-Johnson syndrome/toxic epidermal necrolysis. Acta Derm Venereol 2007;87:144–8.

17. Schneck J, Fagot J-P, Sekula P, Sassolas B, Roujeau JC, Mockenhaupt M. Effects of treatments on the mortality of Stevens-Johnson syndrome and toxic epidermal necrolysis: A retrospective study on patients included in the prospective EuroSCAR Study. J Am Acad Dermatol 2008;58:33–40.

18. Yang Y, Xu J, Li F, Zhu X. Combination therapy of intravenous immunoglobulin and corticosteroid in the treatment of toxic epidermal necrolysis and Stevens-Johnson syndrome: a retrospective comparative study in China. Int J Dermatol 2009;48:1122–8.

19. Chen J, Wang B, Zeng Y, Xu H. High-dose intravenous immunoglobulins in the treatment of Stevens-Johnson syndrome and toxic epidermal necrolysis in Chinese patients: a retrospective study of 82 cases. Eur J Dermatol EJD 2010;20:743–7.

20. Hirahara K, Kano Y, Sato Y, Horie C, Okazaki A, Ishida T, et al. Methylprednisolone pulse therapy for Stevens-Johnson syndrome/toxic epidermal necrolysis: clinical evaluation and analysis of biomarkers. J Am Acad Dermatol 2013;69:496–8.

21. Pasricha JS, Khaitan BK, Shantharaman R, Mital A, Girdhar M. Toxic epidermal necrolysis. Int J Dermatol 1996;35:523–7.

22. Das S, Roy AK, Biswas I. A six-month prospective study to find out the treatment outcome, prognosis and offending drugs in toxic epidermal necrolysis from an urban institution in kolkata. Indian J Dermatol 2013 ;58:191–3.

23. Rai R, Srinivas CR. Suprapharmacologic doses of intravenous dexamethasone followed by cyclosporine in the treatment of toxic epidermal necrolysis. Indian J Dermatol Venereol Leprol 2008;74:263–5.

24. Singh GK, Chatterjee M, Verma R. Cyclosporine in Stevens-Johnson syndrome and toxic epidermal necrolysis and retrospective comparison with systemic corticosteroid. Indian J Dermatol Venereol Leprol 2013;79:686–92.

25. Swanson L, Colven RM. Approach to the Patient with a Suspected Cutaneous Adverse Drug Reaction. Med Clin North Am 2015;99:1337–48.

26. Husain Z, Reddy BY, Schwartz RA. DRESS syndrome: Part II. Management and therapeutics. J Am Acad Dermatol 2013;68:709.e1-9; quiz 718–20.

27. Sidoroff A. Acute generalized exanthematous pustulosis. Chem Immunol Allergy 2012;97:139–48.

28. Oliveira I, Jensen-Fangel S, da Silva D, Ndumba A, Medina C, Nanadje A, et al. Epidemic Stevens-Johnson syndrome in HIV patients in Guinea-Bissau: a side effect of the drug-supply policy? AIDS Lond Engl 2010 ;24:783–5.

29. Birbal S, Dheda M, Ojewole E, Oosthuizen F. Adverse drug reactions associated with antiretroviral therapy in South Africa. Afr J AIDS Res AJAR 2016;15:243–8.

30. Gill S, Sagar A, Shankar S, Nair V. Nevirapine-induced rash with eosinophilia and systemic symptoms (DRESS). Indian J Pharmacol 2013;45:401–2.

31. Walmsley S, Levinton C, Brunton J, Muradali D, Rappaport D, Bast M, et al. A multicenter randomized double-blind placebo-controlled trial of adjunctive corticosteroids in the treatment of *Pneumocystis carinii* pneumonia complicating the acquired immune deficiency syndrome. J Acquir Immune Defic Syndr Hum Retrovirology Off Publ Int Retrovirology Assoc 1995;8:348–57.

32. Montaner JSG, Cahn P, Zala C, Casssetti LI, Losso M, Hall DB, et al. Randomized, controlled study of the effects of a short course of prednisone on the incidence of rash associated with nevirapine in patients infected with HIV-1. J Acquir Immune Defic Syndr 2003;33:41–6.

33. Barreiro P, Soriano V, Casas E, Estrada V, Téllez MJ, Hoetelmans R, et al. Prevention of nevirapine-associated exanthema using slow dose escalation and/or corticosteroids. AIDS Lond Engl 2000 29;14:2153–7.

34. Harman KE, Brown D, Exton LS, Groves RW, Hampton PJ, Mohd Mustapa MF, et al. British Association of Dermatologists' guidelines for the management of pemphigus vulgaris 2017. Br J Dermatol 2017;177:1170–201.

35. Kaplan AP. Clinical practice. Chronic urticaria and angioedema. N Engl J Med 2002;346:175–9.

36. Bernstein JA, Lang DM, Khan DA, Craig T, Dreyfus D, Hsieh F, et al. The diagnosis and management of acute and chronic urticaria: 2014 update. J Allergy Clin Immunol 2014;133:1270–7.

37. Zuberbier T, Aberer W, Asero R, Abdul Latiff AH, Baker D, Ballmer-Weber B, et al. The EAACI/GA2LEN/EDF/WAO guideline for the definition, classification, diagnosis and management of urticaria. Allergy 2018;73:1393–414.

38. Aalto-Korte K, Turpeinen M. Quantifying systemic absorption of topical hydrocortisone in erythroderma. Br J Dermatol 1995;133:403–8.

39. Leclerc-Mercier S, Bodemer C, Bourdon-Lanoy E, Larousserie F, Hovnanian A, Brousse N, et al. Early skin biopsy is helpful for the diagnosis and management of neonatal and infantile erythrodermas. J Cutan Pathol 2010;37:249–55.

40. Trivedi MK, Vaughn AR, Murase JE. Pustular psoriasis of pregnancy: current perspectives. Int J Womens Health 2018;10:109–15.

41. Liu D, Cao F, Yan X, Chen X, Chen Y, Tu Y, et al. Retinoic acid syndrome in a patient with psoriasis. Eur J Dermatol EJD 2009;19:632–4.

42. Seukeran DC, Cunliffe WJ. The treatment of acne fulminans: a review of 25 cases. Br J Dermatol 1999;141:307–9.

Evidence-Based Use of Steroids in Steroid Responsive Dermatoses

Eswari L, Neha Taneja, Neetu Bhari

SUMMARY

- Corticosteroids in all forms—topical, intralesional and systemic, form the backbone of treating majority of the dermatological conditions.
- There are substantial evidences in favour of using corticosteroids in autoimmune blistering disorders, papulosquamous disorders such as psoriasis and lichen planus, dermatitis, vitiligo and alopecia areata.
- Systemic corticosteroids are first-line therapy for the management of pemphigus.
- The pulsed doses help to achieve a more rapid and effective disease control as well as to reduce the cumulative corticosteroid doses and its side-effects.
- Topical corticosteroids are considered as a first-line therapy for mild-to-moderate bullous pemphigoid.
- Systemic corticosteroids should only be used in widespread disease, which can not be managed by topical corticosteroids.
- The goals of topical corticosteroid therapy in atopic dermatitis include progressive reduction to change of the therapy to a topical nonsteroidal agent and at the same time ensuring the absence of relapse after reduction in the frequency of application and/or stepping down to a lower potency steroid.
- Use of systemic corticosteroids is limited in cases of atopic dermatitis with acute and severe exacerbation for a short duration.
- Topical corticosteroids are commonly used as first-line treatment for localized cutaneous lichen planus, psoriasis, vitiligo and alopecia areata. For patients with generalized disease, topical corticosteroids are often used as an adjunct to systemic therapy or phototherapy.
- However, these so called "magic molecules" should be used judiciously and appropriately, in order to limit the short-term and long-term side effects associated with them.

INTRODUCTION

Corticosteroids have an important role in the field of dermatology because of their wide spectrum of actions including their anti-inflammatory and immunosuppressive effects. They can be administered orally, parenterally or intralesionally. This chapter covers the common steroid responsive dermatoses and in whose management, the efficacy of steroids has been proven.

• Most common steroid responsive dermatoses are summarized in Table 9.1.

The use of steroids, both topical and systemic has been graded in this chapter to assist clinical decision making in steroid responsive dermatoses. The grading includes level of evidence (Table 9.2) and strength of recommendation (Table 9.3).

Table 9.1: Common steroid responsive dermatoses	
Dermatitis	• Atopic dermatitis • Seborrheic dermatitis • Allergic and irritant contact dermatitis
Papulosquamous disorders	• Psoriasis • Lichen planus
Pigmentary disorder	Vitiligo
Vesiculobullous disorders	Immunobullous blistering diseases as pemphigus vulgaris and bullous pemphigoid
Autoimmune disorders	• Lupus erythematosus • Dermatomyositis • Morphea • Scleroderma
Others	• Alopecia areata • Lichen sclerosus • Polymorphic eruptions of pregnancy

Table 9.2: Level of evidence	
Level of evidence	Type of evidence
1++	High-quality meta-analyses, systematic reviews of RCTs, or RCTs with a very low risk of bias
1+	Well-conducted meta-analyses, systematic reviews of RCTs, or RCTs with a low risk of bias
1–	Meta-analyses, systematic reviews of RCTs, or RCTs with a high risk of bias
2++	High-quality systematic reviews of case-control or cohort studies, high-quality case-control or cohort studies with a very low risk of confounding, bias or chance and a high probability that the relationship is causal
2+	Well-conducted case-control or cohort studies with a low risk of confounding, bias or chance and a moderate probability that the relationship is causal
2–	Case-control or cohort studies with a high risk of confounding, bias or chance and a significant risk that the relationship is not causal
3	Nonanalytical studies (for example, case reports, case series)
4	Expert opinion, formal consensus

Table 9.3: Strength of recommendation	
Grade	Recommendation
A	Directly based on Level I evidence
B	Directly based on Level II evidence or extrapolated recommendations from Level I evidence
C	Directly based on Level III evidence or extrapolated recommendations from Level I or II evidence
D	Directly based on Level IV evidence or extrapolated recommendations from Level I, II, or III evidence

CORTICOSTEROIDS IN IMMUNOBULLOUS DISORDERS

- The pathogenetic mechanism of immunobullous blistering disorders is abnormal humoral autoimmune response to various molecular components of the basement membrane zone (BMZ).
- The pemphigus group of disorders are characterized by antibodies to desmogleins while the subepidermal autoimmune bullous disorders are associated with antibodies against components of hemidesmosomes, lamina lucida, lamina densa and sub-lamina densa.
- In pemphigus group of diseases, systemic corticosteroids along with steroid-sparing immunosuppressants (cyclophosphamide, azathioprine, or mycophenolate mofetil) are the mainstay of therapy.
- The average mortality in pemphigus vulgaris was up to 75% before the introduction of corticosteroids in the early 1950s, which reduced to 30% after advent of corticosteroids.[1]

Long term randomized controlled trials demonstrating efficacy of corticosteroids are lacking for immunobullous diseases. Most of the data is derived from case reports and small case series with short follow-up. In addition, there are differences in patient's disease profile and subtypes with varied disease definitions and outcome parameters which makes it difficult to compare these results and reach a consensus.

Remission Induction

The main aim of treatment in pemphigus is to initiate the disease control (remission) followed by its maintenance. According to consensus statement by Murrell *et al*, remission in pemphigus has been defined as cessation of development of new lesions and healing of existing lesions.[2] The drug of choice for achieving remission in pemphigus group of diseases is corticosteroid in its oral or parenteral form. Disease activity gets controlled in several weeks (median 3 weeks).[3] Adjuvant therapies have a slower onset of action. The next phase is called consolidation phase which ends when 80% of lesions have healed, with no new lesions for at least 2 weeks.[2] Oral ulceration takes a longer time to heal than cutaneous lesions. Corticosteroids should be tapered at the end of the consolidation phase. Premature tapering is not recommended.

Remission Maintenance

Treatment is gradually reduced to the minimum required for disease control, in order to minimize the side-effects.[2] After the remission is attained, the adjuvant immunosuppressive should be continued for at least 6 to 9 months. Complete remission off therapy is defined as the absence of new and/or established lesions for at least 2 months while the patient is off all systemic therapy.[2]

The main aim for continuing adjuvant drugs is maintenance of remission. They also help in reducing cumulative dose of corticosteroids and its resulting side-effects. A systematic review concluded that adjuvant drugs like azathioprine, cyclophosphamide and mycophenolate mofetil were not helpful in induction of remission but helped in reducing the rate of relapse by 29%.[4]

Oral Corticosteroids
(Strength of Recommendation B; Level of Evidence 1+)

Systemic corticosteroids are first-line therapy for the management of pemphigus. The usual practice is to initiate treatment at the dose of prednisolone 1–2 mg/kg or its equivalent.[5,6] If the disease activity persist for next 5–7 days, the dose should be increased by 0.5 to 1 mg/kg until disease control is achieved.[7] The guidelines by European Dermatology Forum (EDF) and European Academy of Dermatology and Venereology (EADV) recommend initial prednisolone dose at 0.5 mg–1.5 mg/kg/d and if control of the disease is not reached within 2 weeks, a higher prednisolone dose (up to 2 mg/kg) could be administered.[8] If prednisolone dose above 1 mg/kg per day is required for longer duration, pulsed intravenous corticosteroids is usually considered by majority. Many dermatologists now prefer using pulsed intravenous corticosteroids as first line with or without oral steroids. The dose should be tapered after the consolidation phase of disease. There is no established tapering schedule, though a 50% reduction in the dose every 2 weeks is the most commonly used practice.[1] Slower tapering (monthly) after 20 mg is usually followed.

Relapse may occur anytime during tapering of corticosteroids, or stopping of immunosuppressant drugs. Relapse/flare is defined as the appearance of ≥3 new lesions per month that do not heal spontaneously within 1 week, or by the extension of established lesions, in a patient who has achieved control of disease activity.[2] An increase in dose of oral corticosteroids is required to manage a relapse. The dose can be reverted to the previous dose of corticosteroid at which disease control was achieved. The adjuvant should be added to maintain a long-term remission.

Daily dosing schedules usually lead to many corticosteroid induced side-effects such as iatrogenic Cushing syndrome, weight gain, hypertension, diabetes mellitus, peptic ulcer disease, cataract, osteoporosis, avascular necrosis of hip, neuropsychiatric symptoms and septicemia. Protective measures should be taken for those on prednisolone of 7.5 mg/day or more for more than 3 months.[9] This includes use of proton pump inhibitor for gastric protection. Measures should also be aimed at minimizing loss of bone density in postmenopausal women, men more than 50 years, and those with risk of fragile fractures. Patients with PV and other immunobullous disorders such as bullous pemphigoid have lower levels of vitamin D, than controls, suggesting additional risk of bone density loss.[10] Guidelines for the prevention of corticosteroid-induced osteoporosis should be followed.[11,12] Calcium and vitamin D supplementation with a bisphosphonate therapy are effective in preserving bone density, if given from the start of systemic steroid therapy.[13]

Pulsed Intravenous Corticosteroids
(Strength of Recommendation D; Level of Evidence 4)

Pulsed intravenous corticosteroids refers to the administration of supra-pharmacological doses of corticosteroids, usually intravenous methylprednisolone (10–20 mg/kg or 250–1000 mg) or of dexamethasone (100 mg) given on 3–5 consecutive days.[14] The pulsed doses helps to achieve a more rapid and effective disease control as well as to reduce the cumulative corticosteroid doses and its side-effects. Flushing, palpitations, hiccups, asthenia, muscular weakness, numbness in feet, altered taste and hair loss are some of the immediate side effects but these subsides with further pulses. Long-term side-effects have been reported to be significantly lower than with daily corticosteroid.[15] In a randomised controlled trial (RCT) investigating the role of intravenous corticosteroid pulses, one group received monotherapy with oral prednisone in an initial dose of 125 mg/day, whereas the other group was treated with three weekly pulses of intravenous betamethasone (20 mg/day for 4 days) in combination with oral prednisone (50 mg/day) during intervals. The pulse protocol was significantly superior in both, time to resolution of clinical manifestations, including oral lesions, and in safety profile.[16]

Pasricha et al, treated all pemphigus patients with Dexamethasone cyclophosphamide pulse (DCP)/dexamthasone pulse (DP) regimen irrespective of the severity or duration of the disease.[17] Of the 300 patients enrolled for this treatment, 61 patients could not complete the treatment, whereas 12 patients died, some of them due to unrelated causes. Of the remaining 227 patients, 190 patients (84%) completed the treatment and were free of the disease even after complete withdrawal of all treatment. The duration of post-treatment follow-up being more than 5 years in 48 patients, 2 to 5 years in 75 patients, and less than 2 years in 67 patients. The maximum duration of post-treatment follow-up was 9 years. The blood levels of intercellular antibody also decreased as the treatment progressed. The side effects commonly observed during treatment with daily corticosteroids were either absent or insignificant. The relapses of the disease, seen in 59 patients, had been observed mostly in those patients who defaulted during the treatment, but a further course of the DCP regimen led again to complete recovery.

Modified DCP regimens used in several trials have failed to demonstrate consistent superiority over other corticosteroid/adjuvant PV treatment regimens. A nonrandomized trial favoured pulsed cyclophosphamide, which showed a lower cumulative corticosteroid dose when compared with azathioprine although efficacy was similar.[18] Pulsed cyclophosphamide has a superior corticosteroid—sparing effect compared with mycophenolate mofetil.[19]

Recommendations for corticosteroids in pemphigus group of diseases include:

- Oral prednisolone—starts with prednisolone 1 mg/kg per day (or equivalent) in most cases, 0.5–1 mg/kg in milder cases
- Increase in 50–100% increments every 5–7 days if blistering continues
- Consider pulsed intravenous corticosteroids if >1 mg/kg oral prednisolone required, or as initial treatment in severe disease followed by 1 mg/kg per day oral prednisolone
- Taper dose once remission is induced and maintained, with absence of new blisters and healing of the majority of lesions (skin and mucosal). Aim to reduce to 10 mg daily or less.

Topical Corticosteroids

Mild cases of pemphigus can sometimes be controlled by topical therapy alone. However, these are more frequently used as adjunctive therapy in moderate to severe disease. Evidence for the additional benefit of topical treatments is poor. Topical corticosteroids are commonly used in patients with mucosal pemphigus vulgaris and include corticosteroid mouthwashes such as betamethasone sodium phosphate 0.5 mg dissolved in 10 mL of water as a 2–3 min rinse-and-spit solution one to four times a day or topical triamcinolone acetonide 0.1% paste applied twice daily to the lesions.[20]

Intralesional Corticosteroids

Mignogna *et al*, found that perilesional/intralesional triamcinolone acetonide injections in mucosal pemphigus achieved a rapid remission and obtained better patient compliance compared to topical corticosteroids.[21] These are usually used to control mild pemphigus presenting with only a few lesions, to treat recalcitrant lesions such as scalp and oral lesions and to treat new lesions in patients whose systemic therapy is being tapered off.

Pemphigus in Pregnancy

Oral corticosteroids are the main stay of treatment. Current evidence suggests that there is no significant increased risk of stillbirth, preterm delivery or congenital malformations from using prednisolone.[22] Prednisone (FDA pregnancy category B) is preferred as it is 90% inactivated by the placenta, whereas betamethasone and dexamethasone are far less inactivated having a greater effect on the fetus. Azathioprine, in combination with corticosteroids, has been used successfully for pemphigus in pregnancy with very low risk of teratogenicity, but should be used only in severe and recalcitrant disease.[23]

Pemphigus in Children

Systemic corticosteroids are the treatment of choice in both children and adolescent with pemphigus, but extra precautions are required as children are more susceptible to the potential adverse effects of systemic corticosteroids. Growth retardation and cushingoid features are the most important adverse effects in children receiving long-term oral corticosteroids.[24,25]

Corticosteroids in Bullous Pemphigoid

The aim of treatment in bullous pemphigoid (BP) is to suppress the clinical signs of BP sufficiently to make the disease tolerable to an individual patient (reduction of blister formation, urticarial lesions and pruritus). Remission of disease is usually not desired. Patients with BP are usually elderly, often on multiple therapies and at high risk of adverse drug reactions and side-effects. High doses of immuno-suppressants may put these patients at risk of life-threatening adverse effects. Thus, the treatment is aimed at controlling symptoms with minimum adverse effects possible.

There are usually two approaches to the initial control of the disease, and currently there is insufficient evidence to consider one approach over the other. Some dermatologists favour the use of minimum doses of systemic therapy to control the disease, individualizing treatment and accepting that in the occasional patient more aggressive therapy may be needed. Other dermatologists believe in controlling all patients with high-dose initial therapy. Treatment is tapered once control of the disease has been achieved.

Systemic Corticosteroids
(Strength of Recommendation A; Level of Evidence 1+)

Efficacy of systemic corticosteroids in BP is well established. The most commonly used drugs are prednisone and prednisolone. There is rapid suppression of inflammation and blistering, within 1–4 weeks, after which the dose is gradually reduced. However, serious dose dependent metabolic and immunosuppressive adverse effects have been recognized involving systemic steroids in the treatment of BP. Hence, these should only be used in widespread disease, which cannot be managed with topical corticosteroids. Recommended starting dose of prednisolone (prednisone) that would be maximally effective and minimally toxic is 0.75–1 mg/kg for patients with severe involvement, 0.5 mg/kg for moderate disease, 0.3 mg/kg for mild or localized disease. These doses have been shown to be effective within 1–4 weeks in about 60–90% of cases. If after 4 weeks of therapy, the new inflammatory lesions or blisters are few or absent, the dose of steroid should then be gradually tapered depending upon the response. A reduction of the daily dose of prednisolone at fortnightly intervals, initially by about one-third or one-quarter down to 15 mg daily, then by 2.5 mg decrements down to 10 mg daily, is suggested.

The dose could then be reduced by 1 mg each month.[26] In about 50% of cases relapse will occur at some point during the dose-reduction period, indicating that the previous dose is likely to be the minimal effective dose for that patient. The duration of systemic steroid treatment in BP may be for many months.

Intravenous methylprednisolone, either 1 g daily, or 15 mg/kg daily, or dexamethasone (100 mg) daily for 3 days, along with prednisone 30–40 mg daily, has been suggested to be used in patients who respond poorly to oral prednisolone 1 mg/kg or in relapse cases.[26] Adjuvant immunosuppressives may be added for steroid sparing effects in these cases.

Topical Corticosteroids
(Strength of Recommendation A; Level of Evidence 1+)

Topical corticosteroids are considered as first-line treatment for both localized as well as moderate disease. Joly P *et al*,[27] compared topical clobetasol propionate 0.05% cream (20 g) applied all over twice daily with oral prednisone (1 mg/kg) daily and found topical steroids to be better with regards to disease control, adverse events and mortality. In 2009, the same group compared clobetasol propionate cream 0.05% cream (20 g) twice a day (standard regimen) with cream 10–30 g per day depending on disease severity and body weight and found that the median cumulative doses of steroid cream was 5760 g in the standard regimen *vs* 1314 g in the mild regimen, which is a 70% reduction in cumulative doses and there was no significant difference in effectiveness between them.[28] The severe side-effects were diabetes mellitus, cardiovascular and neurovascular disorders and cutaneous side-effects, included purpura, severe skin atrophy and striae. When used as an adjunct therapy, they are mostly applied on the lesions, rather than whole skin. Concluding, very potent topical steroids (clobetasol propionate) are an effective treatment for BP, however, their use in extensive disease may be associated with systemic absorption and adverse events.

Scope for Research

- Systemic steroids
  - Optimum starting dose of oral prednisolone—0.3, 0.5 or 1.0 mg/kg/day
  - Dosing according to severity
  - Protocol for weaning of oral steroids
  - When should a second drug or a change in treatment be considered?
- Topical corticosteroids
  - Should they be used as a monotherapy or as adjuncts?
  - Should they be applied to the whole skin surface or to lesional skin only?
  - For what severity of disease might the above approach be recommended?

CORTICOSTEROIDS IN ATOPIC DERMATITIS

Topical Corticosteroids
(Strength of Recommendation A; Level of Evidence 1+)

Topical corticosteroids are one of the most efficient treatment for atopic dermatitis, though emollients should be liberally used multiple times per day in conjunction with topical corticosteroids. The goals of topical corticosteroid therapy in atopic dermatitis include progressive reduction to change of the therapy to a topical non-steroidal agent and at the same time ensuring the absence of relapse after reduction in the frequency of application and/or stepping down to a lower potency steroid.

For patients with mild atopic dermatitis, a low potency corticosteroid cream or ointment (e.g. desonide 0.05%, hydrocortisone 2.5%) applied once a day for 2 to 4 weeks gives favorable response. Emollients can be applied before or after topical corticosteroids.[29] Patients with moderate and severe disease usually require medium to high to super high potency corticosteroids (e.g. fluocinolone 0.025%, triamcinolone 0.1%, betamethasone dipropionate 0.05%). In patients with acute flares, super high or high potency topical corticosteroids can be used for up to two weeks and then replaced with lower potency preparations until the lesions resolve. The face and skin folds are at higher risk for atrophy with corticosteroids, hence initial therapy in these areas should start with a low potency steroid or topical calcineurin inhibitor (pimecrolimus or tacrolimus) to prevent steroid related side-effects. The finger-tip unit should be used as a guide for external dose application technique. A cream base should be used if lesions of atopic dermatitis are acute (weepy and inflamed), an ointment base is appropriate for chronic lesions (dry or lichenified), and a lotion base is recommended for hairy areas. A systematic review of randomized controlled trials (consisting of 83 studies) of topical corticosteroids for atopic dermatitis indicated a large therapeutic efficacy of topical corticosteroids used for 4 weeks, compared with placebo.[30] No clear benefit has been demonstrated with more than once daily application.[31]

Long-term use of topical corticosteroids, especially high or super high potency preparations, on large body areas leads to adrenal suppression and steroid related adverse effects, hence such use is avoided.[32] Wet wraps improve the efficacy of topical steroids, though large prospective RCTs evaluating wet wraps are lacking. Wet wraps consist of a bottom wet layer and top dry layer on top of topical corticosteroids and emollients. It is usually left in place for up to 2 hours or more, as tolerated by the patient, once or twice daily for 2 to 14 days. Adverse effects include increased systemic absorption of topical corticosteroids, general discomfort, chills, and folliculitis. So, wet wraps should be done for short courses with diluted low- to mid-potency corticosteroids. After induction of remission with continuous use of corticosteroids, maintenance proactive therapy with intermittent use of a moderate to high potency topical corticosteroid or a topical calcineurin inhibitor has been shown to help prevent flare-ups and relapse. Further, this intermittent therapy does not lead to the side-effects that occur with long term continuous use of steroids. In a meta-analysis of four randomized trials, topical fluticasone propionate (once daily for two consecutive days per week for 16 weeks) reduced the risk of a subsequent flare by 54%.[33] "Weekend" steroid therapy is significantly more effective in maintaining an improvement in comparison with placebo. Flares of atopic dermatitis that occur during intermittent treatment may be treated by resuming continuous use of topical corticosteroids or calcineurin inhibitors that have been effective for the patient in the past. Probable side effects of topical corticosteroid therapy include skin atrophy, telangiectasias, striae, steroid-induced acne and/or rosacea, hypertrichosis, and systemic absorption leading to HPA suppression. Usually, they are seen with high potency topical corticosteroids and more so when applied to the skin around the eyes and face. Therefore, strategies for withdrawal of topical corticosteroids should be in place for all children who require prolonged treatment such as, gradual substitution by emollients, weekend-only use, or sequential therapy with nonsteroidal agents.

Topical steroid-antibiotic combinations are effective at reducing *S. aureus* than topical steroids alone, but this does not translate to clinical benefit. Rapid recolonization occurs on cessation of treatment, and hypersensitivity and bacterial resistance may develop. Hence, their use is usually limited to short-term (<2 weeks) for clinically infected eczema.[34]

Guidelines and recommendations for use of topical corticosteroids in atopic dermatitis by Indian Society for Pediatric Dermatology task force, 2016 include:[35]

- Topical corticosteroids should be used as first-line therapy along with appropriate use of moisturizing agents.
- These are best used until acute skin flares are under control.
- During maintenance treatment, they can be applied twice weekly (weekend therapy) to "hot spots" for up to 6–8 weeks. Face, flexural surfaces, and diaper area should be avoided.
- Adequate and suitable quantities of topical corticosteroids to be used should be discussed with the patient attendant/care giver. They should be counselled regarding finger-tip unit use.
- Topical corticosteroids can be applied to areas of broken down skin including severely inflamed skin after suitable cleansing of the part to reduce oozing.
- The choice of potency, frequency, and duration of use of topical corticosteroids should be based on clinical judgment depending on the location, severity, and chronicity of eczema, and the age of the patient.
- Initial use of moderately potent topical corticosteroid for short period (5–7 days) followed by mild corticosteroid to avoid tachyphylaxis and other side effects of potent steroid is recommended.
- Combination of topical steroid with antibacterial should be avoided.

The majority of studies of corticosteroids in atopic dermatitis have been of short duration with wide variety of clinical scoring system, thus no consensus is available regarding the doses and duration of this therapy.

Systemic Corticosteroids
(Strength of Recommendation B; Level of Evidence 2)

Systemic corticosteroids are commonly used in short bursts (a few weeks) in order to get over severe atopic eczema into remission. They are also recommended in patients with moderate to severe atopic dermatitis that is not controlled with optimal topical therapy. Although frequently used in clinical practice for the treatment of severe atopic dermatitis in children and adults, there are no high-quality studies evaluating their role in the management of atopic dermatitis. The European Task Force on Atopic Dermatitis/European Academy of Dermatology and Venereology Task Force position statement on the treatment of atopic dermatitis suggests that a systemic corticosteroids such as methylprednisolone 0.5 mg/kg per day for one to two weeks tapered over one month can be used in cases with acute and severe exacerbation.[36] Though, in a RCT of adults with severe atopic dermatitis comparing 0.5–0.8 mg/kg prednisolone for 2 weeks followed by placebo for 4 weeks against 2.7–4.0 mg/kg ciclosporin for 6 weeks, ciclosporin was found to be superior than prednisolone in achieving initial disease remission.[37]

Rebound flaring and/or worsening of disease are common upon discontinuation of systemic corticosteroids.[38] Also, their long term use results in steroid related side-effects such as weight gain, immunosuppression, impaired glucose tolerance, hypothalamic-pituitary-adrenal axis suppression, gastrointestinal upset, myopathies, fractures, growth retardation, impaired wound healing, cataracts and secondary infections. In conclusion, systemic corticosteroids can be used in adult atopic dermatitis with acute, severe exacerbations and as a bridge therapy to another steroid-sparing agent.[39] However, their use in pediatric atopic dermatitis is not recommended because of their propensity to cause growth retardation.

CORTICOSTEROIDS IN ALLERGIC AND IRRITANT CONTACT DERMATITIS

Although avoidance of the offending allergen is the mainstay of management of allergic and irritant contact dermatitis, treatment is required in most cases to achieve rapid control of symptoms. The treatment of contact dermatitis follows the general principles of treatment of any dermatitis. Topical corticosteroids are the first line treatment for localized contact dermatitis, with the strength of the topical corticosteroid appropriate to the body site and severity of dermatitis. Most frequently, acute and chronic contact dermatitis are treated with topical corticosteroids (classes II–III, most usually mometasone furoate or betamethasone). The tapering of frequency and potency of topical steroid is required once the control of disease is achieved.[40] In areas with thin skin, such as face and intertriginous areas, topical calcineurin inhibitors (e.g. tacrolimus, pimecrolimus) should be used for maintenance therapy after a short course of steroids to reduce inflammation. Topical corticosteroids may be used as continuous application of milder (class 1 or 2) topical corticosteroids or as short bursts of strong (class 3 or 4) topical corticosteroids (for example, twice weekly, or at weekends only). One RCT has shown the efficacy of weekend application of clobetasol proprionate in maintenance of remission in hand eczema.[41]

Oral corticosteroids are considered as the first line treatment for allergic and irritant contact dermatitis which is severe and/or involving >20% of the body surface area or for acute contact dermatitis involving the face, hands, feet or genitalia if quick relief is desired (e.g. involvement of the eyelids).[42] Oral corticosteroids for contact dermatitis have not been studied in randomized trials. However, in clinical experience, they are frequently beneficial.

Long-term use of systemic corticosteroids to treat allergic contact dermatitis may produce severe morbidity. Thus, adding a steroid sparing adjuvant as azathioprine or methotrexate, once the disease control is achieved, has been found beneficial.[43]

CORTICOSTEROIDS IN LICHEN PLANUS

Lichen planus may affect the skin, mucous membranes (especially the oral mucosa), scalp, nails, and genitalia. Corticosteroids are useful in the treatment of all forms of lichen planus.

Cutaneous Lichen Planus
(Strength of Recommendation B; Level of Evidence 1–)

The treatment of cutaneous lichen planus is focused on accelerating resolution and managing pruritus. There are few data to support evidence-based recommendations for the treatment of lichen planus. Only a few randomized trials have been performed, most of which were small and subject to methodologic error. Topical corticosteroids are commonly used as first-line treatment for localized cutaneous lichen planus. For patients with generalized disease, topical corticosteroids are often used as an adjunct to systemic therapy or phototherapy.

Topical corticosteroids: Although topical corticosteroids are the mainstay of treatment for patients with localized cutaneous lichen planus, the efficacy of these agents has not been evaluated in clinical studies. Localized cutaneous lichen planus on the trunk and extremities is usually treated with once daily application of a high potency or super high potency topical corticosteroid cream or ointment. Because topical corticosteroid-induced cutaneous atrophy is most likely to occur in intertriginous or facial skin, mid-potency or low-potency corticosteroids are preferred when treating these areas. Efficacy is usually assessed after two to three weeks.[44] The tapering of frequency and potency should be considered after 2 weeks based on the clinical evaluation.

Intralesional corticosteroids: The thick lesions of hypertrophic lichen planus are less likely than classic cutaneous lesions to respond well to a topical corticosteroid. Clinical experience suggests that intralesional corticosteroid therapy in a concentration of 10 to 40 mg/ml is usually beneficial for the treatment of hypertrophic lichen planus. Cutaneous atrophy and hypopigmentation may occur as a result of intralesional corticosteroid therapy.[45]

Systemic corticosteroids: Patients with cutaneous lichen planus who cannot be treated adequately with topical corticosteroids (e.g. generalized disease or refractory disease) may benefit from oral corticosteroid. Short courses of systemic corticosteroids are usually recommended for moderate to severe cutaneous LP, though, recurrences are possible after treatment withdrawal. Betamethasone 5 mg orally, on two consecutive days in a week has shown excellent clinical response with minimal side effects in patients with cutaneous lichen planus.[46]

Oral Lichen Planus
(Strength of Recommendation B; Level of Evidence 1–)

The primary goals of treatment of oral lichen planus are the alleviation of symptoms and minimization of scarring from erosive lesions. Patients with asymptomatic reticular oral LP do not require treatment.

Topical corticosteroids: Topical corticosteroids are the first-line treatment for oral lichen planus. High potency or medium potency topical corticosteroids are typically used. In a 9 week trial evaluating topical corticosteroids, 40 patients with reticular and/or erosive oral lichen planus were treated with either topical corticosteroid (0.025% fluocinonide) or placebo, applied at least six times per day.[47] Among the 20 patients treated with fluocinonide, 20% had complete response and 60% had good or partial response to therapy.

One RCT of 49 patients with moderate to severe oral lichen planus, the efficacy and safety of topical triamcinolone acetonide (0.1%) was compared with oral betamethasone (5 mg/day for 3 months, followed by a slow taper during 3 months).[48] No significant difference in the response was seen in the 2 groups, though betamethasone group showed an early response in early disease. Cushingoid features and oral candidiasis were seen in the patients on oral steroids. High potency topical corticosteroid, such as clobetasol propionate 0.05%, fluocinonide 0.05%, triamcinolone acetonide or betamethasone propionate 0.05% gel or ointment, are frequently used and patients are instructed to dry the affected areas prior to application. The topical corticosteroid is applied three to four times per day using a fingertip or cotton-tipped applicator. Eating or drinking should be avoided for at least 30 minutes after application. As symptoms improve, the frequency of application is reduced as tolerated.

Intralesional corticosteroids: Intralesional injections of triamcinolone acetonide, in concentrations between 10 and 40 mg/mL, have been used successfully for oral lichen planus. A study of 45 patients with ulcerative oral lichen planus in which only one side was treated with an intralesional corticosteroid injection (0.5 mL of triamcinolone acetonide 40 mg/mL) found statistically significant reductions in signs and symptoms of oral lichen planus within two weeks after treatment.[49] On the treated side, the mean sizes of the areas affected by erythema or ulceration were reduced by 78%. In contrast, the untreated areas remained unchanged.

Oral corticosteroids: Although systemic corticosteroids are widely used in oral lichen planus, their efficacy has not been well documented. Based on clinical practice, systemic corticosteroids 0.5–1 mg/kg are recommended as preferred treatment for erosive oral lichen planus not responding to topical corticosteroid treatment and as first-line treatment in severe oral lichen planus. They may be used as daily dosing regimens of prednisolone tapered over 6 to 8 weeks or as oral mini pulse therapy.[50]

CORTICOSTEROIDS IN PSORIASIS

Topical Corticosteroids
(Strength of Recommendation A; Level of Evidence 1+)

Topical corticosteroids are the mainstay in the treatment of localised psoriasis. The efficacy of topical corticosteroids has been well established over the years, and depends on the potency and the formulation used. The efficacy of class I (super potent) corticosteroids ranges from 58 to 92% in various studies.[51] A 2-week, double-blind, vehicle-controlled trial of 204 patients with moderate to severe psoriasis demonstrated that 92% of the patients treated with halobetasol propionate ointment (class I) had improvement compared with 39% of vehicle treated patients.[52] The efficacy of classes II, III and IV topical corticosteroids is slightly less and ranges from 68 to 74% in moderate to severe psoriasis.[51] In two randomized vehicle-controlled studies involving 383 patients with moderate to severe psoriasis, 68 to 69% of patients treated with fluticasone propionate 0.005% ointment (class III) showed significant improvement as compared with 29 to 30% of patients treated with vehicle for 4 weeks.[53] Efficacy of classes V, VI and VII corticosteroids is less as compared to more potent steroids, as evidenced by the systematic review of topical corticosteroids for the treatment of psoriasis.[54] Apart from the class of topical corticosteroids, the effectiveness of the preparation also depends on its formulation.[55] Other factors affecting the efficacy of treatment include the site of application of medication, thickness of the plaque, how well the vehicle delivers the active drug molecule, how well that drug molecule activates corticosteroid receptors, and compliance of the patient. On the scalp and in the external ear canal, potent corticosteroids in a solution vehicle are usually used. Foam formulations and shampoos are also well suited for the treatment of scalp psoriasis. Clobetasol in a shampoo formulation has been shown to be superior to a tar-blend shampoo.[56] On the face and intertriginous areas, a low-potency ointment or cream is used by most dermatologists while thick plaques, especially over the extensors require more potent topical corticosteroids.

The typical regimen consists of once daily application of topical corticosteroids and most patients show a rapid decrease in inflammation with such therapy, but complete normalization of skin or lasting remission is unpredictable. Once clinical improvement occurs, the frequency of application should be reduced. This also helps to decrease chances of tachyphylaxis and/or rebound with topical corticosteroids, which may occur fairly rapidly (i.e. within a few days to weeks) if they are used continuously for longer periods of time. Thus, intermittent treatment schedules (such as once every 2 or 3 days or on weekends) are advised for more prolonged treatment courses during maintenance phase.[57] Therefore, careful instruction to all patients before initiating the treatment and being maintained on it is essential. The addition of non-corticosteroid topical treatments such as coal tar and calcipotriol also facilitate the avoidance of long-term daily topical corticosteroids, thus preventing their side-effects.

Nail psoriasis is difficult to treat and no therapy has been shown to improve the nail changes effectively. In a small study of 10 patients with nail psoriasis, 8% clobetasol nail lacquer, applied once daily, resulted in reduced onycholysis, pitting, and salmon patches within 4 weeks of initiation of therapy. No local or systemic side effects were noted in this study.[58] Another option is to apply super potent and potent topical corticosteroids over the nail folds daily, which may improve the nail changes, though partially.[59]

The American Academy of Dermatology guidelines for topical therapy in psoriasis recommends the following:[51]

- Topical corticosteroids can be used as monotherapy once or twice daily.
- They can be combined with other topical agents, UV light, and systemic agents, depending on the severity of disease, which can enhance their efficacy.
- Class I topical corticosteroids are usually used for 2–4 weeks whereas for less potent steroids, the optimal end point is not known.
- Gradual reduction in usage is recommended following the clinical response. While optimal end point is unknown, unsupervised continuous use is not recommended.
- For clobetasol and halobetasol, maximal weekly use should be 50 g or less.
- Tachyphylaxis, while not demonstrated in clinical trials, may affect the long-term results achieved in a given patient.
- Combination with other topicals and variations in dosing schedules may lessen risk of long-term side effects.
- Because of the increased skin surface/body mass ratio, the risks to infants and children may be higher for systemic effects secondary to enhanced absorption. Growth retardation is also a potential concern. Thus, they should be used judiciously in pediatric patients with psoriasis.

CORTICOSTEROIDS IN ALOPECIA AREATA

The treatment approach for patients with alopecia areata differs based upon the clinical presentation; especially whether the disease is limited or extensive.

Topical Corticosteroids
(Level of Evidence 2+)

Potent topical corticosteroids may be used alone or in conjunction with other treatments, including intralesional corticosteroids. While topical corticosteroids are frequently used to treat alopecia areata, evidence for their effectiveness is limited. They may be used as sole therapy in limited disease or as an adjunct therapy in patients with extensive alopecia areata. Topical corticosteroids are preferred in pediatric patients as they cannot tolerate pain of intralesional therapy. Though the results may be inferior to intralesional therapy.[60] In a trial of 70 patients with patchy alopecia areata, comparing 0.25% dessoximetasone or placebo twice daily for 12 weeks, complete regrowth was higher among the corticosteroid-treated group (58% vs 39%).[61] Clobetasol propionate foam without occlusion is considered more cosmetically acceptable and convenient for the patient compared to other formulations. One hundred and five patients with localised alopecia areata were randomized to treatment with betamethasone valerate 0.1% foam applied twice daily, intralesional triamcinolone acetonide (10 mg/mL) administered every three weeks, or topical tacrolimus 0.1% ointment applied twice daily in the study by Kuldeep et al.[62] More than 75% hair regrowth was noted in 54, 60, and 0% of patients, respectively, suggesting a slightly less efficacy of topical corticosteroids as compared to intralesional steroids. Potent topical corticosteroids are more efficacious than lower-potency corticosteroids as evidenced by the findings of a 24-week randomized trial performed in 41 children with alopecia areata involving at least 10% of the scalp surface area.[63] The study found that treatment with clobetasol propionate 0.05% cream (a high-potency topical corticosteroid) for 2 to 6 weeks cycles separated by 6 weeks was more effective for decreasing the area of scalp hair loss than hydrocortisone 1% cream (a low-potency topical corticosteroid) administered via the same regimen. After 24 weeks, 85% of children treated with clobetasol propionate had at least a 50% reduction in the surface area with hair loss, compared with only 33% of children treated with hydrocortisone. Adverse effects of topical corticosteroids include acneiform eruption of the face (more common with ointment preparations than foam), striae, telangiectasia, and skin atrophy.[64]

Intralesional Corticosteroids
(Level of Evidence 3)

Intralesional corticosteroids are considered a first-line treatment method for limited disease, and can be used as an adjunctive therapy in extensive disease. Intralesional corticosteroids, most commonly triamcinolone acetonide, are considered the treatment of choice for patchy alopecia areata of limited extent and for cosmetically sensitive areas, such as the eyebrows. Tan *et al* reported that 82% of 127 patients with limited alopecia areata showed 50% improvement with intralesional triamcinolone acetonide injections for 12 weeks.[65] Pull test and exclamation point hairs are usually regarded as indicators of inflammation, thus patients with these clinical evidence of active inflammation are better candidates for intralesional corticosteroid therapy.[66] It has been demonstrated that 2.5 mg/mL triamcinolone acetonide confers the same benefit as either 5 or 10 mg/mL inpatients with patchy alopecia areata.[67] Concentration of 2.5 to 5 mg/mL is injected into the lesions on the face (eyebrow or beard involvement) while concentrations of 5 to 10 mg/mL are injected into the scalp lesions. Small volumes (0.1 mL or less) are injected into multiple sites 1 cm apart. The dose per visit is largely determined by the extent of disease and patient tolerance but is usually around 20 mg or less on the scalp. The dose of triamcinolone administered should not exceed 40 mg per treatment session. Hair regrowth is usually visible within six to eight weeks. The treatment may be repeated as necessary every three to four weeks and is stopped once regrowth is complete. In extensive disease, they can be used as an adjunctive to systemic treatment such as oral corticosteroids and Janus kinase (JAK) inhibitors.[68] Side effects include skin atrophy and hypopigmentation at the site of injection, which typically resolves after a few days.

Oral Corticosteroids
(Level of Evidence 3)

Short courses of oral corticosteroids are often sufficient to stimulate hair regrowth. Systemic corticosteroids have a significant benefit in most clinical variants of alopecia areata, with reduced efficacy in ophiasis and alopecia universalis types, suggesting these to be the disease type with poor prognosis.[69] They may be used as daily dosing schedules or as high-dose pulsed corticosteroid treatment. The efficacy of oral prednisone tapered from 40 mg and stopped over the course of 6 weeks was investigated in a prospective study of 32 children and adults with alopecia areata, including 16 patients with alopecia totalis or universalis.[70] After six weeks, 13 patients achieved at least 50% hair regrowth, including four patients with 75 to 99% hair loss at baseline and four patients with alopecia universalis. An open study on sixteen adolescents and adults with alopecia areata/totalis/universalis treated with oral mini-pulse therapy (betamethasone 5 mg given as a single oral dose after breakfast on two consecutive days every week) for a minimum period of six months showed excellent response in 44% patients, good response in 31% patients and unsatisfactory and no response in 12.5% patients each.[71] However, the response to corticosteroids may not be durable, and patients may relapse within 4 to 9 weeks after discontinuing steroids.[72] The side effects of systemic steroids generally preclude their long-term use.[73]

CORTICOSTEROIDS IN VITILIGO

Treatment of vitiligo is aimed at halting the disease progression, allowing repigmentation of lesional areas and preventing relapses. Some areas, such as the face, usually respond well to therapies whereas hands and feet are relatively refractory to treatment.

Topical Corticosteroids
(Grade of Recommendation B; Level of Evidence 1+)

For medical treatment of localised vitiligo, topical corticosteroids have been used as the first-line treatment. Based on comparative studies, topical corticosteroids are the most clinically effective choice for topical therapy. The ease of application, high rate of compliance, and low cost are the advantages of topical corticosteroid therapy for vitiligo. When used with other therapies like narrow band UVB or PUVA, the repigmentation rate is enhanced. Topical corticosteroids have the best results (75% of repigmentation) on sun-exposed areas (face and neck),[74] in dark skin[75] and in recent lesions.[76] Acral lesions respond poorly. However, frequent local side-effects such as skin atrophy, telangiectasia, hypertrichosis, acneiform eruptions and striae, limit the use of topical corticosteroids on face and topical calcineurin inhibitors are better suited at these sites.

In a meta-analysis of nonsurgical therapies for vitiligo, modest, but significant effectiveness was shown with a success rate of 33% *vs* 0% in the placebo groups.[77] Kwinter *et al*, reported response rates of 64% with complete repigmentation rates as high as 49.3%, with moderate to high-potency topical corticosteroids in children.[78] The side effects prohibit long-term use of steroid and merit frequent monitoring and regular steroid holidays. Several recent studies comparing the use of topical steroids to calcineurin inhibitors have found topical steroids (mometasone 0.1% or clobetasol 0.05% daily) similar in efficacy to calcineurin inhibitors (tacrolimus 0.1% or pimecrolimus 1.0% twice daily), both with tolerable adverse drug reaction rates. A study by Kose *et al*, showed mean repigmentation rates of 65% with mometasone and 42% with pimecrolimus after three months of daily treatment, which was not statistically significant.[79] No differences in efficacy have been found between clobetasol and tacrolimus, and between clobetasol or mometasone and pimecrolimus, although topical calcineurin inhibitors might be less effective for extrafacial lesions.[80]

According to the European Dermatology Forum consensus,[80] the treatment guidelines for use of topical corticosteroids in vitiligo are as follows.

- In children and adults, once-daily application of potent topical corticosteroids can be advised for patients with limited, extrafacial involvement for a period no longer than 3 months, according to a continuous treatment scheme or, better, to a discontinuous scheme (15 days per month for 6 months with a strict assessment of response based on photographs).

- Facial lesions can be treated as effectively and with lesser side-effects by topical calcineurin inhibitors.

- As potent topical corticosteroids appear to be at least as effective as very potent ones, the first category should be the first and safest choice.
- Systemic absorption is a concern when large areas of skin, regions with thin skin and children are treated for a prolonged time with potent steroids. Topical corticosteroids with negligible systemic effects, such as mometasone furoate or methylprednisolone aceponate, should be preferred.

Oral Corticosteroids
(Grade of Recommendation B; Level of Evidence 2++)

Systemic corticosteroids are generally used in rapidly progressive cases to help with disease stabilization. In patients with progressive vitiligo, they can be used in combination with NBUVB phototherapy. However, there are no randomized clinical trials confirming that either speed or magnitude of response to phototherapy and photochemotherapy might be potentiated by concomitant administration of steroids. They can be given as daily dosing or in the form of oral pulse therapy. In one study, 81 patients were treated with prednisolone 0.3 mg/kg per day for two months, and then the dose was progressively reduced in the subsequent 3 months.[81] Control of disease progression was achieved in 90% of patients and repigmentation in 74% patients. Lee et al, also reported favorable results with a combination of topical and systemic immunosuppressants, including two patients with focal non-segmental vitiligo who experienced complete remission within 2 to 3 months of treatment with 0.03% topical tacrolimus and oral prednisone (20 mg) daily.[82]

In studies using oral mini pulse in vitiligo, oral betamethasone or dexamethasone 5 mg was given on two consecutive days per week.[83,84] Stabilisation of disease was noted in 89% of patients within 1–3 months of treatment while within 2–4 months of treatment, 80% of patients noted repigmentation. Low dose OMP has also been found to be effective in stopping the progression of vitiligo. In a large, retrospective study, Kanwar et al, found that low-dose oral dexamethasone mini pulse therapy (2.5 mg/day on 2 consecutive days/week) halted progressive vitiligo in 91.8% of subjects at a mean of 13.2 ± 3.1 weeks. Some degree of repigmentation was observed in all lesions at a mean of 16.1 ± 5.9 weeks, and relapse occurred in 12.3% of patients at an average of 55.7 ± 26.7 weeks post-treatment.

REFERENCES

1. Bystryn JC, Steinman NM. The adjuvant therapy of pemphigus. An update. Arch Dermatol 1996;132:203–12.
2. Murrell DF, Dick S, Ahmed AR, et al. Consensus statement on definitions of disease, end points, and therapeutic response for pemphigus. J Am Acad Dermatol 2008;58:1043–6.
3. Czernik A, Bystryn JC. Kinetics of response to conventional treatment in patients with pemphigus vulgaris. Arch Dermatol 2008;144:682–3.
4. Atzmony L, Hodak E, Leshem YA, et al. The role of adjuvant therapy in pemphigus: a systematic review and meta-analysis. J Am Acad Dermatol 2015;73:264–71.

5. Mimouni D, Nousari CH, Cummins DL, et al. Differences and similarities among expert opinions on the diagnosis and treatment of pemphigus vulgaris. J Am Acad Dermatol 2003;49:1059–62.

6. Lyakhovitsky A, Baum S, Scope A, et al. The impact of stratifying initial dose of corticosteroids by severity of pemphigus vulgaris on long-term disease severity. Int J Dermatol 2011;50:1014–19.

7. Lever WF, White H. Treatment of pemphigus with corticosteroids. Results obtained in 46 patients over a period of 11 years. Arch Dermatol 1963;87:12–26.

8. Hertl M, Jedlickova H, Karpati S, et al. Pemphigus. S2 Guideline for diagnosis and treatment-guided by the European Dermatology Forum (EDF) in cooperation with the European Academy of Dermatology and Venereology (EADV). J Eur Acad Dermatol Venereol2015;29:405–14.

9. Albrecht J, Werth VP. Practice gaps. Improving the care of our patients who are receiving glucocorticoid therapy. Arch Dermatol 2012;148:314–15.

10. Marzano AV, Trevisan V, Eller-Vainicher C, et al. Evidence for vitamin D deficiency and increased prevalence of fractures in autoimmune bullous skin diseases. Br J Dermatol 2012;167:688–91.

11. National Institute for Health and Care Excellence. Osteoporosis - prevention of fragility fractures. Available at: http://cks.nice.org. uk/osteoporosis-prevention-of-fragility-fractures#!topicsummary.

12. van Staa TP, Leufkens HG, Cooper C. The epidemiology of corticosteroid-induced osteoporosis: a meta-analysis. Osteoporos Int 2002;13:777–87.

13. Tee SI, Yosipovitch G, Chan YC, et al. Prevention of glucocorticoid induced osteoporosis in immunobullous diseases with alendronate: a randomized, double-blind, placebo-controlled study. Arch Dermatol 2012;148:307–14.

14. Roujeau JC. Pulse glucocorticoid therapy. The 'big shot' revisited. Arch Dermatol 1996;132:1499–502.

15. Abraham A, Roga G, Job AM. Pulse therapy in pemphigus: Ready reckoner. Indian J Dermatol 2016;61:314–7.

16. Femiano F, Gombos F, Scully C. Pemphigus vulgaris with oral involvement: evaluation of two different systemic corticosteroid therapeutic protocols. J Eur Acad Dermatol Venereol 2002;16(4):353–356.

17. Pasricha J S, Poonam. Current regimen of pulse therapy for pemphigus: Minor modifications, improved results. Indian J DermatolVenereolLeprol2008;74:217–21.

18. Shahidi-Dadras M, Karami A, Toosy P, et al. Pulse versus oral methylprednisolone therapy in pemphigus vulgaris. Arch Iran Med 2007;10:1–6.

19. Chams-Davatchi C, Esmaili N, Daneshpazhooh M, et al. Randomized controlled open-label trial of four treatment regimens for pemphigus vulgaris. J Am Acad Dermatol 2007;57:622–8.

20. Harman KE, Brown D, Exton LS, et al. British Association of Dermatologists' guidelines for the management of pemphigus vulgaris 2017. B Br J Dermatol 2017;177(5):1170–1201.

21. Mignogna MD, Fortuna G, Leuci S, et al. Adjuvant triamcinolone acetonide injections in oro-pharyngeal pemphigus vulgaris. J Eur Acad Dermatol Venereol2010;24:1157–65.

22. McPherson T, Venning VV. Management of autoimmune blistering diseases in pregnancy. Dermatol Clin 2011;29:585–90.

23. Kardos M, Levine D, Gurcan HM, et al. Pemphigus vulgaris in pregnancy: analysis of current data on the management and outcomes. Obstet Gynecol Surv 2009;64:739–49.

24. National Institute for Health and Care Excellence. Corticosteroids—oral. Available at: http://cks.nice.org.uk/corticosteroids-oral#! Scenario.

25. Mabrouk D, Ahmed AR. Analysis of current therapy and clinical outcome in childhood pemphigus vulgaris. Pediatr Dermatol 2011;28:485–93.

26. Venning VA, Taghipour K, Mustapa MM, Highet AS, Kirtschig G. British Association of Dermatologists' guidelines for the management of bullous pemphigoid 2012. Br J Dermatol 2012;167(6):1200–14.

27. Joly P, Roujeau JC, Benichou J, et al. A comparison of oral and topical corticosteroids in patients with bullous pemphigoid. N Engl J Med 2002;346:321–7.

28. Joly P, Roujeau JC, Benichou J, et al. A comparison of two regimens of topical corticosteroids in the treatment of patients with bullous pemphigoid: a multicenter randomized study. J Invest Dermatol 2009;129:1681–7.

29. Ng SY, Begum S, Chong SY. Does Order of Application of Emollient and Topical Corticosteroids Make a Difference in the Severity of Atopic Eczema in Children? Pediatr Dermatol 2016;33:160.

30. Hoare C, Li Wan Po A, Williams H. Systematic review of treatments for atopic eczema. Health Technol Assess 2000; 4:1.

31. Green C, Colquitt JL, Kirby J, Davidson P. Topical corticosteroids for atopic eczema: clinical and cost effectiveness of once-daily vs. more frequent use. Br J Dermatol 2005;152:130.

32. Foelster-Holst R, Nagel F, Zoellner P, et al. Efficacy of crisis intervention treatment with topical corticosteroid prednicarbat with and without partial wet-wrap dressing in atopic dermatitis. Dermatology2006;212(1):66–9.

33. Schmitt J, von Kobyletzki L, Svensson A, Apfelbacher C. Efficacy and tolerability of proactive treatment with topical corticosteroids and calcineurin inhibitors for atopic eczema: systematic review and meta-analysis of randomized controlled trials. Br J Dermatol 2011;164:415.

34. NICE. Atopic Eczema in Children: Management of Atopic Eczema in Children from Birth up to the Age of 12 Years, NICE Clinical Guideline 57. London: National Institute for Health and Clinical Excellence, 2007.

35. Parikh D, Dhar S, Ramamoorthy R, Srinivas S, Sarkar R, Inamdar A, et al. 'Treatment guidelines for the atopic dermatitis by ISPD task force, 2016. Indian J Paediatr Dermatol 2018;19:108–15.

36. Wollenberg A, Oranje A, Deleuran M, et al. ETFAD/EADV Eczema task force 2015 position paper on diagnosis and treatment of atopic dermatitis in adult and paediatric patients. J Eur Acad Dermatol Venereol2016;30:729.

37. Schmitt J, Schäkel K, Fölster-Holst R, et al. Prednisolone vs. ciclosporin for severe adult eczema. An investigator-initiated double-blind placebo-controlled multicentre trial. Br J Dermatol2010;162(3):661–8.

38. Forte WC, Sumits JM, Rodrigues AG, Liuson D, Tanaka E. Rebound phenomenon to systemic corticosteroid in atopic dermatitis. Allergol Immunopath 2005;33:301–311.

39. Yu SH, Drucker AM, Lebwohl M, Silverberg JI. A systematic review of the safety and efficacy of systemic corticosteroids in atopic dermatitis. J Am Acad Dermatol 2018;78(4):733-740.e711.

40. Kostner L, Anzengruber F, Guillod C, Recher M, Schmid-Grendelmeier P, Navarini AA. Allergic contact dermatitis. Immunology and Allergy Clinics 2017;37(1):141–52.

41. Möller H, Svartholm H, Dahl G. Intermittent maintenance therapy in chronic hand eczema with clobetasol propionate and flupredniden acetate. Curr Med Res Opin1983;8:640–4.

42. Brasch J, Becker D, Aberer W, Bircher A, Kränke B, Jung K, et al. Guideline contact dermatitis: S1-Guidelines of the German Contact Allergy Group (DKG) of the German Dermatology Society (DDG), the Information Network of Dermatological Clinics (IVDK), the German Society for Allergology and Clinical Immunology (DGAKI), the Working Group for Occupational and Environmental Dermatology (ABD) of the DDG, the Medical Association of German Allergologists (AeDA), the Professional Association of German Dermatologists (BVDD) and the DDG. Allergo J Int 2014;23(4):126–38.

43. De D, Sarangal R, Handa S. The comparative efficacy and safety of azathioprine vs methotrexate as steroid-sparing agent in the treatment of airborne-contact dermatitis due to Parthenium. Indian J Dermatol Venereol Leprol2013;79:240–1.

44. Fazel N. Cutaneous lichen planus: A systematic review of treatments. J Dermatolog Treat 2015;26:280–3.

45. Deshmukh NS, Belgaumkar VA, Mhaske CB, Doshi BR. Intralesional drug therapy in dermatology. Indian J Dermatol Venereol Leprol 2017;83:127–32.

46. Verma KK, Mittal R, Manchanda Y. Lichen planus treated with betamethasone oral mini-pulse therapy. Indian J Dermatol Venereol Leprol2000;66:34–5.

47. Voûte AB, Schulten EA, Langendijk PN, et al. Fluocinonide in an adhesive base for treatment of oral lichen planus. A double-blind, placebo-controlled clinical study. Oral Surg Oral Med Oral Pathol 1993; 75:181.

48. Malhotra AK, Khaitan BK, Sethuraman G, et al. Betamethasone oral minipulse therapy compared with topical triamcinolone acetonide (0.1%) paste in oral lichen planus: a randomized comparative study. J Am AcadDermatol2008;58:596–602.

49. Xia J, Li C, Hong Y, et al. Short-term clinical evaluation of intralesional triamcinolone acetonide injection for ulcerative oral lichen planus. J Oral Pathol Med 2006; 35:327.

50. Carbone M, Goss E, Carrozzo M, Castellano S, Conrotto D, Broccoletti R. Systemic and topical corticosteroid treatment of oral lichen planus: a comparative study with long-term follow-up. J Oral Pathol Med 2003;32:323–9.

51. Menter A, Korman NJ, Elmets CA, et al. Guidelines of care for the management of psoriasis and psoriatic arthritis. Section 3. Guidelines of care for the management and treatment of psoriasis with topical therapies. J Am Acad Dermatol. 2009;60(04):643–59.

52. Bernhard J, Whitmore C, Guzzo C, Kantor I, Kalb RE, Ellis C, et al. Evaluation of halobetasol propionate ointment in the treatment of plaque psoriasis: report on two double-blind, vehicle-controlled studies. J Am Acad Dermatol 1991;25:1170–4.

53. Olsen EA. Efficacy and safety of fluticasone propionate 0.005% ointment in the treatment of psoriasis. Cutis 1996;57: 57–61.

54. Mason J, Mason AR, Cork MJ. Topical preparations for the treatment of psoriasis: a systematic review. Br J Dermatol 2002;146:351–64.

55. Stein L. Clinical studies of a new vehicle formulation for topical corticosteroids in the treatment of psoriasis. J Am Acad Dermatol 2005;53:S39–49.

56. Bovenschen H, Van de Kerkhof P. Treatment of scalp psoriasis with clobetasol-17 propionate 0.05% shampoo: a study on daily clinical practice. J Eur Acad Dermatol Venereol 2010;24: 439–44.

57. Feldman SR. Tachyphylaxis to topical corticosteroids: the more you use them, the less they work? Clin Dermatol 2006;24:229–30.

58. Sanchez Regana M, Martin Ezquerra G, Umbert Millet P, et al. Treatment of nail psoriasis with 8% clobetasol nail lacquer: positive experience in 10 patients. J Eur Acad Dermatol Venereol 2005;19:573–7.

59. Pasch M. C. Nail Psoriasis: A Review of Treatment Options. Drugs 2016;76(6):675–705.

60. Tosti A, Piraccini BM, Pazzaglia M, Vincenzi C. Clobetasol propionate 0.05% under occlusion in the treatment of alopecia totalis/universalis. J Am Acad Dermatol. 2003;49:96–98.

61. Charuwichitratana S, Wattanakrai P, TanrattanakornS. Randomized double-blind placebo-controlled trial in the treatment of alopecia areata with 0.25% desoximetasone cream. Arch Dermatol 2000; 136:1276–1277.

62. Kuldeep C, Singhal H, Khare AK, et al. Randomized comparison of topical betamethasone valerate foam, intralesional triamcinolone acetonide and tacrolimus ointment in management of localized alopecia areata. Int J Trichology 2011;3:20.

63. Lenane P, Macarthur C, Parkin PC, et al. Clobetasol propionate, 0.05%, vs hydrocortisone, 1%, for alopecia areata in children: a randomized clinical trial. JAMA Dermatol 2014;150:47.

64. Takeda K, Arase S, Takahashi S. Side effects of topicalcorticosteroids and their prevention. Drugs1988;36:15–23.

65. Tan E, Tay YK, Goh CL, Chin Giam Y. The pattern and profile of alopecia areata in Singapore a study of 219 Asians. Int J Dermatol2002;41:748–53.

66. Chang KH, Rojhirunsakool S, Goldberg LJ. Treatment of severe alopecia areata with intralesional steroid injections. J Drugs Dermatol 2009;8:909–12.

67. Chu TW, AlJasser M, Alharbi A, Abahussein O, McElwee K, Shapiro J. Benefit of different concentrations of intralesional triamcinolone acetonide in alopecia areata: an intrasubject pilot study. J Am Acad Dermatol2015;73:338–40.

68. Strazzulla L, Avila L, Lo Sicco K, Shapiro J. Image gallery: treatment of refractory alopecia universalis with oral to facitinib citrate and adjunct intralesional triamcinolone injections. Br J Dermatol 2017;176:e125.

69. Friedli A, Labarthe MP, Engelhardt E, Feldmann R, Salomon D, Saurat JH. Pulse methylprednisolone therapy for severealopecia areata: an open prospective study of 45 patients. J Am Acad Dermatol 1998;39:597–602.

70. Olsen EA, Carson SC, Turney EA. Systemic steroids with or without 2% topical minoxidil in the treatment of alopecia areata. Arch Dermatol 1992;128:1467.

71. Khaitan BK, Mittal R, Verma KK. Extensive alopecia areata treated with betamethasone oral mini-pulse therapy: An open uncontrolled study. Indian J Dermatol Venereol Leprol 2004;70:350–3.

72. Michalowski R, Kuczyńska L. Long-term intramuscular triamcinolon-acetonide therapy in alopecia areatatotalisand universalis. Arch Dermatol Res1978;261:73–6.

73. Kern F, Hoffman WH, Hambrick GW, Blizzard RM. Alopecia areata: immunologic studies and treatment with prednisone. Arch Dermatol 1973;107:407.

74. Njoo MD, Spuls PI, Bos JD, et al. Nonsurgical repigmentation therapies in vitiligo: meta-analysis of the literature. Arch Dermatol 1998;134:1532–40.

75. Kumari J. Vitiligo treated with topical clobetasol propionate. Arch Dermatol 1984;120:631–5.

76. Schaffer JV, Bolognia JL. The treatment of hypopigmentation in children. Clin Dermatol 2003;21:296–310.

77. Njoo MD, Spuls PI, Bos JD, et al. Nonsurgical repigmentation therapies in vitiligo: meta-analysis of the literature. Arch Dermatol1998;134:1532–40.

78. Kwinter J, Pelletier J, Khambalia A, Pope E. High-potency steroid use in children with vitiligo: a retrospective study. J Am Acad Dermatol 2007;56:236–41.

79. Köse O, Arca E, Kurumlu Z. Mometasone cream versus pimecrolimus cream for the treatment of childhood localized vitiligo. J Dermatolog Treat 2010;21:133–9.

80. Taieb A, Alomar A, Bohm M, et al. Guidelines for the management of vitiligo: the European Dermatology Forum consensus. Br J Dermatol 2013;168: 5–19.

81. Kim SM, Lee HS, Hann SK. The efficacy of low-dose oral corticosteroids in the treatment of vitiligo patients. Int J Dermatol 1999;38:546.

82. Lee DY, Kim CR, Lee JH, Yang JM. Recent onset vitiligo treated with systemic corticosteroid and topical tacrolimus: need for early treatment in vitiligo. J Dermatol 2010;37:1057–59.

83. Pasricha JS, Khaitan BK. Oral mini-pulse therapy with betamethasone in vitiligo patients having extensive or fast-spreading disease. Int J Dermatol 1993;32:753–7.

84. Radakovic-Fijan S, Furnsinn-Fridl AM,Honigsmann H, Tanew A. Oral dexamethasone pulse treatment for vitiligo. J Am Acad Dermatol 2001;44:814–17.

85. Kanwar AJ, Mahajan R, Parsad D. Low-dose oral mini-pulse dexamethasone therapy in progressive unstable vitiligo. J Cutan Med Surg 2013;17:259–68.

10

Steroid Misuse

Eswari L, Kerkar Sulaksha Surya

SUMMARY

- Steroid-induced dermatosis is an entity emerging globally due to steroid misuse.
- Topical steroid abuse has become a pandemic in India.
- TS damaged face (TSDF) is characterized by severe rebound erythema, burning and scaling of face on attempted withdrawal leading to successive use of more potent TS to avoid the rebound, a condition labelled as steroid addiction.
- The Indian Association of Dermatologists, Venereologists, and Leprologists has formed a task force against topical steroids abuse named ITATSA (IADVL Task Force Against Topical Steroid Abuse).
- In the year 2006, a thread named 'Topical Steroid Misuse Menace' was initiated in the ACAD IADVL group of IADVL and a memorandum was submitted on this issue to the Union Minister of Health and to the Ministry of Chemicals and Fertilizers.
- Effective management of this public health problem requires combined efforts from the government, health authorities, medical professionals, pharmaceutical companies, and chemists and strict compliance on the part of the patients.

INTRODUCTION

Steroids are the most widely used therapeutic agents for the treatment of dermatological disorders due to their anti-inflammatory, immunosuppressive and anti-proliferative properties. The use of the steroids in treating dermatoses should be individualized and the prescribed dosage/duration/method of use (application in case of topicals) require strict compliance on the part of the patient (and prescribing physician) for effective and safe management, because of the side effect profile of these drugs.

TOPICAL STEROID ABUSE—INDIAN SCENARIO

Dermatologists in India are witnessing a pandemic of adverse effects induced by misuse of topical steroids (TS).[1] TS abuse as a fairness cream is widely prevalent in

India due to stigmatization of dark complexion (and hence craze for fairness) and easy availability of TS over the counter (some even less expensive than a moisturiser). This is compounded by lack of awareness about their adverse effects, self-abuse, inefficient regulations resulting in an epidemic of steroid induced dermatoses, which are difficult to treat as the damage induced by these drugs is often irreversible.

TS misuse occurs at various levels, i.e. manufacturing, marketing misuse, prescription misuse, sales misuse and misuse by laymen.[2] According to IMS Health agency, the annual sales of TS in India was ₹ 1400 crores in 2013, accounting for almost 82% of total dermatological product sale in the country, reflecting immense popularity for TS and a tremendous commercial potential for steroid market.[3]

TS use can lead to several adverse effects including atrophy of skin, increased hair, acneiform eruption, striae and telangiectasia. Apart from these and perioral dermatitis, prolonged and indiscriminate use of TS on face can lead to development of TS damaged face (TSDF) characterized by severe rebound erythema, burning and scaling of face on attempted withdrawal leading to successive use of more potent TS to avoid the rebound, a condition labelled as steroid addiction. Moreover, long-term use of potent TS may also lead to systemic side effects such as adrenal suppression and Cushingoid appearance.[1–4]

Studies from Asia (particularly India) and Africa indicate that TS are frequently misused as fairness creams on recommendation of peers/family, beautician and the pharmacist with a lack of/minimal dermatological consultation (Table 10.1).[5–11]

Of late, following an alarming rise in the number of cases of TS misuse on face resulting in steroid dependence, the entity was labelled as "Topical steroid-dependent/damaged face".[1]

Topical steroid dependent/damaged face is defined as the semi-permanent or permanent damage to the skin of the face precipitated by the irrational, indiscriminate, unsupervised, or prolonged use of TCs resulting in a plethora of cutaneous signs and symptoms and psychological dependence on the drug.[1]

This entity is now being reported worldwide.[7–9]

Laws and Regulations

- Steroids are Schedule H drugs (Drug and Cosmetics Act, 1940), which need to be sold strictly upon the prescription of a registered medical practitioner. However, not all steroid molecules are mentioned in Schedule H drugs. The largest selling preparations of TS in various combinations with antifungals and antibacterials can be purchased by the patients without any doctor's prescription, as Schedule H provides exemption for topical or external use preparations from the purview of Schedule H and H1, in the note appended to these schedules.

Table 10.1: Studies on topical steroid misuse

Authors	Setting	Results
Al-Dhalimi et al[5]	Iraq (2001)	Of 1780 pts, 7.9% had misused TS with 66% of these for fairness and 16% for acne. Dermats prescribed TS in only 4%, other physicians in 11%, parameds in 27%, friends in 21% and pharmacists in 19%. AE* in 26.4%.
Saraswat et al[6]	India (2008)	Of 2926 pts of facial dermatoses, 14% were using TS. Maximum usage in rural and sub-urban patients in 2nd decade of life. Patients used TS as a fairness cream (29%) and for melasma (29%). Half the patients were prescribed TS by dermats, and another quarter by a non-dermatphysicians. AE in 90%.
Hameed AF[7]	Iraq (2010)	Of 75 patients diagnosed as steroid dermatitis resembling rosacea, steroids misused on recommendation of nonmedical personnel in 34%, beauticians, in 26%, self-prescription in 24%, pharmacists in 2%. Only 9% had dermat consultation.
Sendrasoa et al[8]	Madagascar (2012)	Of 384 patients, only 26% had obtained TS on physician's prescription, while in 61% TS were recommended by cosmetic retailer, 23% by pharmacists, 12% by beauticians, and 4% from unspecified sources. AE in 99%.
Sinha et al[9]	India (2013)	Of 50 patients, 74% used TS for fairness, 14% for melasma, 8% for acne induced hyperpigmentation and 4% for dark circles with 80% pts obtaining TS OTC**, 8% through advertisements/ on recommendation of friends/family and only 4% consulted a dermat.
Manchanda et al[10]	India (2013)	Of 100 patients, 85% used TS for medical conditions and 15% as face/fairness cream. Only 1% were prescribed TS by dermats, 72% by non-physician sources, 23% through AYUSH practitioners, 4% by non-dermatologists. AE: Pruritus and acneiform eruptions were common.
Jha et al[11]	India (2014)	Of 410 patients, 35.6% used TS as fairness cream, 21.2% for melasma, 20.4% as anti-acne cream and 2.6% for hypopigmentation. Of these, 43% bought TSOTC** without prescription, 8.5% were recommended by beautician, 20% by friends/family members, 18.2% by a non-dermatologist physician and 10.2% by a dermat.

AE*: Adverse effects
OTC**: Over the counter

- A special taskforce group, i.e. **ITATSA** (IADVL Task Force Against Topical Steroid Abuse) was established by IADVL. To prevent OTC sale TS and antibiotics, it was proposed by IADVL to modify schedule H and to amend the footnote which states, 'the salts, esters, derivatives, and preparations containing the above substances excluding those intended for topical or external use (except preparations containing steroids) are also covered by this schedule'.[11]

- The government has considered the proposal to amend abolishing a footnote in the country's rule book on medicines that currently exempts skin creams from being labelled as Schedule H drugs.[12,13]
- Similarly, under Schedule J clause 18 of 'The Drug and Cosmetics Act, 1940', one cannot claim a drug for the fairness of skin.[14]
- Furthermore, according to the 'Drugs and Magic Remedies (Objectionable Advertisements) Act, 1954', Section 4 (Prohibition of Misleading Advertisements Relating to Drugs), no one can advertise a drug which (a) directly or indirectly gives a false impression regarding the true character of the drug or (b) makes a false claim for the drug.[15,16] Hence, there should be proper check on the advertisement of the drugs which claim to promote fairness of the skin.

Knowledge and Awareness Program: India and Abroad

- In the year 2006, a thread named 'Topical Steroid Misuse Menace' was initiated in the ACAD IADVL group of IADVL and a memorandum was submitted on this issue to the Union Minister of Health and to the Ministry of Chemicals and Fertilizers.[2]
- In January 2007, the IADVL Central Council and General Body unanimously passed the proposal 'Stop OTC supply of potent TS'. Subsequent to this proposal dermatologists from various parts of India have been posting cases of TS misuse in the official ACAD IADVL e-group of IADVL.[2]
- A multicentric study on TS dependence and misuse on face was conducted in 12 centers all over India. The condition resulting from such misuse and dependence was named topical steroid-dependent facies (TSDF).[1,2]
- Dermatologists have been raising awareness regarding this menace of topical steroid abuse through social and print media.
- The Indian Association of Dermatologists, Venereologists, and Leprologists has formed a task force against topical steroids abuse named ITATSA, with main aims to raise public awareness, run media campaigns, form study groups for doctors, highlight the problem in journals, and meet with central and state authorities.
- IADVL has conducted various activities all over India to create awareness among general public about adverse effects of topical corticosteroids. Fixed dose combinations are used by qualified dermatologists for a few selected indications (infected eczema or inflamed dermatophytosis) for a very short period of time not exceeding 2–3 weeks. It has been emphasized by ITATSA that its use beyond the designated time and for other indications by unqualified health professionals should be discouraged.
- ITSAN (International Topical Steroid Addiction Network) is a non-profit charity in USA, formed to raise awareness about 'Topical Steroid Addiction or Topical Steroid Withdrawal Syndrome' and support affected individuals.[17]

REFERENCES

1. Lahiri K, Coondoo A. Topical steroid damaged/dependent face (TSDF): An entity of cutaneous pharmaco dependence. Indian J Dermatol 2016;61:265–72.

2. Coondoo A. Topical corticosteroid misuse: The Indian Scenario. Indian Journal of Dermatology. 2014;59(5):451–455.

3. Verma SB. Sales, status, prescriptions and regulatory problems with topical steroids in India. Indian J Dermatol Venereol Leprol. 2014;80:2012–3.

4. Rathi SK, D'Souza P. Rational and ethical use of topical corticosteroids based on safety and efficacy. Indian J Dermatol 2012;57:251–9.

5. Al-Dhalimi MA and Aljawahiry N. Misuse of topical corticosteroids: A clinical study in an Iraqi hospital. Eastern Mediterranean Health Journal 2006;12:847–52.

6. Saraswat A, Lahiri K, Chatterjee M, Barua S, Coondoo A, Mittal A, et al. Topical corticosteroid abuse on the face: A prospective, multicenter study of dermatology outpatients. Indian J Dermatol Venereol Leprol 2011;77:160–6.

7. Hameed AF. Steroid dermatitis resembling rosacea: A clinical evaluation of 75 patients. ISRN Dermatol 2013;2013:491376.

8. Sendrasoa FA, Ranaivo IM, Andrianarison M, et al. Misuse of Topical Corticosteroids for Cosmetic Purpose in Antananarivo, Madagascar. BioMed Research International. 2017;2017:9637083.

9. Sinha A, Kar S, Yadav N, Madke B. Prevalence of topical steroid misuse among rural masses. Indian J Dermatol 2016;61:119.

10. Manchanda K, Mohanty S, Rohatgi PC. Misuse of topical corticosteroids over face: A clinical study. Indian Dermatol Online J 2017;8:186–91.

11. Jha AK, Sinha R, Prasad S. Misuse of topical corticosteroids on the face: A cross-sectional study among dermatology outpatients. Indian Dermatol Online J 2016;7:259–63.

12. Xiao X, Xie H, Jian D, Deng Y, Chen X, Li J, et al. Rebounding triad (severe itching, dryness and burning) after facial corticosteroid discontinuation defines a specific class of corticosteroid-dependent dermatitis. J Dermatol 2015;42:697–702.

13. Drugs and Cosmetics Act 1940 http://www.cdsco.nic.in/writereaddata/2016 Drugs % 20 and % 20 Cosmetics % 20 Act % 2019 40% 20 & % 20 Rules % 2019 45.pdf.

14. Pande S. Steroid containing fixed drug combinations banned by government of India: A big step towards dermatologic drug safety. Indian J Drugs Dermatol 2016;2:1–2.

15. Health Ministry to Bring Steroid-Based Skin Creams Under Schedule H Drugs for Patient Safety. Available from: http://www.pharmabiz.com/NewsDetails.aspx?aid=95397&sid=1.

16. Drugs and Magic Remedies (Objectionable Advertisements) act, 1954' http://www.drugs control.tn.gov.in/pages/application_forms/dmr_drug_objectional_advertisement_act.pdf.

17. ITSAN (International Topical Steroid Addiction Network) www.itsan.org.

Index